HERBAL TOXICOLOGY

HERBAL TOXICOLOGY

By

Dr. Amita Sarkar
Dept. of Zoology
Agra College
Agra (U.P.)
(India)

DISCOVERY PUBLISHING HOUSE PVT. LTD.
NEW DELHI-110 002

Published by:

Namit Wasan

DISCOVERY PUBLISHING HOUSE PVT. LTD.

4383/4B, Ansari Road, Darya Ganj

New Delhi-110 002 (India)

Phone : +91-11-23279245; 23253475; 43596065

E-mail : discoverybooksindia@gmail.com
discoverypublishinghouse@gmail.com
namitwasan9@gmail.com

web : www.discoverypublishinggroup.com

First Published: **2009**

Reprinted: **2021**

ISBN: 978-81-8356-421-2

Herbal Toxicology

Printed at:

Infinity Imaging Systems

Delhi

Preface

The present title *"Herbal Toxicology"* has been compiled for those involved in agriculture, medicine, pharmaceutical, clinical, teaching and research. Scholars associated with this branch and even lay persons are using herbs for centuries. Despite the widespread use of herbal products, information about their safety and efficacy is generally sparse compared with the information available about prescription drugs. The present title provides a comprehensive and summative formats, objective information on herbal supplements from the most reliable sources, with an emphasis on information not readily available elsewhere. It is hoped that this title will also be used to solve clinical or forensic problems involving dietary supplements, promote dialogue between health care professionals and patients, and stimulate intellectual curiosity about these products, fostering further research into their therapeutic and adverse effects.

To make the work more comprehensive and informative, the author has consulted many authoritative books, research journals, abstracts, monographs etc., so there can be no claim to originality except in the manner of treatment.

The author expresses his thanks to his friends and colleagues whose continue inspirations have initiated him to bring out this book.

The author expresses his gratitude to Mr. Wasan and staff of M/s Discovery Publishing House Pvt. Ltd. for their whole hearted cooperation in the publication of this book.

In the mean time, the author will remain sincerely responsible for any shortcomings of the book and be grateful to the readers for their suggestions and constructive criticism for the continuous betterment of the book. He takes this opportunity to appeal to the readers to send their suggestions straightaway to his Publisher.

Author

CONTENTS

1. **Phytotoxicology** 1–23
Importance of Poisonous Plants to Man and Animals, Current Knowledge of Poisonous Plants, Effects of Toxic Principles Elaborated by Plants, External Structure and Mouth, Rumen, or Foregut, Lower Gut, Liver, Circulatory System, Kidney, Heart, Bone, Lung, Thyroid, Eye, Nervous System, Respiratory System, Reproductive System, Hair and Skin.

2. **Bilberry** 24–31
Sources and Chemical Composition, Products Available, Pharmacological/Toxicological Effects, Antiulcer Activity, Vascular Permeability, Antiangiogenic Effects, Antilipemic and Hypoglycemic Effects, Ocular Effects, Pharmacokinetics, Adverse Effects and Toxicity, Interactions, Reproduction, Regulatory Status.

3. **Citrus aurantium** 32–38
Current Promoted Uses, Sources and Chemical Composition, Products Available, Pharmacological/Toxicological Effects, Pharmacology, Cardiovascular Effect, Thermogenic/Lypolytic Effects, Dermatological Effects, Adverse Effects and Toxicity, Case Reports of Toxicity Caused by Commercially Available Products or Traditional Uses by Various Specialty Populations, Pharmacokinetics, Interactions, Regulatory Status.

4. **Cranberry** 39–43
Current Promoted Uses, Products Available, Dosages Used or Recommended in Clinical Studies and Case Reports, Dosages in Lay References, Various Brand Name Products of Cranberry

Available, Pharmacological/Toxicological Effects, Antimicrobial Activity, Gastrointestinal Effects, Renal Effects.

5. Echinacea **44—53**

Current Promoted Uses, Sources and Chemical Composition, Products Available, Pharmacological/Toxicological Effects, Immunological Effects, Antimicrobial/Antiviral Effects, Antifungal Effects, Antineoplastic Activity, Wound Healing, Anti-Inflammatory Effects, Mutagenicity/Carcinogenicity, Antioxidant Effects, Pharmacokinetics, Adverse Effects and Toxicity, Common Adverse Reactions, Case Reports of Toxicity, Drug Interactions, Reproduction, Regulatory Status.

6. Ephedra Alkaloids **54—70**

Current Promoted Uses, Sources and Chemical Composition, Products Available, Pharmacological Effects, Clinical Studies, Bronchodilation, Weight Loss, Athletic Performance, Pharmacokinetics, Adverse Effects and Toxicity, Neurological Disorders, Renal Disorders, Cardiovascular Diseases, Workplace Drug Testing, Postmortem Toxicology, Methamphetamine Manufacture, Drug Interactions, Reproduction, Regulatory Status.

7. Evening Primrose **71—87**

Current Promoted Uses, Sources and Chemical Composition, Products Available, Dosage, Pharmacological/Toxicological Effects, Dermatological Effects, Anti-Inflammatory Effects, Autoimmune, Neurological System Effects, Endocrine System Effects, Cardiovascular System Effects, Cytotoxic Effects, Miscellaneous, Pharmacokinetics, Adverse Effects and Toxicity, Interactions, Reproduction, Regulatory Status.

8. Feverfew **88—97**

Current Promoted Uses, Sources and Chemical Composition, Products Available, Pharmacological/Toxicological Effects, Neurological Effects, Anti-Inflammatory Effects, Mutagenicity/Carcinogenicity/Teratogenicity, Adverse Effects and Toxicity, Case Reports of Toxicity Caused by Commercially Available Products, Drug Interactions, Regulation.

9. Garlic **98—119**

Current Promoted Uses, Sources and Chemical Composition, Products Available, Product Names, Recommended Daily Doses in Humans, Garlic Compounds, Pharmacological/Toxicological

Effects, Cardiovascular Effects, GI Effects, Antimicrobial Activity, Antineoplastic Effects, Immunostimulant Effects, Other Effects, Pharmacokinetics, Absorption, Distribution, Metabolism/Elimination, Adverse Effects and Toxicity, Garlic Allergy, Topical Reactions, Interactions, Regulatory Status.

10. **Ginger** **120—130**

Current Promoted Uses, Sources and Chemical Composition, Products Available, Pharmacological/Toxicological Effects, Gastrointestinal Effects, Anti-Inflammatory Activity, Migraine Prevention, Cardiovascular Effects, Mutagenicity, Pharmacokinetics, Adverse Effects, Case Reports of Toxicity Caused by Commercially Available Products, Drug Interactions, Reproduction, Regulatory Status.

11. **Ginkgo biloba** **131—140**

Current Promoted Use, Products Available, Pharmacological/Toxicological Effects, Nervous System Effects, Cardiovascular Effects, Carcinogenicity/Mutagenicity/Teratogenicity, Endocrine Effects, Drug Interactions, Pharmacokinetics/Toxicokinetics, Absorption, Distribution, Metabolism/Elimination, Adverse Effects and Toxicity, Case Reports of Toxicity Caused By Commercially Available Products, Regulatory Status.

12. **Hawthorn** **141—146**

Current Promoted Uses, Sources and Chemical Composition, Products Available, Pharmacological/Toxicological Effects, Cardiovascular Effects, Neurological Effects, Lethal Dose for 50% of Test Population, Teratogenicity/Mutagenicity/Carcinogenicity, Pharmacokinetics/Toxicokinetics, Adverse Effects and Toxicity, Case Reports of Toxicity Caused by Commercially Available Products, Drug Interactions, Regulatory Status.

13. **Hypericum perforatum** **147—166**

Current Promoted Uses, Sources and Chemical Composition, Products Available, Pharmacological/Toxicological Effects, Neurological Effects, Antimicrobial Effects, Mutagenicity, Neuropathic Pain, Inflammation/Asthma, Atopic Dermatitis, Antioxidant, Premenstrual Syndrome, Tumor Growth Inhibition, Pharmacokinetics/Toxicokinetics, Absorption, Distribution, Metabolism/Elimination, Adverse Effects and Toxicity, Interactions, Reproduction, Regulatory Status.

14. **Kava** 167—177

Current Promoted Users, Sources and Chemical Composition, Products Available, Pharmacological/Toxicological Effects, Neurological Effects, Dermatological Effects, Musculoskeletal Effects, Antimicrobial Activity, Antiplatelet Effects, Cancer Prevention, Pharmacokinetics, Absorption, Metabolism/Elimination, Case Reports of Toxicity Caused by Commercial Kava Products, Toxicity Associated with Traditional Use by Native Populations, Interactions, Reproduction, Regulatory Status.

15. **Panax ginseng** 178—190

Current Promoted Uses, Sources and Chemical Composition, Products Available, Pharmacological/Toxicological Effects, Endocrine Effects, Neurological Effects, Cardiovascular Effects, Hematological Effects, Immunological Effects, Antineoplastic Effects, Case Reports of Toxicity Caused by Commercially Available Products, Drug Interactions, Pharmacokinetics, Absorption, Distribution, Metabolism/Elimination, Regulatory Status.

16. **Saw Palmetto** 191—199

Sources and Chemical Composition, Products Available, Pharmacological/Toxicological Effects, In Vitro/Animal Studies, Human Studies, Adverse Effects and Toxicity, Case Reports of Toxicity Caused by Saw Palmetto Products, Pharmacokinetics/Toxicokinetics, Drug Interactions, Reproduction, Regulatory Status.

17. **Valerian** 200—212

Current Promoted Uses, Sources and Chemical Composition, Products Available, Pharmacological/Toxicological Effects, Insomnia, Anxiety, Musculoskeletal Relaxation, Pharmacokinetics, Adverse Effects and Toxicity, Reproductive System, Cardiovascular System, Cytotoxicity, Case Reports of Toxicity, Interactions, Reproduction, Regulatory Status.

18. **Vitex agnus-castus** 213—223

Current Promoted Uses, Sources and Chemical Composition, Products Available, Dosage, Pharmacological/Toxicological Effects, Prolactin Secretion, Follicle-Stimulating Hormone, Luteinizing Hormone, Progesterone/Testosterone Synthesis, Infertility, PMS and Menopausal Symptoms, Mastodynia, Luteal Phase Length, Premenstrual Dysphoric Disorder, Toxicological Effects, Adverse Effects and Toxicity, Case Reports of Toxicity Caused by

Commercially Available Products, Interactions, Reproduction, Regulatory Status.

19. **Inhibitors of Phospholipase** 224—235

Medicinal Aristolochiaceae, Medicinal Myristicaceae, Medicinal Caprifoliaceae, Medicinal Asteraceae.

20. **Inhibitors of Lipoxygenases** 236—242

Medicinal Myrsinaceae, Medicinal Clusiaceae, Medicinal Asteraceae, Medicinal Apiaceae.

21. **Inhibitors of Elastase** 243—248

Medicinal Asteraceae, Medicinal Droseraceae.

22. **Inhibitors of Nitric Oxide Synthetase** 249—257

Medicinal Asteraceae, Medicinal Lauraceae, Medicinal Solanaceae.

23. **Biochemicals Protecting Herbal Plants** 258—322

Economic and Public Health, Control of Vector-Borne Disease, Agricultural Productivity, Urban Pest Control, Environmental Contamination, Production and Use Statistics, Human Poisonings, Routes of Exposure, Insecticides, Organophosphorus Insecticides, Carbamate Insecticides, Organochlorine Insecticides, Botanical Insecticides, Herbicides, Chlorophenoxy Compounds, Dinitrophenols, Bipyridyl Compounds, Carbamate Herbicides, Substituted Urea, Triazines, Amide Herbicides, Fungicides, Rodenticides, Warfarin, Red Squill, Norbormide, Sodium Fluoroacetate and Fluoroacetamide, Alpha Naphthyl Thiourea (ANTU), Strychnine Sulfate, Inorganic Rodenticides, Fumigants, Special Problems, Interactions, Carcinogenic, Teratogenic, and Mutagenic Properties of Pesticides, Comparative Toxicity.

Index 323—329

1

PHYTOTOXICOLOGY

At the subcellular level, plants and animals display more similarities than differences. Consider the processes of replication of information, genetic recombination, development of subcellular structures, and respiration. Attention should be focused on the fact that, although plants and animals are different, they are evolving branches of a common origin. The study of phytotoxicology, then, is an examination of those products characteristic of one major part of the biota that produce or evoke a specific deleterious reaction when they interact with systems characteristic of the other. This view emphasizes the differences that have evolved between plants and animals despite their common beginnings.

In every plant poisoning case it should be possible to identify precisely the plant product and the animal system involved, the route by which they are brought together, and the specific subsequent events that occur until the animal either dies or recovers. However, according to a recent authoritative statement on this subject, "Probably no field of scientific endeavor exists in which it is more difficult to separate fact from fiction than in the study of poisonous plants. Examination of the pertinent literature will reveal considerable confusion tending to mask an even greater amount of ignorance.... Unbelievable chaos reigns in the area of plant identification and nomenclature as applied by the nonspecialist".

This chapter is directed toward three main topics: (i) the importance of poisonous plants to man and animals, (ii) an assessment of current knowledge of poisonous plants, and (iii) a discussion of the effects of toxic principles elaborated by plants.

Importance of Poisonous Plants to Man and Animals

Although incomplete, the best figures on incidence of human poisoning by plants are those collected from individual poison control centers and analyzed by the National Clearinghouse for Poison Control Centers. Ingestions are grouped by categories in the annual summaries. Plants as a category have consistently ranked in the top seven, accounting for about 4 percent of the reported ingestions until the 1970s. In 1970, plants (excluding mushrooms and toadstools) accounted for 4,059 reported ingestions, representing 4.8 percent of all reported ingestions for that year. This was greater than the number of disinfectant, tranquilizer, insecticide, hormone, acid and alkali, antiseptic, polish, or paint ingestions and was exceeded only by the incidence of ingestion of aspirin and soap-detergents-cleaners. Since the, however, plants as a category has come to the top of the list of "products" most frequently implicated in poisoning of children under 5 years of age. Now, about one out of every ten cases reported by poison control centers is related to plants. This conspicuous rise in importance of plants since 1965 is related to the equally dramatic decrease in cases of poisoning from aspirin. These have fallen from greater than 25 percent of reported incidents in 1965 to just 4.1 percent in 1976. Safety packaging, limited quantities per package, and increased public awareness of hazards—the result of governmental and private compaigns—have been the main contributing factors in reducing the importance of aspirin. Only the latter method of decreasing incidents is easily applicable to the unnecessarily high volume of ingestions involving plants now being experienced at poison control centers. According to reported figures there are approximately 75,000 human ingestions of poisonous plants in the United States each year. According to Canadian figures, ingestions of nonfood plants are more than ten times greater than the number of reported incidents involving venomous bites or stings.

The above figures need to be viewed with a certain amount of caution. First, the majority of the ingestions were of materials, or in amounts, that would not have proved capable of eliciting a toxic response, or else treatment, usually emesis, intervened before such a response occurred. These, strictly speaking, are better defined as ingestions than as poisonings, without implying whether a toxic reaction was or was not possible. Second, many incidents are treated by private physicians who do not report to a poison control center. In addition, some poison control centers fail to report to the National Clearinghouse. Thus, the precise number of toxic responses that occur from plants annually in the human population cannot be determined from these data.

Poisoning of pets and livestock is even more extensive than is poisoning of man. No reliable figures exist, but estimates as to loss of range livestock in western states consistently place the annual figure at more than one million dollars per state or region. Certainly, well-documented instances in which more than 1,500 animals have been killed at a single time, such as losses of sheep to *Halogeton glomeratus*, represent considerable economic impact and do not need to be multiplied by many such events or by many similar plants to assume major importance to the livestock industry. The resulting economic loss includes not only the value of the animals but also the diminution in real value of the range acreage following its infestation with a poisonous weed. Looses of pets and wild animals are so poorly documented that no useful generalizations are possible.

Current Knowledge of Poisonous Plants

Effective consideration of phytotoxicology requires a synthesis across wide academic boundaries and is thus difficult. This, and the diversity of natural phenomena dealt with, perhaps more than other factors, have inhibited a more rapid, rigorous, development of the subject. Comparison of the principal current references dealing with North American poisonous plants shows immediately that fundamental input and analysis are required from botany, physiology, and pathology. In all cases, full development of a particular topic also requires the attention of one or more academic or practical specialists, such as physician, veterinarian, toxicologist, clinician, organic chemist or biochemist, plant physiologist, pharmacologist, pharmacognosist, agronomist, horticulturist, geneticist, and animal husbandman. Consideration must be given to identification and description of a toxic reaction; practical understanding of the history, to aid in diagnosis and in formulating control; secure determination of the etiology; identification and perhaps isolation of a toxic principle; specific description of tis action; the seasonal, ecologic, and genetic control of production of the toxic principle by the plant; and the way in which man or animals were or may be exposed. The latter involves agricultural practices in the case of livestock. In man, a plethora of possibilities exist, from overuse of plant-derived drugs by adults to accidental or experimental ingestions of drugs or whole plant parts by children.

Approximately 700 species of North American plants are considered to be poisonous on the basis of case histories, experimental investigations, or other specific reasons. More will be discovered. This is only a small fraction of the perhaps 30,000 species of plants in the wild and cultivated floras of North America. Nevertheless, it is a large number, and no generalization emerges from a review of their botany, ecology, or management by man to allow systematizing them for easier comprehension. Poisonous species are scattered throughout the plant kingdom from algae, to ferns, to gymnosperms, to angiosperms, and in the latter large groups they appear almost randomly among the plant families. One sometimes hears that certain groups such as the nightshade or potato family (Solanaceae) are particularly dangerous, but such statements are not entirely valid. Such families are the larger ones, and certain poisonous species more or less in relation to their size.

Toxicity usually exists at the level of the genus. If one species of a genus is toxic, some or all others in that genus usually display similar toxicity. This is why species names are sometimes omitted in general discussion of toxicity. This is a mistake. First, exceptions to the generalization are numerous and important. Second, even when similar species display similar toxicity, they may have other important differences. For example, most species of the genus *Asclepias* (milkweeds) are toxic, but the most toxic species (*A. labriformis*) is found only in a limited area of Utah. However, the most troublesome milkweeds (*A. subverticillata*, *A. eriocarpa*) differs in appearance from the former and have significantly less toxicity on a weight basis, but are much more widely distributed geographically. Important distinctions such as these are lost when species names are not used.

In some cases, groups of genera within a single family display similar toxicity. This is true, for example, of the laurel group of the heath family (Ericaceae). At the other extreme, however, are those instances in which closely related species differ in toxicity. *Eupatorium rugosum* is closely related to the numerous other species of *Eupatorium*, but only the former is known to be toxic. Occasionally the same toxic principle is found in plants of great botanical or habitat difference. For example, the only other plant known to contain the same poisonous principle as *Eupatorium rugosum* is *Aplopappus heterophyllus*. These two are in the same plant family (Compositae), but the former is found in woodlands of eastern North America while the latter is limited to the dry ranges of the Southwest. Nicotine, as another example, can be isolated from plants as botanically distant as tobacco (*Nicotiana tabacum*) of the nightshade or potato family of angiosperms, and from club moss (*Lycopodium* spp.) of the primitive, spore-bearing lycopods.

The content of a given poisonous principle, and even to some extent its molecular structure, can vary widely in some species with the environmental conditions under which the plant grew. This is particularly true of many glycosides. In other cases, certain alkaloids for instance, elaboration of the poisonous principle in a given species in under reasonably tight genetic control and varies little with growing conditions. Even when under strict genetic control, the content of a poisonous principle in a given plant may vary with stage of growth; it may concentrate in particular parts of the plant, or it may vary with the particular variety or strain of plant.

Exemplifying the last point, one of the nightshades exists in two distinct populations, which fortunately do not normally interbreed. The botanic distinctions between them are so small that the two populations were originally recognized as a single species (*Solanum nigrum*). One kind, however, is quite toxic. The other, now set off taxonomically as *Solanum intrusum*, is not known to be toxic. In fact, *S. intrusum* has entered trade as "garden huckleberry" or "wonderberry" and is sometimes recommended to home gardeners for its edible fruits. Poinsettia (*Euphorbia pulcherrima*) may represent a similar example. Its listing as toxic was found originally on a reported case of human mortality in Hawaii in 1919. Recent feeding experiments, prompted by the belief of horticulturists that the poinsettia is really not poisonous, showed no toxic effect in rodents fed large quantities of the red bracts. However, poison control centers continue to report instances of gastric distress in children after ingestion of poinsettia. A possible explanation for the apparent conflict in these several observations is the very great horticultural manipulation that has in recent years been devoted to breeding showier, longer-lasting, and differently colored poinsettias. It is reasonable to suppose that the ability to form a toxic principle may have been consciously selected against at the same time that desirable floral characteristics were sought. If this is the case, older varieties of poinsettia, or ones distinctly different from those experimentally fed to the rodents, may still be capable of eliciting a toxic reaction. These examples could be extended to demonstrate that toxicity can vary not only with species, sex, age, and even individuality of plants and animals but also with environmental factors. The examples quoted above should suffice to convey an idea of the complexity of phytotoxicology.

A major factor in much of the present confusion regarding poisonous plants is the problem of adequate identification of the plant material involved. A physician or veterinarian faced with a case of plant poisoning is, in a sense, like a chemist conducting experiments by guesswork from a stockroom of unlabeled reagents. Accurate identification of the plant is prerequisite to making use of existing pertinent toxicologic information.

The layman rarely appreciates the difficulties involved in the accurate identification of plant materials. Not only are the reagents unknown, but some of them may not be identifiable with the material and tests at hand. Botanic identification often requires a particular part of the plant—usually the mature reproductive parts (which evolve most slowly and hence show relationships best). This means the flower, and the flower is often a very transitory event in the life of a plant. Flowers often are not present when the berries of a plant attract children. Also, flowers do not generally survive well in the gut, so that examination of vomitus or of ruminal or stomach contents will rarely yield identifiable flowering stages, even if initially present.

Most actual cases of poisoning of man and livestock involve the identification of plant material by common name alone. This can be disastrous. Serious errors in reputable reports in the medical and veterinary literature can be traced to erroneous use of common names or failure to appreciate the lac of precision in such usage. All plant materials involved in toxicologic examinations of any kind should be identified by genus and species. If this requires the help of a taxonomic botanist, it should be obtained. If experimental work resulting in a published report is done with plant materials, voucher specimens should be prepared and deposited in a major herbarium, and the fact should be noted in the publication. One or more such herbaria exist in every state, usually at the department of botany in the state university, but sometimes at the state museum or at a major private university. Herbaria function, somewhat like libraries, as depositories of materials that can be recalled in good condition at a later date if it prove necessary to reassess the botanic materials involved in a particular investigation. Despite the obvious benefit of such a practice and its relative simplicity, it is rarely done.

The foregoing discussion presents reasons why current practices make it difficult to deal with poisonous plants. There are historic reasons as well. At the risk of oversimplification, they may be summarized as follows.

The Greeks and Romans were astute and recorded, in some detail and with commendable accuracy, their conclusions concerning the useful, medicinal, or toxic characteristics of the natural world. For most areas of knowledge, these collected observations went into eclipse during the Dark Ages, surviving largely as manuscripts copied from generation to generation without significant addition or modification. This was not the case with poisonous materials, for the practice of poisoning to obtain succession of royalty or ecclesiastic authority, inheritance of wealth, or defeat of armies became a highly developed art. Persons able to get results commanded high fees. In order to protect their hard-won trade secrets, these artisans compounded recipes with many esoteric ingredients, thereby obscuring the identity of the actual active principle. A perhaps overdrawn, but nonetheless illuminating example is the several-stanza list of ingredients that went into the witches' cauldron in Shakespeare's *Macbeth*; only two could be expected to do the job.

With the Renaissance, it became necessary to separate fact from fiction, something that was only imperfectly accomplished. Further confusion resulted from an innocent attempt to relate the reports of the classic authors, who dealt mainly with Mediterranean plants, to the flora of central and northern Europe. Keep in mind that the science of naming plants originated with Linneaus' *Species Plantarum* of 1753; before that time all names applied to plants had no more authority than the common names used today.

Herbals supplanted classic manuscripts around 1470; floras and tomes on materia medica supplanted herbals around 1670; all contained frequent reference to toxic capacities of plants. Monographs devoted solely to poisonous plants began to appear shortly before 1700. All of these works were European, and interested educated persons were expected to know the literature of their subject well enough so that citation of authority for particular statements was not deemed necessary. Hence, for the most part, the first books dealing with poisonous plants do not say where the information came from. Most later writers on poisonous plants have apparently been reluctant to eliminate anything that sounds reasonable, in spite of their inability to verify the information. Some patently unreasonable things are also perpetuated. Even today, books may appear in which medieval error is repeated unconsciously but with devastating effect if taken as scientifically accurate documents.

In 1814 M.J.B. Orfila published the first edition of his substantial work on toxicology, to which the use of an experimental approach in toxicology is generally traced. Orfila experimented with a number of plants, describing their effects and attempting to trace the distribution of the poisonous principle in the body. His chief experimental animal was the dog, an animal that vomits readily, and Orfila frequently found it necessary to excise and tie off the esophagus to ensure absorption when dealing with plants or plant materials administered orally. Although Orfila recognized the difficulties this caused in interpreting his results, it remains problematic to separate the effects of the toxic principle from the effects of this relatively drastic procedure.

The flora of North America east of the Mississippi is essentially similar to that of Europe, while west of that river it becomes increasingly foreign. Thus, the early settlers of the United States were able to bring with them not only their livestock but also their practical experience in dealing with the plants they found here. The few persons interested in pursuing investigations of poisonous plants could look up appropriate information in European compendia and apply it with some usefulness to local conditions. The dawn of scientific agriculture in North America can be traced to events a score of years apart: the founding of the Department of Agriculture and the passage of the Morrill Land Grant Act in support of agricultural experimentation and experiment stations in 1887.

These events meant, in practical terms, that as settler moved their livestock west into an increasingly foreign flora and began to put pressure on it, they could no longer turn to experience or to European knowledge to cope with the poisonings that occurred. On the other hand, as each state organized it took advantage of federal programs to establish a college of agriculture and an experiment station, and it was to these agencies that the problems were referred. Increasingly sophisticated experimentation ensured, and by 1900 all but three states west of the Mississippi had published work dealing in a practical way with poisonous plants. At the same time, reports of experimental work from eastern states remained almost nonexistent.

Looking at the results of these influence at the present time, one sees that about a third of thee existing body of information derives from case histories in man and animals, about a third derives from experimental investigation, mostly from a veterinary point of view, and about one third entered our literature from European source. At the same time, the excellence of mush of the recent experimental work with poisonous plants, and the continuous long-term record of productivity of such laboratories as the federal poisonous plants investigational program at Logan, Utah, contrast sharply with the fact that apparently current information being used to treat human poisonings today may in fact be traced to experiments of Orfila and even to Dioscorides.

Given so many potentially harmful plants and the variety of syndromes they may provoke under particular circumstances, a common first reaction of those who must learn to deal practically with the problem of plant poisoning in man is to seek a list of the few most dangerous or troublesome ones.

The National Clearinghouse for Poison Control Centers published a detailed review of the collected reports of plant ingestions for 1965 that were treated as poisoning emergencies. If reporting were accurate, this list should contain the most troublesome plants of the United States. It is not difficult, however, to show that the clearinghouse list is actually of little value for this purpose. Assuming that the personnel of most poison control centers are competent, concerned, conscientious, and medically trained, this list represents a summation of their frustrations in obtaining useful histories, identifying plants, finding or interpreting appropriate literature, discovering that useful or recent experimental results do not exist for the plant in question, or finding that no tested treatments have been recommended for particular circumstances, as was suggested earlier in this chapter.

Taking the plants in order as named:

Standard botanical manuals for the United States list at least three different genera to which the name "pokeweed" or "pokeroot" is commonly applied. All three (*Phytolacca americana* [=*P. decandra*], *Veratrum viride*, and *Symplocarpus foetidus*) have histories of toxicity, but the syndromes differ greatly, as would appropriate treatments. All three are discussed later in this chapter. (*Symplocarpus foetidus*, also called skunk cabbage, is an aroid or member of the plant family Araceae.)

"Yew" is another common name that can cause trouble. It normally refers to a species of *Taxus*. One of these species, *T. canadensis*, is more commonly called "ground hemlock" in some areas. Thus, it is easy for the uninitiated to transfer inadvertently in the literature from "yew" to "hemlock," especially since the latter is a well-known name associated with toxic plants. However, "hemlock" is applied as a common name to at least four genera of plant, only one of which is not lethal. Again the syndromes and appropriate treatments vary.

"Philodendron" is both a scientific name and a common name. As the later, it is applied by the public, and nearly as loosely by many florists, to almost any viny, leafy, nondeciduous (not shedding) potted plant, with or without holes in the leaf blade. A survey of plants with these characteristics, made with the help of the staff at Cornell's Hortorium, resulted in a tally or several score species of plants in nine genera. Only a plant specialist could accurately identify the plant involved when a call comes to a poison control center that a child has eaten "philodendron," and then probably only by seeing the actual plant.

The name "bittersweet" is commonly applied to two entirely different plant genera, one of which has only an ancient European record of putative toxicity. The other is a species of *Solanum* (*dulcamara*), thus a "nightshade." "Nightshade" is perhaps the worst possible designation for a poisonous plant. Usually it refers to one of the multitude of species of *Solanum*. However, it can apply to more than one genus (for example, *Atropa belladonna* is commonly called "nightshade") and is also regularly used to designate the family that contains these plants, the Solanaceae. This is one of the larger plant families and contains such useful plants as potato (*Solanum tuberosum*) and tomato (*Lycopersicon esculentum*). Any member of the family can be called a "nightshade") in a general way, and many are poisonous ("deadly nightshade") under some circumstances including potato and tomato, despite their widespread daily use as food. The last plant named is also a nightshade (Jerusalem cherry = *Solanum pseudocapsicum*), but is at worst only mildly poisonous according to the available information. In conclusion, "nightshade" and "deadly nightshade" are words many parents know. They are likely to come up when a child has eaten a wild plant whose identity is not known by the distraught mother. Under these circumstances, the usefulness of "nightshade" for indicating the identity of a species of plant is virtually nil.

"Holly" is applied to a dozen species of the genus *Ilex*. Many are native American plants and have no record to toxicity. English holly (*I. opaca*) figures in a wealth of Middle Ages mythology. The only definite published reference to the toxicity of *Ilex* is in a second-hand French report from 1889, with authority not stated. Although this has been carried forward in texts to the present, and may even have some validity to it, the present-day physician would be unwise to base his treatment on this kind of information.

"Honeysuckle" refers to more than a score of species of plants in eight genera belonging to four different plant families. The plant commonly referred to in the East as "honeysuckle" is not known to be toxic.

"Pyracantha" is a scientific name and, although several common names are available for this shrub. Without a species name this particular plant is identified only partially, although probably better than with only a common name. The berries of *Pyracantha*, however, have been shown by experiments to be nontoxic in four species of laboratory animals. At present there is no reason to assume that *Pyracantha* berries are poisonous to man.

"Castor bean" is a satisfactory (i.e. unambiguous) common name designation for a single plant species. *Ricinus communis*. The seeds of this plant are well known to be lethal if ingested in small to moderate amount. However, the plant has been subjected to horticultural manipulation so that two main commercial selections now exist. One is grown for production of oil; the other, as a showy, ornamental hedge or garden plant. The unselected native type grows wild in Florida. Whether these three types have equivalent toxicity is not known.

Greater impetus for detailed experimentation with poisonous plants might develop if more investigators realized the important discoveries that have come from such research in the past. Some, such as ergot, digitalis, belladonna, and morphine, are classic. The discovery of dicoumarol as an anticoagulant and the development of warfarin as a rodenticide came directly from an experiment station investigation of why cattle fed moldy sweetclover hay (*Melilotus* spp.) bled to death. More recently investigation of the toxicity of cyads (*Cycas* spp.) has yielded important information about carcinogenesis of bracken fern (*Pteridium aquilinum*), about avitaminosis B_1 in nonruminants; of pokeweed (*Phytolacca americana*), about mitogenesis in leukocytes of hellebore (*Veratrum californicum*) and lupine (*Lupinus sericeus*), about teratogenesis; and of groundsels (*Senecio* spp.) about liver function.

Other sources of sophisticated information on the effects of plants on animals are the pharmaceutical industry and feed manufacturers, or academic laboratories functioning in these areas. The pertinence of investigations of natural drug products is obvious. Less obvious, perhaps, is the work that has been done to analyze and determine nutritional insufficiencies or minor toxicities associated with utilizing large amounts of particular crops for feedstuffs. A good example is the detailed analysis of gossypol, the toxic component of cottonseed (*Gossypium* spp.) that makes cottonseed meal potentially poisonous to livestock.

Effects of Toxic Principles Elaborated by Plants

Poisonous principles of plants range from single elements or simple salts accumulated by some species under certain circumstances (e.g., selenium in cereal crops or oxalates in *Halogeton glomeratus*) to the elaboration of complex molecules of high toxicity (the phytotoxin abrin, a protein, in *Abrus precatorius*, the infamous Rosary pea or Jequirity bean). The specific action of a toxic principle in an animal as presently understood may range from simple irritation of mucous tissues to disruption of an enzymatic process at the microsomal or mitochondrial level. Thus, it is difficult to organize the available information along lines of either molecular structure or fundamental physiology. This difficulty is compounded by the fact that precise knowledge of the toxicity of the 700 species of plants known to be toxic is lacking for more than half. Different authors use various more or less successful schemes based on physiology, pathology, chemistry, or some combination. Any attempt to categorize poisonous principles of plants on chemical grounds suffers not only from the fact that the exact chemistry is rarely known but also that the common categories employed for such purposes (alkaloids, glycosides, saponins, etc.) are not parallel and therefore not mutually exclusive.

Information on poisonous principles and actions is organized below according to observed responses to average toxicologic exposures, and this in turn is considered in sequence of major target organ or tissue as the poison passes through the body, assuming initial exposure by ingestion. Poisons and responses they elicit are so numerous and varied that what follows is more of a summary than a discussion. Only one example is given for each situation, although numerous examples may exist, and subsidiary effects or consequences in additional organs or tissues are ignored, although they are often clinically important. The discussion is also limited to effects of plants ingested as such, not to overdoses of drugs of plant origin, and does not include consideration of differential diagnosis, clinical signs, pathology, or treatment, except as specially important to the point singled out for attention.

External Structure and Mouth

The sap of some plants is acrid and irritating to skin and mucous membranes. The mown stubble of a field of spurge (*Euphorbia esula*) has caused inflammation and loss of hair on the legs of horses used to mow it. Some plants taken into the mouth cause intense stomatitis by direct irritation. The foliage or berries of the ornamental shrub daphne (*Daphne mezereum*), for example, cause corrosive lesions of the mouth, if chewed or eaten. Animals will taken such distasteful materials into the mouth out of curiosity, and most poisonings occur when prunings or clippings are thrown into a pasture or stall. Children exhibit similar curiosity and will swallow distasteful material as readily as they spit it out, just to get it out of the mouth. Either of these plants, and many others of course, will produce intense irritation of the esophagus and, if swallowed, the gut. The exact nature of the irritant is usually unknown. Many aroids (members of the plant family Araceae) cause a similar intense burning sensation in the mouth. Perhaps the most notorious is dumbcane (*Dieffenbachia* spp.) These plants contain needle-like crystals of calcium oxalate that may cause some mechanical as well as chemical irritation. The severity of the reaction has been traced, however, to the presence of a proteolytic enzyme in the plant that attacks the oral tissues. This reaction is often accompanied by swelling and glottic edema and has been fatal in man when the breathing passages have been blocked as a consequence.

Degree of mastication of seeds and fleshy or thick plant parts may determine the severity of the subsequent reaction, or whether it takes place at all. Seeds of precatory bean (*Abrus precatorius*), for example, are highly toxic if chewed, but will pass through the gut undigested if the seed coat is left intact.

Rumen, or Foregut

Ruminants may react to plant poisons quite differently from nonruminants due to differences in digestive structure and function between these two major groups of animals. Ability to vomit effectively is one difference. Some plants stimulate a strong vomit reflex. The vomiting disease of swine, for example, requires ingestion of only a very small amount of barley grain parasitized by a mold fungus (*Gibberella* sp.). Cardioactive glycosides such as those in foxglove (*Digitalis purpurea*) similarly provoke vomiting in most species of animals, even when administered parenterally. Many simple-stomached animals (e.g., man and dog) vomit easily. Ruminants can vomit, but the reflex is not as easily stimulated and the degree to which vomiting is effective in removing poisonous material from the gut is much less than in nonruminants. Vomiting in ruminants is not equivalent to normal eructation. Horses can vomit, but the structure of the oral cavity leads to complications if vomiting occurs. In horses, vomitus is directed into the trachea. Pneumonitis is a common result, and this can develop into pneumonia and result in death. In severe cases, death may result directly from asphyxiation after vomiting.

Many glycosides, as they exist in plants, are not toxic to animals. Toxicity comes from breakdown of the glycoside to release a toxic component. Breakdown often occurs more readily or more rapidly in the rumen than in the digestive tract of monogastric animals. Also, small molecules can be absorbed at the rumen and thus enter the circulation rapidly. Breakdown of cyanogenic glycosides, such as amygdalin, from members of the rose family (Rosaceae) is an example. The ruminant is more likely to achieve toxic levels of cyanide in the blood in the balance between breakdown of the glycoside, absorption of cyanide, and its detoxification and excretion, than is the nonruminant. Occasionally, unexpected events occur. Sheep on dry range pasture may die of cyanide poisoning shortly after drinking water. The loss of life from ingestion of poison suckleya (*Suckleyea suckleyana*) is an example. It is hypothesized that the ruminal contents are too dry for effective breakdown of the glycoside until the animal drinks, whereupon the reaction is intense. Sometimes such instances are erroneously diagnosed as poisoning from the water itself. Many of the symptoms are similar to those of nitrate poisoning.

Ingestion of abnormally large amounts of various forages or grains, or sudden massive change in diet, can provoke unusual reactions in the rumen that have toxicologic consequences. These can range from a simple pH shift to the elaboration of specific highly toxic molecules. For example, it has been suggested that, under unusual circumstances, silage of high nitrate content can undergo a reaction in the rumen that yields nitrogen oxide gases. Taken into the lungs, small amounts of nitrogen oxides cause severe, irreversible pulmonary emphysema. The same thing happens when nitrogen oxides are formed in silage made from forage (usually corn, *Zea mays*) of high nitrate concentration. Being heavier than air, the nitrogen oxides accumulate around the base of the silo. Breathed by man, they cause a similar syndrome, which is called "silo-filler's disease."

A syndrome of cattle, associated clinically with reduced levels of magnesium in the blood, is characterized by staggering that develops shortly after they are placed on lush pasturage. It has been postulated that, under these pasturage conditions, sufficient ammonia is formed in the rumen to react with, and tie up enough, magnesium (as hydroxide) to produce dietary insufficiency.

Some plants cause ruminal stasis. When this happens, a low-grade toxemia commences that becomes more severe with time. Also, signs of starvation appear. Mesquite bean (*Prosopis juliflora*) poisoning, recognized on southwestern ranges in cattle, is an example. Stasis is complete or nearly so. Mesquite beans have been found in the rumen on postmortem examination of animals that had not had access to this plant for as long as nine months. Under these conditions, the seeds have sometimes sprouted and begun to grow in the rumen.

Ruminants are more susceptible to bloat (the foamy entrapment of gases) than are monogastric animals. Bloat, if unrelieved, can have lethal consequences. Some plants promote bloat. These include some common leguminous forage crops and certain wild plants. Among the latter is the wild larkspur (*Delphinium* spp.) of western ranges. Under range conditions bloat may not be observed in time to be treated effectively.

Just as the rumen can promote the release of a toxic compound from an innocuous precursor, so can it sometimes aid in the detoxification of an initially poisonous compound. Sheep fed high-calcium alfalfa hay, for example, are protected to some degree against the toxic effects of halogeton (*Halogeton glomeratus*), which contains soluble oxalates. It is postulated that calcium is precipitated by the oxalate ions in the rumen, thus making the oxalate unavailable for absorption from the gut.

Another situation in which the ruminant has the advantage over the nonruminant occurs in the case of ingestion of plants containing a thiaminase, such as field horsetail (*Equisetum arvense*). In the horse, continued exposure to such plants causes destruction of the thiamine in the diet and the development of a definite and eventually lethal B_1 deficiency with classic signs of polyneuritis. This is one of the few instances where the ultimate biochemical lesion, disruption of carboxylation in the Krebs cycle, is known. In a ruminant, the microflora of the rumen manufacture copious quantities of thiamine, which apparently is carried intact in the bacterial cell to a point in the gut beyond which the thiaminase is inactivated or destroyed. There it is released by digestion of the bacterial cell and absorbed by the ruminant. In any event, ruminants do not suffer from thiamine deficiency despite having a level of thiaminase in the diet that would kill a horse.

The initial distribution of ingested materials in the ruminant is determined partly by density. Seeds tend to pass quickly through the rumen and to concentrate in the abomasum. Here irritant substances may be released from seeds in concentrated form and promote irritation and hemorrhage of the abomasal wall seeds of members of the mustard family (Cruciferae) are examples.

Lower Gut

Two important actions, irritation and absorption, may occur in the stomach and intestines. Many plants cause irritation, varying in severity from mild to ulcerative, and the principal signs or symptoms in many cases of poisoning are simply those of gastroenteritis. Pokeroot (*Phytolacca americana*), for example, experimentally produces hemorrhagic gastritis, and ulcers are found in postmortem examination at locations where pieces of root lie against the mucosa of the gut. Pokeweed poisoning in cattle results in copious, almost explosive diarrhea that may contain signs of hemorrhage. In contrast, although blood-tinged feces are characteristic of oak (*Quercus* spp.) poisoning of cattle, the gastroenteritis is usually accompanied by constipation.

Absorption of toxins into the bloodstream normally takes place in the lower gut. Some toxic principles are large molecules, not readily absorbed. Saponins, such as those of the cockles (*Saponaria* spp.), are examples. As irritants, however, they promote their own absorption. Cardioactive glycosides are saponic in physical properties. It has been shown that the nature of the sugar portion of the intact glycoside is important in determining the solubility of these molecules and, therefore, their physiologic availability.

Liver

Poisonous principles absorbed into the circulatory system pass first to the liver. Here many different things can happen. A number of plant substances are severely poisonous to hepatic tissue, causing rapid destruction and necrosis where contact is made. A common finding on necropsy is a pathologic liver, but the exact pathology varies considerably. In many cases, the assault is somewhat chronic, and the appearance and function of the liver represent whatever current balance exists between destructive and regenerative changes.

A great deal of recent work has gone into elucidation of the exact hepatotoxic effects of pyrrolizidine alkaloids. Alkaloids of this configuration are found in a number of genera of higher plants (such as *Senecio* spp.). The primary lesion is a characteristic megalocytosis accompanied by venous obstruction or occlusion. Some plants. (e.g., *Trifolium subterraneum*, subterranean clover) accumulate copper from soils of high copper content. Copper then accumulates in and produces degenerative changes of the liver. In akee (*Blighia sapida*) poisoning of man, a hypoglycemic poisonous principle in the plant reduces the glycogen content of the liver to nearly zero.

One of the types of liver dysfunction that commonly occurs in plant poisonings is the reduced ability to eliminate certain pigmented molecules in the bile. These, instead, enter general circulation. When they reach the capillaries of the skin, they react with light and cause the capillaries to leak serum. This reaction and its consequences constitute the syndrome of photosensitization. If edematous swelling is severe, the involved tissues die and are sloughed off. Thus, in range sheep, the disease known as bighead is characterized initially by erythema, then by edematous swelling, and ultimately by necrosis of portions of the ears, cheeks, and lips, if severe Animals that have lost the lips are unable to forage effectively and die of starvation. The identity of all pigments involved in photosensitization is not yet known, but several have been established. One or more are breakdown products of chlorophyll and are normally present in the hepatic portal circulation. In other cases, the photosensitizing pigment is contained in the plant itself and passes unchanged through digestion, absorption, and the normal liver. Photosensitization caused by the first type of pigment, always accompanied by signs of liver damage, and usually by icterus, is termed secondary. Photosensitization involving a normal liver and lacking any signs of liver dysfunction is termed primary. A range plant commonly provoking secondary photosensitization (bighead) is horsebrush (*Tetradymia* spp.). Primary photosensitization is less common, but can be caused by ingestion of St. Johnswort (*Hypericum perforatum*).

Circulatory System

The discussion of photosensitization has taken us from the liver to the general circulation. A number of other disease syndromes may occur in the circulatory system or involve the blood itself. The toxic principle of sweet pea (*Lathyrus odoratus*), β-aminopropionitrile, causes dissecting aneurysm of the aorta in small animals. A number of plants contain toxins that provoke lysis of red blood cells and consequent hemolytic anemia. Among them are cultivated onion (*Allium cepa*) and rape forage (*Brassica napus*). Saponins and phytotoxins cause lysis of red blood cells *in vitro*. Their role *in vivo* is less clear.

Coumarin, contained in sweetclover hay (*Melilotus* spp.), is converted to dicoumarin by molds under certain conditions. This compound interferes with prothrombin synthesis and results in a hemorrhagic disease when molded sweetclover hay is ingested over a period of time. Animals bleed to death from minor injuries or, in advanced cases, bleed to death internally. Large subdermal hemorrhages are usually found in these cases. Soluble oxalates in the diet can result in the precipitation of calcium ions in the circulating blood. The resulting ionic imbalance has neurologic consequences. Hypomagnesemia and its consequences have already been mentioned.

Kidney

Once a toxin is in the blood, all organs are exposed to its effect unless a membrane barrier intervenes. Many plant toxins are destructive to parenchymatous organs in general. Digenerative effects are seen primarily in liver and kidneys on postmortem examination. In some cases described above, the liver is the primary target organ. In a few others, the kidney shows the major pathology. The latter includes the effects of tannins in oak (*Quercus* spp.) poisoning, and the crystallization of oxalates in kidney tubules in oxalate poisoning as by halogeton (*Halogeton glomeratus*).

Heart

In many lethal poisonings, the immediate cause of death is heart failure. Heart dysfunction can be brought about by malfunction of innervation or of the heart's conducting tissues, or it may be a result of a more direct effect on the heart musculature. Ingestion of foxglove (*Digitalis purpurea*) is similar to an overdose of the drug digitalis, which acts by stimulating the vagus center. At toxic levels, cardioactive glycosides produce cardiac irregularities and heart block. The alkaloid of yew (*Taxus cuspidata*) depresses the conducting tissue of the heart and stops it, often very quickly, in diastole. Hypotensive alkaloids, such as in false hellebore (*Veratrum viride*), cause a marked slowing of the heart rate.

Bone

Bracken fern (*Pteridium aquilinum*) contains two toxins. One is a thiaminase. The other, more slowly acting, has its target the bone marrow. Thus, ruminants exposed to a steady diet of bracken for many weeks develop a blood dyscrasia, characterized particularly by diminished counts of leukocytes and platelets, which may be traced in origin to severe destruction of bone marrow. Clinical signs of this disease are unusual for a poisoning and consist chiefly of hemorrhaging throughout the body due to thrombocytopenia, and invasion of the body by ordinarily nonpathogenic bacteria due to leukocytopenia, and the concomitant development of an elevated temperature. This disease is basically indistinguishable from radiation poisoning.

Pokeweed (*Phytolacca americana*), in contrast, contains an active principle that promotes the division of white blood cells. The pokeweed mitogen is also associated with the stimulation of production of interferon.

Some unusual plant toxins act on the skeletal structure itself. Sweet pea (*Lathyrus odoratus*) poisoning in laboratory animals consists primarily of disturbance of the normal deposition and resorption of bone in such a way that cartilage proliferates. The gross effect includes a twisting of the vertebral column. The poisonous principle is the same as that causing dissecting aneurysms in other animals. "Crooked-calf disease" is associated with lupines (*Lupinus sericeus*).

Lung

Under some circumstances, ingestion of rape (*Brassica napus*) forage results in lesions of the lung. Edematous swelling and emphysema are followed by rupture of the alveoli and passage of air from the lungs to collect subdermally on either side of the backbone, where it may be palpated. Somewhat similar lesions are produced by nitrogen gases, as described above.

Thyroid

Many members of the cabbage family (Cruciferae) contain glycosides that release goitrogenic factors (thiocyanates and thiooxazolidone) when digested. The thyroid responds to these compounds by enlarging, and other signs of goiter appear. These goitrogens are iodine responsive.

Eye

The eyes are sometimes involved in signs of poisoning. Severe mydriasis that may provoke visual disturbance is a common sign of poisoning by alkaloids of the tropane configuration, such as atropine found in jimsonweed (*Datura stramonium*). Blindness accompanies a number of poisonings in which other signs may be primary. Often the eye appears normal in structure and function, and blindness may be ascribed to malfunction in the central nervous system. An example of a plant that causes functional blindness is tansy mustard (*Descurainia pinnata*). In man, ingestion of poppy (isoquinoline) alkaloids as from prickly poppy (*Argemone mexicana*) often causes generalized edema and has been held responsible for producing glaucoma.

Nervous System

Nervous signs are perhaps second in frequency only to gastroenteric signs in case of plant poisoning. Nervous involvement and the consequent specific signs are extremely varied and may depend as much on species of animal as on the poisonous principle itself. When nervous tissue is the principal target, lesions are usually absent. There are exceptions. Cerebral demyelination has been reported in lambs born to ewes fed heavily on seaweeds. Liquefactive necrosis of cerebellar areas has been associated with molded forage and with ingestion of sensitive fern (*Onoclea sensibilis*) by horses. More recently, focal necrosis in the anterior globus pallidus of the cerebrum and substantia nigra of the mesencephalon has been described as the primary lesion in "chewing disease" of horses fed on yellow star thistle (*Centaurea solstitialis*). Pigs born to sows that have fed heavily on white clover (*Trifolium repens*) may under some circumstances display demyelination of the spinal cord and be unable to suckle . The exact signs associated with lesions of cranial and spinal nervous tissue vary widely and depend on exactly what areas are involved. An example of a type of poisoning in which obvious lesions of the nervous tissue do not occur is the convulsive syndrome characteristic of water hemlock (*Cicuta maculata*) poisoning.

In many cases a nervous syndrome may be characterized grossly as excitatory or depressive. An example of the former is the hyperexcitable condition produced in animals after ingestion of Dallis grass (*Paspalum dilatatum*) parasitized by an ergot (*Claviceps paspali*). In contrast, weakness and paralysis are characteristic of the effect of poisons that interfere with the normal action of the voluntary musculature through its innervation. For example, guajillo (*Acacia berlandieri*) provokes a classic syndrome of ascending posterior paralysis. In this case, the identity of the poisonous principle, N-methyl-β-phenylalanine, has been worked out. Coniine, the alkaloid of poison hemlock (*Conium maculatum*), the first alkaloid to be synthesized, has an action that is essentially similar in gross effect. Sleepy grass (*Stipa robusta*), found in a limited area of the American Southwest, provokes drowsiness in horses in small amounts and deep sleep in larger doses. The active principle is unknown.

Additional nervous symptoms can be described in man. Paresthesias and hallucinations are associated with particular types of poisoning. The alkaloid aconitine (e.g., from monkshood, *Aconitum napellus*) causes the former, and jimsonweed (*Datura stramonium*) in moderate amount gives rise to the latter.

In gangrenous ergotism, chronic ingestion of ergot (usually *Claviceps purpurea* on rye—*Secale cereale*) causes constriction of the musculature of arterioles. This results in a predisposition to thromboses or other occlusions of the circulation, particularly in the extremities where blood pressure is minimal. The tissue distal to the occlusion dies, becomes septic, and eventually is lost.

Respiratory System

Respiration can be inhibited or prevented at any level, from the mouth to the respiring cells themselves. Cases involving the oral cavity, the lungs, and the cardiovascular system have already been mentioned. In addition to these, respiration can be blocked by the inability of blood to carry oxygen, as in nitrate poisoning, or of the cells to use it, as in cyanide poisoning. Many plants can take up dangerously high levels of nitrogen under conditions of heavy fertilization; a few (such as corn—*Zea mays*) are predisposed to do so. Treatment of crops with 2,4-D can upset nitrogen metabolism with similar results. Nitrate in plants is largely converted to nitrite in the gut. This reacts with hemoglobin to form methemoglobin. The ability of the blood to carry oxygen is impaired in proportion to conversion. Cyanide, released from cyanogenetic glycosides of various kinds elaborated in a large number of plants (e.g., wild cherries—*Prunus* spp.), blocks the action of cytochrome oxidase and thereby interferes with the uptake of oxygen into cellular respiration. In both cases the general signs are those associated with asphyxiation.

Reproductive System

Some plants can elaborate estrogenic factors under certain conditions. Certain forage legumes are known to do so. Corn (*Zea mays*) molded by an unknown fungus has provoked a similar syndrome. Poisoning is characterized by vaginal swelling and prolapse in female animals. Some effects may also be observed in male animals.

Some plants, ingested by pregnant animals, have a pronounced teratogenic effect on the developing embryo. Perhaps the best example is the cycloptic lambs born to ewes that have been exposed to ingestion of hellebore (*Veratrum californicum*) on the fourteenth day of gestation. At that time the embryo is sensitive in development of facial structure. A massive exposure to the plant results in severely inhibited facial development. While the lower jaw remains more or less normal, the upper jaw disappears nearly entirely, and both eyes occupy a single orbit in the center of the forehead, or there may be but one central eye.

Some poisonous principles (fortunately few) are readily excreted in milk. These include especially those of high fat solubility, which may be concentrated in the butterfat. While excretion of toxic principles is beneficial to the animal doing so, the consumption of milk from poisoned animals can induce poisoning in man or nursing animals. The secondary poisoning can be more severe than that in the lactating animal because of the concentration of the poison and the lesser ability of the nonlactating consumer to eliminate it. Perhaps the best example is given by white snakeroot (*Eupatorium rugosum*). The poisonous principle (tremetol) it contains provokes a disease in cattle called trembles. Ingestion of milk from poisoned cattle causes a serious debilitating disease, "milksickness," in man.

Farmers commonly associate abortion in livestock with ingestion of weeds. The actual causes of abortion are many. Some plants in toxic amounts (e.g., broomweed—*Gutierrezia microcephala*) undoubtedly can lead to abortion in pregnant animals, but the mechanism is undetermined.

Hair and Skin

The effect of photosensitization on the skin has been mentioned above. Thickening of the skin (hyperkeratosis), usually accompanied by loss of hair, can result from a variety of causes but is often related to a deficiency of vitamin A. It has been shown that some isolates of the imperfect fungus *Aspergillus* can induce the formation of a factor in the substrate that produces well-developed cases of hyperkeratosis in experimental animals.

Some forage plants, particularly legumes, grown on high molybdenum soils accumulate enough molybdenum to become toxic to grazing animals. One of the chief signs of poisoning is depigmentation of the hair. The incidence of this disease in cattle at pasture can be mapped by airplane. Depigmentation, which develops slowly, is ascribed to the inability of tyrosinase to mediate the formation of melanin in the absence of copper, the availability of which in the body is reciprocally related to the bodily concentration of molybdenum.

Loss of long hair and hoof deformity accompany one type of selenium poisoning. On certain seleniferous soils, grain crops may develop concentrations of selenium, in organic combination, of 5 ppm or more. At this level, continued ingestion of grain or forage produces the syndrome known as "alkali disease." It appears that selenium substitutes for sulfur in amino acids. Hoof deformity and sloughing will become severe enough in time that affected animals will graze from a kneeling position and eventually starve to death. The amino acid mimosine (as in koa haole, *Leucaena glauca*) is held responsible for causing a similar syndrome when ingested.

Poisonous plants are numerous, ubiquitous, troublesome, and poorly studied. No general botanic, ecologic, or geographic relationship exists among them to bring order to an understanding of the diversity of toxic principles contained in plants, viewed either chemically or physiologically, and in the syndromes provoked by them in man and animals. Syndromes in which a plant poison is the prime etiologic factor may involve the integument and hair, the mouth and any portion of the digestive system (with a major distinction possible between ruminant and simple-stomached animals), the parenchymatous organs (especially the liver and kidney), the circulatory system (including the heart, vascularization, and blood itself), the skeletal system, the lungs and respiratory system (including cellular respiration), various glands (especially the thyroid), the central and autonomic nervous systems, the eye, and the reproductive system. Full elucidation of a poisonous plant syndrome usually requires the efforts of a team of research specialists. Some past investigations have yielded results of great medical or economic importance. Results are needed even more urgently so that reaction to poisoning by plants, its treatment, and prevention can be more intelligently founded than at present.

2

BILBERRY

Vaccinium myrtillus L. (Ericaceae) is a shrub found in the mountains of Europe and North America. It is related to the North America's blueberry and huckleberry. The shrub produces a blue-black or purple berry with purple meat from July through September, depending on the elevation. This berry is the part of the plant of interest. In addition to its use as a food, it was documented as being used to treat kidney stones, biliary problems, scurvy, coughs, and tuberculosis in the 1500s. It has also been used to make a traditional tea to treat diabetes, and purportedly has a hypoglycemic effect. Little is known about bilberry's active constituents and their pharmacology, although it has been studied since at least 1964 for ophthalmological and vascular disorders. Most of these studies were performed in Europe, and many are published in non-English or obscure journals. Stories of British Royal Air Force pilots eating bilberry jam during World War II to improve their night vision may have prompted some of these studies.

Orally, bilberry is used for improving visual acuity including night vision, degenerative retinal conditions, varicose veins, atherosclerosis, venous insufficiency, *chronic fatigue syndrome* (CFS), and hemorrhoids. It is also used orally for angina, diabetes, arthritis, gout, dermatitis, and prevention and treatment of gastrointestinal (GI), kidney, and urinary tract symptoms and diseases. Topically, it is used for mild inflammation of the mouth and throat mucous membranes.

SOURCES AND CHEMICAL COMPOSITION

Tegens is a standardized Italian bilberry product that contains Myrtocyan (*V. myrtillus* L., fresh fruits, 25% anthocyanidins and 35% anthocyanosides).

Products Available

In the United States, bilberry is usually sold in capsule form as an antioxidant and to promote eye health. It is sometimes combined with other vitamins or herbs purported to be beneficial to the eye, such as lutein or eyebright.

Pharmacological/Toxicological Effects

Bilberry's ability to stimulate synthesis of connective tissue glycosaminoglycans may be the mechanism underlying its beneficial effects in several pathologies. Its gastroprotective, vasoprotective, and healing properties may all be tied to this action.

Antiulcer Activity

A bilberry extract containing 25% anthocyanidins (Myrtocyan) demonstrated antiulcer activity in several rat models. Efficacy was measured using an "*index of ulceration*" and means were compared using the Mann- Whitney U test. Minimum doses producing statistically significant benefit were 100 mg/kg for ulcers induced by pyloric ligation, 25 mg/kg for reserpine ulcer, and 100 mg/kg for phenylbutazone ulcers ($p < 0.01$ compared to control). For acetic acid ulcers, efficacy was determined by measuring the ulcer surface area. The minimum effective dose was 50 mg/kg ($p < 0.01$ compared to control, Dunnett *t*-test). For restraint ulcer, efficacy was determined by comparing the number of ulcers in the control vs bilberry groups. The minimum effective dose was 100 mg/kg ($p < 0.01$ compared with control, Mann-Whitney U-test). Effects on volume or pH of gastric secretion were ruled out as a mechanism of action. Histological examination of the gastric mucosa showed increased mucus production in treated rats. Bilberry's beneficial effects were attributed to an increase in production of mucopolysaccharides.

Based on the promising results of this study, the antiulcer activity of the individual anthocyanidins was studied. One anthocyanidin, 3,5,7-trihydroxy-2-(3 ,4-dihydroxyphenyl)-1-benzopyrylium chloride showed particular promise, and so it was produced synthetically so that its effects on several animal models of acute and chronic stomach ulcers could be studied further. IdB 1027 administrered orally or intraperitoneally was able to inhibit acute gastric ulceration induced by pyloric ligation, stress (cold plus restraint), phenylbutazone, indomethacin, reserpine, ethanol, and histamine, as well as duodenal ulceration induced by cysteamine and chronic gastric ulcers induced by acetic acid. Results of additional experiments suggest the mechanism of action involves stimulation of protective gastric mucosal secretions.

A drawback of this study is that the severity of ulceration caused by phenylbutazone, indomethacin, ethanol, and histamine was assessed using nonvalidated ordinal scales.

Vascular Permeability

In a rat model of hypertension, animals pretreated with *V. myrtillus* dry extract "rich in anthocyanin glucosides" at a dose of 50 mg/100 g body weight for 12 days prior to aortic ligation and for 14 days thereafter showed less permeability of the aorta, blood- brain barrier, and blood vessels of the skin to a tracer dye (1% tryptan blue solution), compared to untreated animals on day 7 after ligature. The effect was most pronounced in the brain and least pronounced in the blood vessels of the skin. The investigators proposed, based on previous experiments, that anthocyanins in bilberry extract interact with collagen to make it more resistant to the effects of collagenase, thus preserving the integrity of the basal lamina and its control of vascular permeability.

In a subsequent experiment, intraperitoneal injection of Myrtocyan ameliorated histamine-induced capillary permeability measured by permeability to Evans blue. The minimum effective dose was 50 mg/kg ($p < 0.01$ compared to control, Dunnett *t*-test). At a dose of 200 mg/kg Myrtocyan was effective in improving capillary resistance to vacuum-induced petechiae in rats fed a flavonoid deficient diet ($p < 0.01$ compared to baseline, Dunnett *t*-test).

Antiangiogenic Effects

Billberry extract was able to inhibit vascular endothelial growth factor expression by human keratinocytes in vitro. This suggests that bilberry or its constituents may have a role in cancer prevention or treatment.

Antilipemic and Hypoglycemic Effects

Because bilberry has traditionally been used to treat diabetes, which is associated with alteration of lipid metabolism, the effects of a bilberry leaf extract on plasma glucose and triglycerides were studied in various rat models. The study preparation was made by percolation of bilberry leaf powder with ethanol 40% (Indena, Milano, Italy). All statistical comparisons were done using unpaired *t*-tests.

In Sprague-Dawley rats made diabetic with streptozocin, plasma glucose levels were 26% lower ($p < 0.05$) 4 days after streptozocin administration, and 26.6% lower ($p < 0.01$, unpaired *t*-test) 3 weeks after streptozocin administration in rats treated with bilberry extract at a dose of 3 g/kg twice daily for five doses compared with untreated diabetic rats. Triglycerides were also 38.8% ($p < 0.05$) lower in the treated rats. The extract did not affect glucose levels in control animals, and did not affect weight.

In rats with diet-induced hyperlipidemia, triglycerides were lower in rats treated with the extract at doses of 1.2 g/kg ($p < 0.05$) and 3 g/kg ($p < 0.01$) than in untreated rats. Weight was not affected. In genetically hyperlipidemic Yoshida rats, and in rats with alcohol-induced hypertriglyceridemia, triglycerides were 31.8% ($p < 0.05$) and 61.5% ($p < 0.01$) lower, respectively, in bilberry-treated rats than in untreated rats.

The antilipemic effect of bilberry may be caused by improved breakdown of triglyceride-rich lipoproteins, as evidenced by findings of a third part of this study. Rats were administrered Triton WR-1339 to induce hypertriglyceridemia. This agent has an acute effect of blocking lipoprotein clearance, and a secondary effect of stimulation of liver lipoprotein synthesis. Bilberry was able to attenuate only the acute effect of Triton on triglycerides, suggesting that bilberry improves lipoprotein clearance, but does not affect lipoprotein production.

Although bilberry's effect on triglycerides is similar to that of the fibric acid derivatives (e.g., gemfibrozil, fenofibrate) used therapeutically to treat hypertriglyceridemia, bilberry did not affect thrombus size or composition, suggesting that it does not possess antithrombotic activity, as has been demonstrated with some fibric acid derivatives.

Oxidized *low-density liporpotein* (LDL) is known for its ability to stimulate inflammatory processes involved in the formation of atherosclerotic plaques. For this reason, there has been interest in the use of antioxidants such as bilberry to protect against LDL oxidation.

In an in vitro study, the ability of a bilberry extract containing 74.2 ± 4.9 mg/g polyphenols with 17.3 ± 3.3% catechin (mean ± standard deviation [SD] of 10 preparations) to attenuate copper-mediated LDL oxidation was studied. LDL was taken from six volunteers with normal lipid levels, and markers of oxidation were measured in the presence of bilberry extract at concentrations of 0, 5, 10, 15, 20, and 30 μg/mL. All comparisons were made using the Mann-Whitney test. Compared with control, bilberry was able to prolong the time to conjugated diene formation at concentrations of 20 and 30 μg/mL ($p < 0.01$), decrease production of lipoperoxides and malondialdehyde at concentrations of 10 μg/mL or higher for at least 1 hour and 0.5 hour ($p < 0.05$), respectively, and attenuate change in the net negative charge of LDL at concentrations of at least 15 μg/mL ($p < 0.01$).

Ocular Effects

Bilberry was reported to have beneficial effects on retinal vascular permeability and tendency to hemorrhage in 31 patients with retinopathy in a German study. Benefits were particularly pronounced in patients with diabetic retinopathy, according to the abstract, which was the only part of the study published in English. A study published in Italian showed ophthalmoscopic improvement in 11 and angiographic improvement in 12 of 14 patients with retinopathy caused by diabetes and/or hypertension, according to a review article.

Bilberry jam purportedly improved night vision in Royal Air Force pilots within 24 hours of eating bilberry jam, and at least five European studies showing the beneficial effect of bilberry on night vision were published prior to 1970. A 1997 Israeli study published as an abstract found negative results, as did a more recent study performed in 15 Navy Seals. In this trial, Muth and colleagues studied the effect of bilberry extract (25% anthocyanocides) 160 mg taken three times daily for 3 weeks on night visual acuity and night contrast sensitivity in subjects with visual acuity correctable to at least 20/20. An independent laboratory verified the composition of the extract used. Eight subjects were given placebo and seven were given the extract in double-blind fashion. After a 30-day washout, the subjects were crossed over the alternate treatment arm. Nighttime visual acuity and contrast sensitivity were measured under lighting conditions simulating full moonlight (i.e., a luminescence of 0.005 candelas/m^2). To measure visual acuity, subjects were presented with Landolt C targets (computer-generated black Cs on a white background) with the opening of the C facing one of eight directions. Each subject was given five tries to correctly identify the direction of the C. If the subject was correct three out of five times, the subject was presented with another five targets of smaller size. Three incorrect responses ended the test. Contrast sensitivity was measured in the same fashion, except that instead of decreasing the size of the targets, the contrast between the target and the background was decreased. Baseline visual acuity and contrast sensitivity were measured three times during the first week of the study; 24–36 hours after beginning treatment, 4–6 days after beginning treatment; once between days 12–14; and once between day 19–21. Testing was performed once each week during the 4-week washout. After the second treatment phase, measurements were again taken weekly for 4 weeks. Repeated measures analysis of variance was used to compare the median of the three pretreatment visual acuity and contrast sensitivity measurements to the mean of those obtained during each of the two treatment periods, and to the last measurement taken in each of the two treatment periods. Subjects were also placed into one of four categories depending on whether they showed improvement with both treatments, neither treatment, placebo only, or bilberry only. These results were compared using McNemar's test. No difference between bilberry and placebo was detected. The investigators describe a previous French study in which improvement in five of 14 subjects with poor pretreatment night vision was noted. A larger sample size or use of subjects with poor night vision at baseline may have yielded more promising results.

In a subsequent review, the results of two other early studies published in French are described. These studies showed that bilberry improved night visual acuity, adaptation to darkness, and recovery of visual acuity after glare. Other articles published during the late 1960s in Italian and German showed beneficial effects of bilberry on retinitis pigmentosa and quinine-induced hemeralopia, according to this review. The review also mentions a study published in an Italian journal that purportedly showed that a single dose of bilberry anthocyanosides 200 mg improved electroretinographic findings in eight patients with glaucoma, purportedly by stabilizing the collagen of the trabecular network, thus improving aqueous humor outflow.

A review by Head describes a study published in Italian in which bilberry extract (25% anthocyanosides) 180 mg and *d,l*-tocopheryl acetate 100 mg twice daily for 12 weeks stabilized cataract growth in 96% of 25 treated patients vs 76% of 25 controls (n = 50).

Pharmacokinetics

The anthocyanins present in bilberry are thought to cross the blood-brain barrier. To date, no human studies have been published regarding the pharmacokinetics of the anthocyanins present in bilberry. However, studies have been conducted using other sources of anthocyanins, such as blueberries, elderberries, and blackcurrant juice. Mazza and colleagues studied the absorption of anthocyanins from a freeze-dried blueberry preparation in five human subjects. Following administration of 100 g of blueberry supplement containing 1.2 g of anthocyanins, serum concentrations of 11 anthocyanins were measured at 1, 2, 3, and 4 hours postdose. Serum concentrations of each of the anthocyanins ranged from 0.23 to 3.68 ng/mL, suggesting very low absorption of anthocyanidins from this preparation. However, urinary excretion was not measured, precluding an accurate assessment of absorption. The concentration of total anthocyanins ranged from 6.6 ng/mL at 1 hour to 9.6, 12.1, and 13.1 ng/mL at 2, 3, and 4 hours, respectively.

In a more complete pharmacokinetic study, Cao et al. studied the plasma and urine pharmacokinetics of 720 mg of anthocyanins from an elderberry extract in four elderly women. Blood and urine samples were collected over 24 hours. These investigators found primarily two anthocyanins (cyanidin 3-sambubioside and cyanidin 3-glucoside) present in both blood and urine. The time to maximum concentration (t_{max}) of total anthocyanidins was approx 1 hour and the C_{max} was 97 nmol/L. The average half-life for total anthocyanidins was approx 130 minutes, with the mean half-life of cyanidin 3-sambubioside being 170 minutes and that of cyanidin 3-glucoside being 100 minutes. In concurrence with the results of Mazza et al., less than 0.001% of the dose of anthocyanins was recovered in the urine within 24 hours, again indicative of poor absorption of these compounds. However, no attempts were made to analyze for potential glucuronide or sulfate conjugate metabolites of these compounds, and thus a more complete absorption picture is not available.

Another study in six healthy volunteers studied the pharmacokinetics and bioavailability of anthocyanidin-3-glycosides from either blackcurrant juice or elderberries. As with other studies listed previously, these investigators found very little (~0.04% from blackcurrant juice to 0.4% from elderberry extract) of the dose recovered in the urine, suggesting low bioavailability. Though the half-life of the anthocyanidins was similar regardless of preparation, the area under the curve and amount of anthocyanidins excreted were approx 10-fold higher in the subjects administered the elderberry extract as compared with those receiving blackcurrant juice. The half-life (~1.7 hours) was comparable to that in the aforementioned study by Cao et al., but the recovery of anthocyanins in the previous study by Cao et al. administering elderberry extract was substantially lower (~400-fold lower) than that observed in this study. The reason for this discrepancy in amount recovered is unclear from the information given in the articles, but may relate to how the elderberry extract is formulated.

Adverse Effects and Toxicity

The lethal dose of 50% of the population (LD_{50}) of Myrtocyan in rodents is over 2000 mg/kg, and in dogs the only adverse effect from a dose of 3000 mg/kg was dark urine and feces. There is no evidence of mutagenicity, or of teratogenicity or impaired fertility in rats. According to unpublished data of 2295 patients taking Tegens, most of whom took 160 mg twice daily for 1–2 months, 94 subjects complained of adverse effects involving the GI, dermatological, and nervous system.

There are currently no reported adverse effects from the consumption of bilberry or related compounds. When the fruit is consumed in amounts normally contained in foods, bilberry falls under the "Generally Recognized as Safe" category according to the US Food and Drug Administration. However, death has been reported with the chronic consumption or high doses of the leaf (1.5 g/[kg · day]).

Interactions

Bilberry extract 200 mg/(kg · day) administered intraperitoneally to euthyroid rats increased radiolabeled triiodothyronine (T3) transport into the brain, compared to vehicle only. Postulated mechanisms include central or peripheral inhibition of L-thyroxine's (T4) deiodination to T3; inhibition of T3 protein binding; or enhanced T3 binding to carrier proteins in the brain capillary wall. Whether bilberry could interact with thyroid replacement therapy remains to be seen.

Studying a diabetic rat model, Cignarella and colleagues found that administration of an extract from the leaves of blueberry plants caused a 26% reduction in plasma glucose. This was also accompanied by a 39% decrease in plasma triglycerides. Whether this reduction in glucose levels might result in a clinically significant interaction in patients taking antidiabetic agents is unknown, because the glucose lower effects have not been studied in humans. Likewise, whether the triglyceride-lowering effects of hypolipidemic agents used in humans would be enhanced by coadministration of anthocyanidins is unknown.

Reproduction

There is insufficient information to determine the safety of bilberry consumption during pregnancy or lactation.

Regulatory Status

Bilberry is classified as a dietary supplement.

3

Citrus aurantium

It is generally thought that the Citrus originated in Southeast Asia. There are a number of Citrus types, but within oranges the principal members are the sweet orange and the bitter orange. The horticultural mapping of *Citrus* is notoriously difficult, with large discrepancies between writings of number of variants of all types of Citrus. Despite this, there are three properly recognized bitter orange fruits and two other closely related fruits. One of these relatives is the bergamot, the oil of which is famous for giving the distinct taste in Earl Gray tea. Bitter orange fruit is too sour for general consumption, although it is eaten with salt and chili in Mexico and raw in Iran. The peel of the fruit has a distinctive taste that is highly valued in marmalade, its most widespread culinary use. *Citrus aurantium* is used in several alcoholic beverages. When dried, the peel is used in a distinctive Belgian beer called Orange Muscat. The oil from *C. aurantium* is a standard ingredient in other liquors such as Triple Sec, Cointreau, and Curacao. The oil is also common in perfumes and as a flavoring agent in sweets.

The bulk primary usage of *C. aurantium* is for medicinal purposes. In China, Japan, and Korea, when dried, the entire unripe fruit is used to treat digestive problems. The dried fruit is used to stimulate gastric acid secretion and appetite in Western countries.

Current Promoted Uses

C. aurantium is still used in traditional culinary ways as described previously. It has also been investigated for a number of other medicinal uses in addition to gastrointestinal disturbances. As a dermatological agent, it has been used as an antifungal and exhibits some evidence of fungicidal and fungi-static activity. Other uses cited are as a stimulant, a sedative, and for the treatment of anemia, frostbite, general feebleness, retinal hemorrhage, bloody stools, duodenal ulcers, and prolapsed uterus or anus, among other things.

Recently, the most predominant use of *C. aurantium* has been as a weight loss aid or as an energy-boosting supplement. After the ban of phenylpropanolamine owing to increased risk of hemorrhagic stroke, ephedra use in supplements increased substantially. In April of 2004, the Food and Drug Administration (FDA) banned the sale of ephedra because of the dangers of this alkaloid. Since then, alternatives to this popular supplement have been sought and bitter orange has emerged as the mostly predominantly used substitute. Although *C. aurantium* has been reviewed for this use, lack of studies make this difficult—as evidenced by a 2004 Cochrane Collaboration Database that identified only one eligible randomized placebo controlled trial. Despite this relative lack of data, since the banning of ephedra, *C. aurantium* has been used extensively in a variety of products—from weight loss pills to two patents for weight-loss toothpaste.

Sources and Chemical Composition

C. aurantium, synonyms *Citrus amara*, *Citrus bigarradia*, *Citrus vulgaris*. Also known as *Aurantii pericarpium*, Chisil, *Fructus aurantii*, Green Orange, Kijitsu, Neroli Oil, Seville Orange, Shangzhou Zhiqiao, Sour Orange, Synephrine, Zhi Qiao, Zhi Shi.

Products Available

C. aurantium is available in a wide variety of products in multiple dosage forms.

Pharmacological/Toxicological Effects

Pharmacology

C. aurantium contains the adrenergic amines synephrine, octopamine, and tyramine, and many flavones and glycosylated flavanones. These sympathomimetic molecules can be found in normal human plasma and are known to be involved in alternate metabolic pathways of common biogenic amines. Of the three active adrenergic molecules in *C. aurantium*, synephrine is present in amounts at least 100-fold greater than either octopamine or tyramine found in the fresh fruit, dried extracts, or herbal medicines.

The locations of the substituents on the phenylethylamine backbone play an integral role in determining the observed pharmacological effects of sympathomimetic molecules. Substitution of a hydroxyl group on the β-carbon tends to increase activity toward both α and β receptors, but decreases activity in the central nervous system (CNS). Substitution of hydroxyl groups in any place in the phenylethylamine structure increases the hydrophilicity, and thus decreases the propensity of the molecule to enter the CNS.

Ephedrine, for example, is a weaker CNS stimulant than amphetamine but is a stronger bronchodilator and has greater effect on increasing heart rate and blood pressure. The relatively polar epinephrine is essentially devoid of CNS activity aside from anxiety related to other systemic effects. Hydroxyl groups at both the 3 and 4 position provides the most α and β activity. Also, substitution at the amino position generally enhances the effect on β receptors. This accounts for the strength of epinephrine for β_2 receptor subtype relative to that of norepinephrine and is probably important in interpreting the potential cardiovascular effects of *C. aurantium*.

Although the effects of synephrine and *C. aurantium* differ slightly in hemodynamic studies, the relative content of synephrine compared to octopamine and tyramine (at least 100 times more synephrine) in *C. aura ntium* products substantially outweighs the effects of octopamine and tyramine. Although synephrine is found endogenously in the adrenal glands, the function is still unclear.

There seems to be general agreement that synephrine is an active agonist of β_1, β_2, and β_3 adrenergic receptors. There are conflicting reports, however, as to whether synephrine possesses any β_1- or β_2-receptor-agonist activity. The effects observed in studies and case reports of *C. aurantium* use are consistent with that of both α- and β-receptor activation. Also, the published study demonstrating lack of β-adrenergic activation was conducted in guinea pig atria/trachea, whereas the study demonstrating activation of β receptors was conducted in cloned human β_2 adrenergic receptors. Drugs such as phenylephrine, which primarily exhibit α-agonist activity, induce a rise in blood pressure and a dose-related increase in peripheral vascular resistance. Associated with these actions is a sinus bradycardia caused by vagal reflex. Epinephrine, on the other hand, exhibits both α- and β-agonist activity. Effects seen with norepinephrine infusion are tachycardia, a moderate increase in systolic blood pressure, a rise in cardiac output, and shorter and more powerful cardiac systole. The β_2 effect relaxes skeletal muscle vasculature, leading to a lowering of peripheral resistance and diastolic blood pressure.

Cardiovascular Effect

There are limited animal and human data on the cardiovascular effects of *C. aurantium*. When administered to rats, *C. aurantium* and synephrine both raised blood pressure in a dose-dependent manner. In another study in rats, repeated oral *C. aurantium* extract led to dose-dependent cardiovascular toxicity and mortality. Two studies using synephrine or *C. aurantium* in rats with induced portal hypertension (by portal vein ligation) have been conducted. In these studies, both synephrine and *C. aurantium* significantly reduced portal venous pressure. Interestingly, *C. aurantium* had a greater effect on portal hypertension than synephrine alone.

In one of two human clinical studies to date, intravenous synephrine was injected into 12 healthy male volunteers. The parameters recorded were transthoracic echocardiography (ECG), cardiac index, arterial blood pressure, and peripheral vascular resistance. Volunteers were given a continuous infusion of 4 mg/minute synephrine. Systolic blood pressure increased by a mean of 27 mmHg ($p < 0.005$) and mean arterial blood pressure increased by 9 mmHg ($p < 0.005$). The cardiac index increased from 3.6 to 4.6 L/(minute · μ_2) ($p < 0.001$) whereas peripheral vascular resistance was decreased ($p < 0.01$). The heart rate and diastolic pressure remained unchanged. By ECG, left ventricular contractility parameters also increased significantly—as shown by systolic shortening fraction ($p = 0.001$) and maximal velocity of shortening of the left ventricular diameter ($p = 0.005$). These data are consistent with predominant stimulation of α-adrenergic receptors, but also stimulation of both β_1/β_2 receptors.

In another study, the effects of ingestion of Seville orange (*C. aurantium*) juice on blood pressure were studied. A group of 12 normotensive adults were given an 8-oz glass of juice (approx 13–14 mg synephrine) 8 hours apart. Blood pressure and heart rate were measured every hour for 5 hours after the second glass. The study was conducted in a crossover design and subjects returned in 1 week to repeat the test with water control. The administration of *C. aurantium* juice did not result in the change of any hemodynamic parameters.

Thermogenic/Lypolytic Effects

Synephrine and octopamine have been shown to stimulate β_3 receptors, the stimulation of which is thought to contribute to lypolysis and thermogenesis. Stimulation of the α_2-adrenergic receptor is also reported to have this effect. To date, one placebo-controlled, randomized, double-blind study evaluating the effects of a *C. aurantium*-

containing weight loss product has been conducted. A total of 20 healthy adults received either the active pill ($n = 9$), a placebo ($n = 7$), or nothing ($n = 4$). The treatment group was given a daily pill for 6 weeks containing 975 mg *C. aurantium* extract (6% synephrine alkaloids), 528 mg of caffeine, and 900 mg of St. John's wort. Subjects followed an 1800 kcal/day diet and engaged in a 3-day/week training program under the guidance of an exercise physiologist. Measurements of weight, blood pressure, fat loss, and mood were taken at baseline, 3 weeks, and 6 weeks. At week 6, the treatment group lost significantly more fat (average of 3.1 kg) compared with other groups and also lost a significantly greater amount of body weight (average of 1.4 kg). No significant changes in blood pressure were seen at weeks 3 or 6, although it is unclear whether or not the treatment group took the medication prior to measurement on those days.

Dermatological Effects

Oil of bergamot (*C. aurantium* spp. *bergamia*) was a relatively frequent cause of dermatitis prior to the banning of this aromatic substance from cosmetics. The phenomena of "*Berloque dermatitis*" has been extensively reviewed and is thought to be caused mainly by the furocoumarin bergapten (5-methoxypsoralen). This photomutagenic and photocarcinogenic substance has been largely removed from the cosmetic industry, but the extract is still prevalent in aromatherapy. Recently cases have been reported of bullous reactions after contact or aerosolization exposure followed by sun exposure or tanning.

Adverse Effects and Toxicity

Case Reports of Toxicity Caused by Commercially Available Products or Traditional Uses by Various Specialty Populations

One case of an acute lateral wall *myocardial infarction* (MI) was reported in a woman after daily ingestion of Edita's Skinny Pill (containing 300 mg bitter orange plus caffeine and guarana) for 1 year. The 55-year-old Caucasian woman developed chest discomfort after eating Chinese food. After workup at the hospital, the woman was diagnosed with acute lateral-wall MI and smoking addiction. Her ejection fraction was 0.45. Prior to this incident, she had no known coronary artery disease, hypertension, or hyperlipidemia.

In another case, a 52-year-old woman experienced tachycardia shortly after taking a dry herbal extract of unripe *C. aurantium* fruit. The patient took no medications except for a 10-year history of thyroxine (50 μg/day) treatment. The woman had ingested a dietary supplement for weight loss and consumed 500 mg of *C. aurantium* titrated at 6% synephrine (30 mg). Later in the same day of her first dose, she experienced unrelenting tachycardia and was admitted to the emergency room. She stated that she had never experienced prolonged tachycardia in the past. She was released from the ER after the tachycardia subsided, and felt well. After approx 1 month of feeling well, the woman took another dose of the supplement. Again, later in the day after ingestion of the supplement, she experienced a new episode of prolonged tachycardia. She was seen at the same hospital and released without incident. At the time of publication, she had not taken any more of the supplement and had no reports of tachycardia or other medical problems.

An article in the Canadian Adverse Reaction Newsletter published their reporting of adverse effects caused by products containing *C. aura ntium* from January 1, 1998 to February 28, 2004. The article lists 16 reports of synephrine associated with cardiovascular events including tachycardia, cardiac arrest, ventricular fibrillation, transient collapse, and blackout. In one case, bitter orange was the sole suspected culprit. In seven others the products also contained caffeine, and in eight cases the product contained both caffeine and ephedrine. Health Canada has issued an advisory stating that synephrine may have effects similar to ephedrine and caution should be used if taking it.

Pharmacokinetics

No current information exists on the pharmacokinetics of exogenously administered synephrine.

Interactions

Juice of the Seville orange is known to inhibit intestinal CYP3A4 and has been used for this purpose experimentally. This effect is similar to that observed with grapefruit juice in that it only affects intestinal CYP3A4 and has no effect on hepatic CYP3A4. Many drugs may be potentially affected by coadministration with Seville orange juice, including antifungals (ketoconazole, itraconazole), calcium channel blockers (diltiazem, nicardipine, verapamil), chemotherapeutic agents (etoposide, paclitaxel, vinblastine, vincristine, vindesine), dextromethorphan, felodipine, fexofenadine, glucocorticoids, losartan, midazolam, and others. The effects of Seville orange juice on cyclosporine disposition has been evaluated in several studies with mixed results. In one study, the C_{max} of cyclosporine was increased by 64% after ingestion of *C. aurantium*. Another study demonstrated no effect of *C. aurantium* on cyclosporine concentrations. A third study looked at the effect of long-term administration of *C. aurantium* extract on CYP3A4 activity. The study found no effect of the extract on CYP3A4 activity. The authors proposed a novel explanation for the discrepancy in results from that of Seville orange juice. They suggest that although juice retains the poorly soluble furanocoumarins, most hot-water prepared extracts (including those used in the study) do not.

There are theoretical drug interactions with caffeine and monoamine oxidase inhibitors. Caffeine could increase risk of cardiovascular events when taken with *C. aurantium*. The case report of MI and several of the Canadian reported adverse events included caffeine. Synephrine, tyramine, and octopamine are all substrates of monoamine oxidase. Taking a monoamine oxidase inhibitor with *C. aurantium* could increase concentrations of these sympathomimetics, and thus should be avoided.

Regulatory Status

Citrus oils are found on the list of items on the FDA's Generally Recognized as Safe list. Because of this, manufacturers are only required to include the term, "*natural flavoring*" on the package label when referring to *C. aurantium*. Canada has issued warnings about synephrine and has not allowed cross-border shipment of one synephrine-containing supplement.

4

Cranberry

Cranberry (*Vaccinium macrocarpon*) is a small evergreen shrub that grows in mountains, forests and damp bogs from Alaska to Tennessee. Native Americans introduced the Europeans to cranberry as a food, dye, and medicine. In the 1920s, canned cranberry sauce was introduced, and in the 1940s, cranberry juice became commercially available. Cranberry has been used to prevent and treat urinary tract infections since the 19th century.

Current Promoted Uses

Cranberry juice has been widely used for the prevention, treatment, and symptomatic relief of urinary tract infections. Also, cranberry juice has been given to patients to help reduce urinary odors in incontinence. Another potential benefit of the use of cranberry is a decrease in the rates of kidney stone formation.

Products Available

Cranberry is available in a variety of forms such as fresh or frozen cranberries, cranberry juice cocktail, other cranberry drinks, cranberry sauce, and powder in hard or soft gelatin capsules. Cranberries are approx 88% water and contain flavonoids, anthrocyanins (odain), cetechin, triterpinoids, γ-hydroxybutyric acid, citric acid, malic acid, glucuronic acid, quinic acid, benzoic acid, ellagic acid, and vitamin C. Fresh or frozen cranberries are a good source of cranberry because they contain pure fruit; however, because of their high acidity and extremely sour taste, they are less readily used in clinical practice. Pure cranberry juice is tart like lemon juice because of the high citric and quinic acid content. Cranberry juice cocktail is more palatable, but is only 25–33% juice and contains corn syrup as a sweetener, whereas other cranberry juice drinks contain as little as 10% juice. These sweetened beverages are relatively high in calories (approx 140 kcal per 8-oz serving) and could cause weight gain in a patient consuming the juice for medicinal purposes. Another drawback to sweetened beverages is that, theoretically, the sugar could act as a source of food for uropathogens. Cranberry sauce consisting of sweetened or gelled berries at a concentration one-half that of cranberry juice cocktail is also readily available to consumers. Cranberry capsules are a sugar-free source of cranberry. Hard gelatin capsules contain more crude fiber and organic acids than cranberry juice cocktail, whereas the soft gelatin capsules contain soybean oil and have only 8% of the total organic acids found in fresh cranberries. It takes 12 capsules of cranberry powder to equal 6 fluid oz of cranberry juice cocktail. In the various studies and consumer references, many dosages and dosing regimens have been reported for the use of cranberry in prevention of renal calculi, prevention of urinary odor, and prevention and treatment of urinary tract infections.

Dosages Used or Recommended in Clinical Studies and Case Reports

Prevention of urinary tract infection: 8 oz of cranberry juice four times a day for several days, then twice daily; 300 mL/day as cranberry juice cocktail.

Treatment of urinary tract infection: 6 oz cranberry juice of daily for 21 days; cranberry juice 6 oz twice daily.

Reduction of urinary odors: 16 oz of cranberry juice daily; 3 oz of cranberry juice daily, then increased by 1 oz each week to a maximum of 6 oz daily.

Prevention of urinary stones: 1 qt of cranberry juice cocktail daily; 8 oz of cranberry juice four times a day for several days, then 8 oz twice daily.

Dosages in Lay References

Prevention of urinary tract infection: 3 oz daily as a cocktail. Treatment of urinary tract infection: 12–32 oz daily as a cocktail.

Various Brand Name Products of Cranberry Available

Nature's Resource contains 405 mg of standardized cranberry juice concentrate per capsule. The recommended dose is two to four capsules three times a day with water, at meals. The label also recommends drinking a full glass of water when taking the capsules and drinking 6–8 oz of liquids per day.

Spring Valley contains 475 mg of cranberry fruit per capsule. The recommended dose is two to four capsules three times a day, preferably with meals.

Cranberry Fruit Sundown Herbals contain 425 mg of cranberry fruit per capsule. The recommended dose is two to four capsules up to three times a day as needed.

Celestial Seasonings Cranberry contains 400 mg of cranberry extract standardized to more than 35% organic acids. The recommended dose is one capsule every day as needed with a full glass of water.

Ocean Spray Cranberry Juice Cocktail is 27% cranberry juice. It contains filtered water, high fructose corn syrup, cranberry juice concentrate, and ascorbic acid.

PHARMACOLOGICAL/TOXICOLOGICAL EFFECTS

Antimicrobial Activity

Controversy exists on the pharmacological mechanism of cranberry. In the mid-19th century, German researchers discovered hippuric acid in the urine of people who ate cranberries. From the 1920s through the 1970s, many researchers thought that hippuric acid produced a bacteriostatic effect by acidifying the urine. The ability of cranberry to prevent renal calculi has also been attributed to its ability to decrease urine pH and inhibit bacterial growth. Not all studies documented a change in urinary pH with cranberry administration, so a parallel line of thinking suggested that hippuric acid, which was structurally similar to mandelic acid, inhibited bacterial multiplication. It was found that the concentration of hippuric acid in the urine rarely reached a concentration necessary for bacteriostatic effects. Because hippuric acid is a weak acid, it exists in equilibrium with its conjugate base, and requires a urine pH of at least 5.0 to produce the minimum bacteriostatic hippuric acid concentration. Thus, these researchers felt that both urine pH and hippuric acid concentration were important for the bacterio static effect of cranberry. More recently, however, studies have shown that the mechanism of action of cranberry is the inhibition of bacterial adherence to mucosal surfaces. One study proposed that there are two substances in cranberry juice cocktail, fructose and a glycoprotein, responsible for inhibiting adherence of *Escherichia coli* to mucosal cells.

E. coli is responsible for 85% of urinary tract infections. Virtually all *E. coli* express type 1 fimbrae, and most uropathogenic *E. coli* express P fimbriae, which are responsible for mediating the adherence of the bacteria to uroepithelial cells. Fructose is responsible for inhibiting the adherence of type-1-fimbriated *E. coli*, whereas a polymeric compound inhibits P-fimbriated *E. coli*. Recently, a study identified this polymeric compound as condensed tannins (proanthocyanidins) based on the ability of proanthocyanidins purified from cranberries to inhibit the ability of P-fimbriated *E. coli* to attach to isolated uroepithelial cells at concentrations of 10–50 μg/mL. Blueberries, another member of the *Vaccinium* genus, may be a more palatable source of proanthicyanidins.

Epidemiological data and data from a double-blind, placebo-controlled trial support the use of cranberry juice to prevent urinary tract infections, although in the latter study differences in baseline characteristics between study groups may have influenced the results. Cranberry extract in capsule form was more effective than placebo in preventing recurrent urinary tract infections in a small study.

Another potential benefit to the use of cranberry is its antiviral effect. One study evaluated the ability of various commercial juices and beverages to inactivate poliovirus type I (Sabin) in vitro. Cranberry juice had some antiviral activity that was noted to be enhanced at pH 7.0. The antiviral effect of commercial juices is thought to be caused by polyphenols, including tannins, which form complexes with viruses.

Gastrointestinal Effects

The ingestion of large amounts of cranberry (>3–4 L/day) may result in diarrhea and other gastrointestinal symptoms.

Renal Effects

Ammoniacal fermentation, or alkalinization and decomposition of urine, is responsible for the foul odor of urine. The results of one study found that a single dose of 16 oz of cranberry juice lowered the urine pH of six men with chronic urinary tract disorders, and decreased ammoniacal odor and turbidity. The urine pH of five of six men free of urinary tract infections was also lowered with this dose. In another study, hospital personnel noted a decrease in urine odor in the geriatric wards of a nursing home, but a change in urine pH or change in ammonia levels in the air could not be detected. Other subjective comments by nursing home personnel included a decrease in complaints among patients who had experienced burning upon urination, and more frequent voiding.

Another potential effect of the use of cranberry is in the management of calculus formation because of the association between alkalinization of the urine and stone formation. A specially prepared sweetened cranberry juice consisting of 80% juice was administered to 41 people who were randomly assigned to ingest 150, 180, 210, or 240 mL of the juice with each meal for 1 week. Each subject served as his or her own control. Urine pH was measured by the subjects at each voiding, and a urine sample was collected daily after the evening meal. Mean urine pH was decreased to a statistically significant extent with cranberry juice ingestion compared to baseline. The decrease was not dose-related. Cranberry juice had some effect in lowering daily fluctuations in urine pH, but this effect again was not dose-related. The effect of cranberry juice on urine pH persisted throughout the experimental period (i.e., the kidney did not compensate for changes in pH). Side effects included weight gain and increased frequency of bowel movements.

In another study of cranberry's effect on urinary pH, two 6-oz servings of cranberry juice daily for 20 days were able to lower urinary pH more than orange juice in eight patients with multiple sclerosis, but were unable to lower pH consistently to below 5.5.

5

ECHINACEA

Echinacea is a group of American coneflowers in the Family Asteraceae/Compositae. There are nine species of the plant included in the genus. Three of these are typically seen in herbal preparations: *Echinacea purpurea*, *Echinacea angustifolia*, and *Echinacea pallida*. Common preparations consist of freshly pressed or ethanolic extracts of the roots, leaves, and flowers as well as dried portions of the plants. *E. purpurea* is the most commonly used species, although it is often seen in combination with *E. angustifolia*.

Echinacea was first used by Native Americans for treatment of many conditions. These included pain relief, cough and sore throat, fever, smallpox, mumps, measles, rheumatism, arthritis, and as an antidote for poisons and venoms. As early as 1762, Echinacea was mentioned for use on saddle sores on horses. Until 1885, no further study is documented in the literature. That year marked the beginning of the rise of Echinacea into mainstream medicine. H.C .F. Meyer, a Nebraska physician, began promoting the product for conditions such as syphilis, hemorrhoids, and rabies, among many other claims. This same year the Lloyd Brothers pharmaceutical company was finally persuaded to produce and market an Echinacea product. They began producing a number of products containing Echinacea and had a great deal of success with their line of products. In a survey conducted on preference and use of phyto-pharmaceuticals early in the 20th century, 6000 physicians ranked Echinacea 11th overall out of a list of several hundred products. Antibiotics and the push for patentable medicines led to the fall of Echinacea and herbal medicine in the United States and Europe. In recent years, Echinacea has made a comeback in the United States and, in 2002, it was the second-best-selling herbal product.

Current Promoted Uses

In the United States, Echinacea is marketed primarily in oral dosage forms (tablet, capsule, and liquid) as an immune stimulant used to help with the symptoms of *upper respiratory infections* (URIs). It has also been promoted as a general immune stimulant to help fight various other infections. Topical preparations are also available for treatment of wounds and inflammatory skin conditions.

Sources and Chemical Composition

E. purpurea (L.) Moench, *E. angustifolia* D.C., *E. pallida* (Nutt.); American Coneflower, Black Sampson, Black Susan, *Brauneria angustifolia*, *Brauneria pallida*, Cock-Up-Hat, Comb Flower, Coneflower, Echinaceawurzel, Hedgehog, Igelkopfwurzel, Indian Head Lyons, Kansas Snakeroot, Missouri Snakeroot, Narrow-Leaved Purple Cone Flower, Pale Coneflower, Purple Kansas Coneflower, Purpursonnenhutkraut, Purpursonnenhutwurzel, Racine d'echinacea, Red Sunflower, Rock-Up-Hat, Roter Sonnenhut, *Rudbeckia purpurea*, Schmallblaettriger Kegelblumenwurzel, Schmallblaettriger Sonnenhut, Scurvy Root, Snakeroot, and Sonnenhutwurzel.

Products Available

Numerous forms of Echinacea are available in the United States. Dried herb and concentrated extracts in oral dosage forms make up the bulk of the products available. There are also available fresh, freeze-dried, and liquid alcoholic extracts, which come in a variety of forms including tablets, capsules, lozenges, liquids, teas, and salves. A good number of these products are combined with other herbs such as ginseng, goldenseal, and various other supplements to enhance the efficacy of Echinacea.

Consumer Reports analyzed 19 different Echinacea products in its February 2004 issue to determine content and potency. As a primary standard they used the phenolic content as a measure of potency. The products varied with their phenolic content, some from bottle to bottle of the same manufacturer. Some of the combination products that were tested were found to have unacceptable lead levels according to California standards. Only three of the products were deemed to have adequate labeling with regards to precautions.

Pharmacological/Toxicological Effects

Immunological Effects

The majority of literature published about Echinacea focuses on its activity as an immunostimulant. Many of the studies focus on the activity of macrophages and Echinacea's ability to activate and stimulate immune function.

One constituent of Echinacea, the polysaccharide arabinogalactan, has been identified as a macrophage activator in vitro, causing macrophages to attack tumor cells and microorganisms. When injected into mice intraperitoneally, arabinogalactan was able to activate macrophages. Macrophage production of tumor necrosis factor (TNF)-α, interleukin (IL)-1, and interferon-B_2 was increased in vitro, and production of oxygen free radicals was increased both in vitro and in vivo.

Three of the main active components of Echinacea, cichoric acid, polysaccharides, and alkylamides, were separated and tested at various doses in rats for phagocytic activity in alveolar macrophages and splenocytes. The alveolar macrophages from the group of rats treated with the alkylamides were the only cells to show any significant increases in phagocytic activity, phagocytic index, TNF-α, and nitric oxide. None of the components tested had any activity on splenocytes.

Echinacea was fed to aging male rats and was found to cause an increase in total white cell counts during the first 2 weeks of the administration and increases in IL-2 levels in the final 5 weeks. Differential white counts were altered during the entire 8-week study, with mononuclear cells significantly increased, whereas granulocytes decreased.

Antimicrobial/Antiviral Effects

The focus of Echinacea research most recently has been for the treatment and prevention of URIs of varying causes. There are a number of studies using Echinacea products in the treatment of URI. Many of these show positive results with reduction of symptoms and duration of URI. Studies evaluating the preventative role of Echinacea in URI have shown less impressive results. A few reasons for the differences in efficacy may have to do with the quality of the Echinacea used in the study and study design. The treatment studies demonstrating effectiveness tend to start treatment early in the course of a URI.

A double-blind, placebo-controlled, randomized trial evaluating Echinacea for the treatment of colds involved 559 adult patients and three different Echinacea products (Echinaforce [*E. purpurea* 95% herb and 5% root], *E. purpurea* concentrate, and *E. purpurea* root preparation). In the patients that were treated, two of the Echinacea products produced a statistically significant reduction in symptoms compared to placebo and the *E. purpurea* root preparation. In another study evaluating the prophylactic role of Echinacea, 302 patients were enrolled in a three-armed, randomized, double-blind, placebo-controlled trial. Each of the groups was given ethanolic extract of *E. purpurea* roots, *E. angustifolia* roots, or placebo for 12 weeks. They did not find a significant reduction in occurrence of URI in either treatment group; however, they speculated from their results and the results of two other similar studies that there was a 10 to 20% relative risk reduction for URI. It was concluded that larger sample sizes were needed to confirm their observation.

A randomized, double-blind, placebo-controlled study was done in 48 healthy patients given *E. purpurea* extract or placebo for 7 days and then inoculated with rhinovirus type 39. Treatment was continued for 7 more days after the inoculation. They did not find a statistically significant decrease in the rate of infection. Because of the small sample size, power analysis did not detect any differences in the frequency and severity of the illness that ensued after inoculation. However, their findings did show a trend of reduced symptoms consistent with previous studies relative to prevention of URI.

Eight different varieties of Echinacea were found to have antiviral activity against *Herpes simplex virus* (HSV) Type I in vitro. The two most potent inhibitors found were ethanol extracts of *E. pallida* var. *san guinea* and n-hexane extracts of *E. purpurea.*

In another study, to evaluate the prophylactic action of Echinacea on Influenza virus Type A, a mixture of four herbal extracts, which included *Thujae occidentalis* herb, *Baptisiae tinctoriae* root, *E. purpurea* root, and *E. pallida* root, were given to mice. After 6 days the mice were inoculated with Influenza virus Type A. They found a statistically significant increase in survival rate, survival time, reduced lung consolidation, and virus titer.

A single center, prospective, double-blind, placebo-controlled, crossover trial investigated the activity of Echinacea in humans for the treatment of recurrent genital herpes. The 1-year study involved 50 patients who were each given the product Echinaforce for 6 months and placebo for 6 months. The study found no statistically significant benefit in using Echinaforce vs placebo for frequently recurrent genital herpes.

Antifungal Effects

Acetylenic isobutylamides and polyacetylenes occurring in Echinacea have been shown to inhibit the growth of yeast strains of *Saccharomyces cerevisiae*, *Candida shehata*, *Candida kefyr*, *Candida albicans*, *Candida steatulytica*, and *Candida tropicalis*. This growth inhibition occurred to a greater extent under ultraviolet irradiation than without it. There are other compounds in Echinacea that are suspected to be phototoxic to microbes, but this has yet to be demonstrated.

Pretreatment with a polysaccharide *E. purpurea* extract was found to decrease morbidity and mortality in mice infected by *C. albicans* immunosuppresed with cyclophosphamide and cyclosporine A. They found that macrophages in the Echinacea group produced an increased amount of TNF-α. The authors state that this led to an increased resistance toward *Listeria monocytogenes*, *C. albicans*, and the intracellular parasite *Leishmania enrietti*.

Antineoplastic Activity

An investigation details the isolation of (Z)- 1 ,8-pentadecadiene from *E. angustifolia* and *E. pallida*. This root oil constituent has inhibitory effects against Walker carcinosarcoma 256 and P-388 lymphocytic leukemia in the mouse and rat, respectively.

An examination of mature and precursor cells in the bone marrow and spleen was conducted to determine the activity of Echinacea in these cell's development. After an extract of Echinacea was given to mice for 1- and 2-week periods, populations of natural-killer cells and monocytes were increased in both organs, whereas other hemopoietic and immune cell populations remained at control levels. This study confirmed Echinacea' s effectiveness as a nonspecific immune stimulant and suggested a prophylactic role for Echinacea in treating virus-based tumors and infection.

An investigation into the effects of Echinacea in mice with leukemia was performed to determine the antineoplastic activity. Two groups of mice were used; one group of mice was given a vaccine of killed erytholeukemia cells and then given live tumor cells to induce leukemia, the other group received live tumor cells. It was found that the mice that had been given the vaccine and Echinacea survived longer than the control group and the group given the vaccine alone. They found significant elevations in natural killer cells in these mice. It was concluded that combination therapy of Echinacea and vaccine prolonged the life more than the group that had received the vaccine alone. In an earlier study by the same investigator, it was shown that leukemic mice treated with Echinacea had a much higher survival rate than the control. The treatment group showed a 2.5-fold increase in natural killer cells in their spleens. All other major hemopoietic and immune cell lineages remained normal in the treatment group at 3 months after tumor onset. The authors concluded that the positive effects observed suggest a potential use of Echinacea in treatment of leukemia.

Wound Healing

Echinacea has been used topically for wound-healing. The exact mechanism is unknown but is likely caused by antihyaluronidase activity of echinacoside. A study investigating this activity found that *E. pallida,* which is known to contain echinacoside, had more anti-inflammatory and wound- healing activity in rats after topical application. The effects were much greater with *E. pallida* compared with *E. purpurea* and control.

Anti-Inflammatory Effects

Alkylamides from the roots of *E. purpurea* have been shown to have anti-inflammatory activity in vitro. In a study by Clifford et al., they demonstrated 36–60% and 15–46% of cyclooxygenase (COX)-I and COX-II, respectively.

Two in vitro studies have demonstrated anti-inflammatory activity by various Echinacea preparations. Speroni et al. showed anti-inflammatory activity attributed to echinacosides in *E. pallida* in rats. Another in vitro study used *E. purpurea* in mice that had induced paw edema. Only the higher dose used in the study downregulated COX-2 expression. The authors suggested that the anti-inflammatory properties of Echinacea are related to this inhibition.

Mutagenicity/Carcinogenicity

E. purpurea gave negative results in mammalian cells and bacteria in vitro and in vivo in mice mutagenicity tests. Hamster embryo cell carcinogenicity studies revealed no morphological transformations.

Antioxidant Effects

In an analysis of the different components of the extracts of the roots and leaves of *E. purpurea*, *E. angustifolia*, and *E. pallida*, all possessed antioxidant properties in a free-radical scavenging assay and in a lipid peroxidation assay.

Pharmacokinetics

To date, only one study has evaluated the pharmacokinetics of the alkamides contained in the Echinacea products administered to humans. Subjects ($n = 11$) received a single oral 2.5-mL dose of the 60% ethanolic extract from *E. angustifolia* roots or placebo (60% ethanol). Six different alkamides were analyzed: (i) Undeca-2D/Z-ene-8,10-diynoic acid isobutylamides; (ii) Dodeca-2D,4Z-diene-8,10-diynoic acid isobutylamide; (iii) Dodeca-2E-ene-8,1 0-diynoic acid isobutylamide; (iv) Dodeca-2E,4E,8Z,10E/Z-tetraenoic acid isobutylamides; (v) Dodeca-2E,4E,8Z-trienoic acid isobutylamide; and (vi) Dodeca-2E,4E-dienoic acid isobutylamide. The extract contained approx 2.5 mg of (iv), and approx 0.5 mg of all other components. The C_{max} and area under the curve (AUC) for (iv) were approx 10-fold that achieved with each of the other components. Thus, despite a fivefold higher amount per dose, the 10-fold greater C_{max} and AUC achieved with (iv) suggest it exhibits a greater bioavailability than the other components.

Adverse Effects and Toxicity

Common Adverse Reactions

Side effects that have been observed with administration of Echinacea are generally mild and uncommon. Infrequent adverse effects include abdominal upset, nausea, unpleasant taste, and dizziness. Rarely seen effects are anaphylaxis, exacerbation of asthma, and angioedema.

There is a potential for interaction in patients with immunosuppression, especially those on medications designed to suppress an autoimmune disorder or prevent transplant rejection. In a study looking at the use of herbal medications in a population of patients that had liver transplants, the researchers found that of five patients that had taken Echinacea, two of them had elevated aminotransferase levels, which returned to normal after stopping the product.

In Germany from 1989 to 1995, there were 13 adverse events possibly associated with the use of Echinacin (pressed juice from *E. purpurea* herb). Only four of these, all allergic skin reactions, were thought to be related to use of the product. During this time period, several million people were thought to treat themselves or obtain a prescription for an Echinacea product.

In a study of Australian adverse events thought to be caused by Echinacea, 26 separate cases were studied. Four of these cases developed anaphylaxis, 12 were acute asthma attacks, and 10 were urticaria/angioedema. Four of the 26 reacted after their first ever dose of Echinacea. More than 50% of the patients were found to have some form of atopic disease. In a study of 100 patients with atopic disease, 20 demonstrated positive *skin-prick testing* (SPT) to other plants in the Family Asteraceae (ragweed, daisies, and others), and specifically Echinacea. Only three of this group of 100 had ever taken an Echinacea supplement. Five of these patients were studied more closely and had what was believed to be immunoglobulin E-mediated reactions to Echinacea products. All had SPT and four of five had *radioallergosorbent testing* (RAST) performed. Three of the five had positive skin-reaction SPT and three of four had positive RAST results. The authors concluded that atopic patients should exercise caution when using Echinacea.

Case Reports of Toxicity

Echinacea has been thought to have potential for liver toxicity because of the presence of pyrrolizidine alkaloids, and some authors have warned about its concurrent use with known hepatoxic drugs. The importance of this purported toxicity has been questioned, as Echinacea lacks the 1,2-unsaturated necrine ring system that is associated with the hepatoxicity of pyrrolizidine alkaloids.

A case report describing a 41-year-old male who took Echinacea routinely at the start of influenza-like illness recalled taking it before each of four clinical episodes of erythema nodosum. These episodes lasted anywhere from a few days to 2 weeks and each time they resolved when the Echinacea was stopped. He was followed a year later and had not had any more recurrences of erythema nodosum. He had other bouts of intermittent influenza illness similar to the previous episodes, which he treated with Echinacea, but the patient was unwilling to rechallenge with Echinacea. The authors concluded that the erythema nodosum could have been caused by a number of pathways but were more convinced that Echinacea had brought on his symptoms because each recurrence of his disease resolved after stopping his Echinacea use.

Another case report identified a 51-year-old woman who had been taking Echinacea for 2 months and was found to have a depressed white blood cell count (WBC). After stopping the Echinacea, she was retested and her WBC returned to normal. After 1 year, she returned for a routine check up and 2 months earlier started taking Echinacea again. Her WBC was found to be depressed again and similar increases into the normal range were found after discontinuing the Echinacea 2 months later. The authors could not be certain that Echinacea decreased the WBC in this patient, but suggested a type IV allergic response to Echinacea may be responsible.

A 36-year-old patient started taking a combination of herbal products including Echinacea, and 2 weeks later she presented with generalized muscle weakness that limited her ambulation and ability to use her hands. She was found to have distal renal tubular acidosis and was extremely hypokalemic (K^+ of 1.3). Over 4 days she received 1200 mEq of sodium bicarbonate and 400 mEq of potassium chloride along with other electrolyte supplements to correct the imbalances. After her serum electrolytes were corrected, her muscle weakness improved rapidly. She was diagnosed and treated for Sjögren's syndrome and her condition rapidly improved. The researchers suggested that her use of the immunostimulant Echinacea could have contributed to the activation of her autoimmune disease, which ultimately caused her severe metabolic disturbances. Because she had remained symptom free for more than 3 years, the authors concluded that, after review, her disease was relatively mild and was exacerbated by Echinacea.

In a study to determine the LD_{50} of express juice of *E. purpurea* in rats and mice, one researcher was unable to kill either rat or mouse at oral doses greater than 15 g/kg body weight and intravenous doses greater than 5 g/kg body weight. Injected concentrates of polysaccharide fractions produced an LD_{50} of 2.5 g/kg body weight in mice. Echinacea has a wide margin of safety considering a typical oral dose in a 50–80 kg human is 200–2000 mg of Echinacea or 2.5–40 mg/kg body weight.

Drug Interactions

Analysis of dilutions of extract of *E. angustifolia* and *E. purpurea* showed medium to high levels of inhibition of cytochrome P450 3A4 in vitro. Testing of chicoric acid and echinacoside alone showed low to very low inhibition. The authors did not speculate on what other compounds may be present in either *Echinacea* sp. that caused the more significant enzyme inhibition.

Caffeine, tolbutamide, dextromethorphan, and oral and intravenous midazolam were given to 12 healthy subjects. This was followed with a course of *E. purpurea*, 400 mg four times a day for 8 days, then these drugs were given again and the subjects were assessed for cytochrome P450 activity. They found that the Echinacea significantly reduced the activity of hepatic CYP 1A2 and intestinal CYP 3A and induced hepatic CYP 3A activity. They advised caution when giving drugs that are metabolized by these same enzyme systems.

Reproduction

In a prospective, controlled study, 206 women who reported use of Echinacea during their pregnancy were compared to a group of 206 women who were matched to the study group with regards to maternal age, alcohol, and cigarette use. In comparing the rates of major and minor malformation, it was found that there were no statistical differences in number of live births, spontaneous abortions, therapeutic abortions, or major malformations. This study suggests that use of Echinacea during organogenesis is not associated with any detectable increased risk for any major malformations.

In a study of human sperm, Echinacea was found to inhibit the motility of the sperm only at high concentrations and after 24 hours. One potential effect of Echinacea is thought to be the inhibition of hyaluronidase activity. Hyaluronidase is localized on the sperm head and helps the sperm to penetrate the oocyte. This potential inhibition could prevent sperm from fertilizing oocytes, but further studies are needed to confirm this potential interaction.

Another study of human sperm and oocytes showed that Echinacea at high concentrations had adverse effects on oocytes and suggested that Echinacea damages reproductive cells.

Regulatory Status

Echinacea is regulated as a dietary supplement in the United States. The Homeopathic Mother tincture is a Class C over-the-counter drug official in the *Homeopathic Pharmacopoeia of the United States*, Official Compendium (1992). *E. angustifolia* powdered and powdered extract, *E. pallida* powdered and powdered extract, *E. purpurea* root, powdered root extract, and powdered extract have monographs for their identity, quality, and other properties in the United States Pharmacopeia National Formulary (USP-NF). *E. purpurea* herb is being reviewed and will likely be added to the next USP-NF.

6

EPHEDRA ALKALOIDS

Ephedra, and other medicinal plants have been identified at European neanderthal burial sites dating from 60,000 BCE. Thousands of years later, Pliny accurately described the medicinal uses of ephedra. But thousands of years before Pliny, traditional Chinese healers used ephedra extracts. Chinese texts from the 15th century recommended ephedra as an antipyretic and antitussive. In Russia, around the same time, extracts of ephedra were used to treat joint pain; and though recent laboratory studies confirm that ephedra might be useful for that purpose, additional trials and studies have not been forthcoming. In the 1600s, Indians and Spaniards in the American South-west used ephedra as a treatment for venereal disease. That idea might also have had some merit, as some studies show that ephedra contains compounds with antibiotic activity called *transtorines*. Whether the transtorines will prove to be clinically useful has not been determined.

In 1885, Nagayoshi Nagi, a German-trained, Japanese-born chemist, isolated and synthesized ephedrine. Nagi's original observations were confirmed by Merck chemists 40 years later. Merck's attempts at commercializing ephedrine were unsuccessful, at least until 1930, when Chen and Schmidt published a monograph recommending ephedrine as the treatment of choice for asthma. During the 1920s and 1930s, epinephrine was the only effective oral agent for treating asthma. Epinephrine, which had been available since the early 1900s was (and still is) an effective bronchodilator, but it has to be given by injection, or administered with special nebulizers. Ephedrine was nearly as effective as epinephrine, and could be taken orally. As a result, ephedrine became the first-line drug against asthma. It was displaced from that front during the late 1970s and early 1980s, when aerosolized synthetic β-agonists were introduced.

Unlike most of the other alkaloids contained in ephedra (methylephedrine and cathinone are both psychoactive, but the amount contained in unadulterated ephedra is too low to be of clinical significance), ephedrine is also a potent *central nervous system* (CNS) stimulant. Injections of ephedrine, called *philopon* (which means "love of work") were given to Japanese kamikaze pilots during World War II. A major epidemic of ephedrine abuse occurred in postwar Japan, when stockpiles of ephedrine accumulated for use by the Army were dumped on the black market. Abusers in Tokyo, and other large Japanese cities, injected themselves with ephedrine (then referred to as hirapon), in much the same way that methamphetamine is injected today. In the Philippines, a mixture of ephedrine and caffeine called *shabu* was traditionally smoked for its stimulating effect. In the late 1980s, shabu smoking gave way to the practice of smoking methamphetamine ("ice"). In what is perhaps a tribute to the past, some "ice" is sold under the philopon name.

The chemistry and nomenclature of these compounds are somewhat confusing, and are best understood by reference to the synthetic route used by plants to make ephedrine. All ephedra plants contain phenylalanine-derived alkaloids. Plants use phenylalanine as a precursor, but incorporate only seven of its carbon atoms. Phenylalanine is metabolized to benzoic acid, which is then acetylated and decarboxylated to form pyruvic acid. Transamination, results in the formation of forms (–)-cathinone.

Reduction of one carbonlyl group leads to the formation of either (–)- norephedrine (phenylpropanolamine is the name used to refer to the synthetic mixture of ± norephedrine), or norpseudoephedrine (called *cathine*). N-methylation of (–)-norephedrine results in the formation of (+)-ephedrine. N-methylation of cathine leads to the formation of (+)-pseudoephedrine.

Current Promoted Uses

Physicians routinely used intravenous ephedrine for the prophylaxis and treatment of hypotension caused by spinal anesthesia particularly during caesarean section. In the past, ephedrine was used to treat Stokes–Adams attacks (complete heart block), and was also recommended as a treatment for narcolepsy. Over the years, ephedrine has been replaced by other, more effective agents, and the advent of highly selective β-agonists has mostly eliminated the need to use ephedrine in treating asthma.

European medical researchers have, for several years, used ephedrine to help promote weight loss, at least in the morbidly obese, and nutritional supplements containing naturally occurring ephedra alkaloids are sold in the United States for the same purpose. Clinical trials confirm that, taken as directed, use of these supplements does result in weight loss, though whether such losses are sustained has not been determined.

Prior to its banning by the Food and Drug Administration (FDA) in 2004, ephedra was found in many "*food supplements*," used by bodybuilders. Generally, it was compounded with other ingredients such as vitamins, minerals, and amino acids in products, which are said to increase muscle mass and enhance endurance. Performance improvement secondary to ephedrine ingestion has been established in a controlled clinical trials, and use of ephedrine has been prohibited by the International Olympic Committee.

Ephedra was also sold in combination with many other herbs in obscure combinations. Labels frequently listed 10 or 15 different herbs, but, analysis usually disclosed only the ephedra alkaloids and caffeine as present in sufficient quantities to be physiologically active. After several well-publicized accidental deaths, products clearly intended for abuse, such as "*herbal ecstasy*," and other "look-alike drugs" (products usually containing ephedrine or phenylpropanolamine designed to look like illicit methamphetamine, but in concentrations higher than recommended by industry or the FDA) were withdrawn from the market. Labels on these products were frequently misleading. For example, one might suppose that a product called "Ephedrine 60" contained 60 mg of ephedrine when, in fact, the actual ephedrine content was 25 mg.

Sources and Chemical Composition

Ephedra is a small perennial shrub with thin stems. It rarely grows to more than a foot in height, and at first glance, the plant looks very much like a small broom. Different, closely related species are found in Western Europe, southeastern Europe, Asia, and even the Americas. Some of the better known species include *Ephedra sinica* and *E. equisentina* from China (collectively known as ma haung), as well as *E. geriardiana*, *E. intermedia*, and *E. major*, which grow in India and Pakistan, and countless other members of the family Ephedraceae that grow in Europe and the United States (*E. distachya*, *E. vulgaris*).

Ephedra species vary widely in their ephedrine content. One of the most common Chinese cultivars, known as "China 3," contains 1.39% ephedrine, 0.361% pseudoephedrine, and 0.069% methylephedrine. This mix is fairly typical for commercially grown ephedra plants. Noncommercial varieties of ephedra may contain no ephedrine at all, while others may contain more pseudoephedrine than ephedrine. Depending on the variety, trace amounts of phenylpropanolamine, (–) norephedrine, and methylephedrine may also be present, however (+) norephedrine does not occur naturally, and its presence is proof of adulteration.

Labels on herbal supplements listed total ephedra alkaloid content, usually 10 or 11 mg per serving. Depending on the raw materials used, different production runs of the same product contained ephedrine and pseudoephedrine in varying proportions. Occasionally, supplement makers were accused of adulterating their product by adding synthetic ephedrine or pseudoephedrine. Unlike with (+)-norephedrine, these compounds occur naturally and product adulteration should not have been alleged just because alkaloids other than ephedrine were detected in trace amounts, or because the ratio of ephedrine to pseudoephedrine was close to, or even greater than, 1:1. Of course, if one of the minor alkaloids, such as methylephedrine, were found to be present in concentrations approaching those of ephedrine, the ratio could only be explained by adulteration.

Products Available

Prior to its ban in 2004, no one government agency was tasked with tracking production of ephedrine-containing products. Nor were these products indexed by any industry or trade organization. Ephedrine-containing supplement products were mostly purchased at health food stores or over the Internet. Claims made by some of the Internet vendors were quite outrageous and totally unsupported by any scientific research.

The large supplement makers, of course, had web pages, many of which contained, or had links to, the most recent peer review studies. But in addition to the established names, hundreds of other, smaller manufacturers also advertised and sold over the Internet. These companies came into and went out of existence so rapidly that a detailed listing of their web sites would likely be outdated before the links were published. Even today, a simple search using the word "*ephedrine*," will disclosed numerous off-shore vendors, along with numbers of attorneys soliciting for ephedra-related class action legal cases.

In addition to selling their own proprietary mixture, many of these same web sites sold the same popular products as the herbal and general retail outlets, such as a previous Twin Labs best seller "Ripped Fuel," which contained ephedrine in the form of ma huang, combined with guarana, L-carnitine, and chromium picolinate. Metabolife 356TM contained guarana (40 mg caffeine), 12 mg ephedrine as ma huang, chromium picolinate 75 mg, and several other ingredients. Ever since ephedrine became the precursor of choice for making methamphetamine, federal regulators have severely restricted bulk sales of ephedrine, but these restrictions have been bypassed in some cases by illegally ordering from a foreign web site.

In most products, ephedrine content ranged anywhere from 12 to 80 mg per serving, with the majority of products falling into the lower range. Industry standards called for a total dose of ephedrine of less than 100 mg/day. The FDA, however, allowed a maximum daily dose of 150 mg/day of synthetic ephedrine. Unless fortified, the expected ephedrine content of ma huang capsules was generally less than 10%. Thus, a capsule said to contain 1000 g of ephedra would probably have contained no more than 80 mg of ephedrine.

In the United States, (+)-norpseudoephedrine, in its pure form, is considered a Schedule IV controlled substance. However, because of the small amounts of this alkaloid in ephedra plants or extracts, the Drug Enforcement Administration (DEA) had never stated or proposed that ephedra products were subject to the scheduling requirements of the Controlled Substances Act. Quite the contrary, DEA published a proposed rule in 1998 that stated DEA's intent to exempt legitimate ephedra products in finished form from regulation even as "chemical mixtures." Other regulatory sanctions and actions on ephedra rendered action on this regulation moot.

Pharmacological Effects

Studies have shown that resultant effects are similar, regardless of whether pure synthetic ephedrine or naturally occurring ephedra is ingested. There are, however, significant enantioselective differences between the enantomers in both pharmacokinetic and pharmacodynamic effects. All of the ephedra alkaloids have important effects on the cardiovascular and respiratory systems, but not to the same degree.

Ephedrine, the predominant alkaloid in ephedra, is both an α and β stimulant. It directly stimulates α_2 and β_1; receptors and, because it also causes the release of norepinephrine from nerve endings, it also acts as a β_2 stimulant. The resultant physiological changes are variable, depending on receptor distribution and receptor regulation. Tolerance to ephedrine's β agonist actions emerges rapidly, which is why ephedrine is no longer the preferred agent for treating asthma; receptor downregulation quickly occurs and the bronchodilator effects are lost.

Receptor distribution probably explains why ephedrine has no effect on diastolic pressure, and only minimal effect on systolic. β_2 Stimulation of vessels in peripheral muscles results in peripheral vasodilation and "*diastolic runoff*," which more than cancels ephedrine's other inotropic effects. The absence of any significant effect on blood pressure was firmly established during the late 1970s and early 1980s in dozens of double-blind, placebo-controlled studies performed to compare the effectiveness of ephedrine with that of newly synthesized adrenergic agents. The pharmacokinetic and toxicokinetic behavior of any isomer cannot be used to predict that of any other ephedrine isomer. The (+) isomer of methamphetamine, for example, is a potent CNS stimulant, but the (–)-isomer is merely a decongestant. There is a tendency in the literature to lump together all "*ephedrine alkaloids*" and use the term "*class effect*" to assume that all the different drugs in that class exert the same effects on the same biological targets. In fact, some of the drugs in the class will be similar in some regards and different in others.

The affinity of the various ephedrine isomers for human β-receptors has been measured and compared (as indicated by the amount of cyclic adenosine monophosphate produced compared to that of isoproterenol) in tissue culture. Activity of the different isomers is highly stereoselective, i.e., the different isomers had very different receptor-binding characteristics. For β_1-receptors, maximal response (relative to isoproterenol = 100%) was greatest for ephedrine (68% for 1R, 2S-ephedrine and 66% for the 1S, 2R-ephedrine isomer). Both of the pseudoephedrine isomers had much lower affinities (53%). When binding to 32-receptors was measured, the rank order of potency for 1R, 2S-ephedrine was 78%, followed by 1R, 2R-pseudoephedrine (50%), followed by 1S, 2S-pseudoephedrine (47%). The 1S, 2R-ephedrine isomer had only 22% of the activity exerted by isoproterenol, but was the only isomer that showed any significant agonist activity on human β_3-receptors (31%). Stimulation of β_3-receptors, which are thought to be located only in fat cells, may account for ephedrine's ability to cause weight loss.

Ephedrine is also an α agonist and, as such, is capable of stimulating bladder smooth muscle. At one time, it was used to promote urinary continence. In animal models, when compared to norepinephrine, ephedrine is a relatively weak α-adrenergic agonist, possessing less than one-third the activity of norepinephrine. Ephedrine's usefulness as a bronchodilator is limited by the number of β-receptors on the bronchi. The number of β-receptors located on human lymphocytes (which correlates with the number found in the lungs) decreases rapidly after the administration of ephedrine; the density of binding sites drops to 50% after 8 days of treatment and returns to normal 5 to 7 days after the drug has been withdrawn.

Clinical Studies

Bronchodilation

Banner et al. summarized studies where the effects of ephedrine and ephedra were compared to placebo in controlled studies in humans. None of the controlled trials disclosed any evidence of cardiovascular toxicity when ephedrine was given in doses as high as 1 mg/kg, even when it was administered to severe asthmatics with known cardiac arrhythmias. The trial reported by Banner et al. studied the respiratory and circulatory effects of orally administered ephedrine sulfate, 25 mg, aminophylline, 400 mg, terbutaline sulfate, 5 mg, and placebo in 20 patients with ventricular arrhythmia by a double-blind crossover method. The study was comprised of 20 patients, with an average age of 60 years and a preexisting history of both asthma and heart disease (as evidence by the presence of frequent premature ventricular contractions). The bronchodilator effect of terbutaline was similar to that of aminophylline over 4 hours but superior to ephedrine at hour 4. Both terbutaline and ephedrine exhibited chronotropic effects, with the effect of terbutaline greater than that of ephedrine at hour 4. The effect of aminophylline on heart rate (HR) did not differ from placebo. Only terbutaline was associated with an increase in ventricular ectopic beats. Ventricular tachycardia occurred in three patients treated with terbutaline and in one patient with ephedrine (which occurred before he was given ephedrine). There were no significant changes in blood pressure. Orally administered terbutaline should not be regarded as safer than orally administered ephedrine or aminophylline in patients with arrhythmias.

In 1992, Astrup studied the effects of ephedrine and caffeine in a group of obese patients. In a randomized, placebo-controlled, double-blind study, 180 obese patients were treated by diet (4.2 mJ/day) and either an ephedrine/caffeine combination (20 mg/200 mg), ephedrine (20 mg), caffeine (200 mg), or placebo three times a day for 24 weeks.

Withdrawals were distributed equally in the four groups, and 141 patients completed the trial. Mean weight losses was significantly greater with the combination than with placebo from week 8 to week 24 (ephedrine/caffeine, 16.6 ± 6.8 kg vs placebo, 13.2 ± 6.6 kg [mean ± standard deviation {SD}], $P = 0.0015$). Weight loss in both the ephedrine and the caffeine groups was similar to that of the placebo group. Side effects (tremor, insomnia, and dizziness) were transient and after 8 weeks of treatment they had reached placebo levels. Systolic and diastolic blood pressure fell similarly in all four groups.

Weight Loss

The most recent of the studies examining weight control were designed to address concerns about long-term safety and efficacy for weight loss using a mixture containing 90 mg of ephedrine (from ephedra) and 192 mg of caffeine, derived from cola nuts. A 6-month randomized, double-blind, placebo-controlled trial was performed, in which a total of 167 subjects (body mass index 31.8 ± 4.1 kg/m^2) were randomized to receive either placebo ($n = 84$) or herbal treatment ($n = 83$). The primary outcome measurements were changes in blood pressure, heart function, and body weight. Secondary variables included body composition and metabolic changes. It was found that herbal vs placebo treatment decreased body weight (–5.3 ± 5.0 vs –2.6 ± 3.2 kg, $P < 0.001$), body fat (–4.3 ± 3.3 vs –2.7 ± 2.8 kg, $P = 0.020$), and low- density lipoprotein cholesterol (–8 ± 20 vs 0 ± 17 mg/dL, $P = 0.013$), and increased high-density lipoprotein cholesterol (+2.7 ± 5.7 vs –0.3 ± 6.7 mg/ dL, $P = 0.004$). Herbal treatment produced small changes in blood pressure variables (+3 to –5 mmHg, $P \sim 0.05$), and increased HR (4 ± 9 vs –3 ± 9 beats per minute, $P < 0.001$), but cardiac arrhythmias were not increased ($P > 0.05$). By self-report, dry mouth ($P < 0.01$), heartburn ($P < 0.05$), and insomnia ($P < 0.01$) were increased and diarrhea decreased ($P < 0.05$). Irritability, nausea, chest pain, and palpitations did not differ, nor did numbers of subjects who withdrew. *Conclusions*: In this 6-month placebo-controlled trial, herbal ephedra/caffeine (90/192 mg/day) promoted body-weight and body-fat reduction and improved blood lipids without significant adverse events.

Athletic Performance

In a series of studies, Bell et al. assessed the effects of ephedrine mixtures on performance, and found measurable improvement. One and one half hours after ingesting a placebo (P), caffeine (C) (4 mg/ kg), ephedrine (E) (0.8 mg/kg), or caffeine and ephedrine, 12 subjects performed a 10-km run while wearing a helmet and backpack weighing 11 kg. The trials were performed in a climatic suite at 12–13°C, on a treadmill where the speed was regulated by the subject. VO_2, VCO_2, V(E), HR, and rating of perceived exertion were measured during the run at 15 and 30 minutes, and again when the individual reached 9 km. Blood was sampled at 15 and 30 minutes and again at the end of the run and assayed for lactate, glucose, and catecholamines. Run times (mean ± SD), in minutes, were for C (46.0 ± 2.8), E (45.5 ± 2.9), C + E (45.7 ± 3.3), and P (46.8 ± 3.2). The run times for the E trials (E and C + E) were significantly reduced compared with the non-E trials (C and P). Pace was increased for the E trials compared with the non-E trials over the last 5 km of the run. VO_2 was not affected by drug ingestion. HR was elevated for the ephedrine trials (E and C + E), but the respiratory exchange ratio (a measure of maximal exertion) remained similar for all trails. Caffeine increased the epinephrine and norepinephrine response associated with exercise and also increased blood lactate, glucose, and glycerol levels. Ephedrine reduced the epinephrine response but increased dopamine and free fatty acid levels. Bell concluded previously that the effects of caffeine, when taken with ephedrine, were not additive, and that all of the observed improvement could be accounted for by the presence of ephedrine.

Pharmacokinetics

Phenylpropanolamine is readily and completely absorbed, but pseudoephedrine, with a bioavailability of only approx 38%, is subject to gut wall metabolism, and absorption may be erratic. Pure ephedrine is well absorbed from the stomach, but absorption is much slower when it is given as a component of ma huang, rather than in its pure form. Ephedrine ingested in the form of ma huang has a t_{max} of nearly 4 hours, compared to only 2 hours when pure ephedrine is given. Like its enantiomers, ephedrine is eliminated in the urine largely as unchanged drug, with a half-life of approx 3–6 hours.

The rate at which any of the enantiomers is eliminated depends upon the urinary pH. At high pHs, excretion time is prolonged. At low pH ranges, excretion is accelerated. In controlled laboratory studies, where volunteer subjects were given either bicarbonate or ammonium chloride, the higher the urine pH, the more slowly the ephedrine and pseudoephedrine were excreted. Conversely, when the urine pH is low, excretion is accelerated. The importance of these observations is hard to assess, because without the addition of bicarbonate, urine pH values in the general population rarely approach 8.0. A study of pseudoephedrine pharmacokinetics in 33 volunteers who were not treated with drugs to alter urine pH found that these parameters could not be correlated to urine pH, mainly because there was little difference in pH between the different participants. Excretion patterns may be much more rapid in children, and a greater dosage may be required to achieve therapeutic effects. Patients with renal impairment are at special risk for toxicity.

Peak concentrations for the other enantiomers, specifically phenylpropanolamine and pseudoephedrine, occur earlier (0.5 and 2 hours, respectively) than for ephedrine, but all three drugs are extensively distributed into extravascular sites (apparent volume of distribution between 2.6 and 5.0 L/kg). No protein-binding data in humans are available. Peak ephedrine levels after ingestion of 400 mg of ma huang, containing 20 mg of ephedrine, resulted in blood concentrations of 81 ng/mL—essentially no different than the peak ephedrine levels observed after giving an equivalent amount of pure ephedrine. In another study, 50 mg of ephedrine given orally to six healthy, 21-year-old women produced mean peak plasma concentrations of 168 ng/mL, 127 min after ingestion, with a half-life of slightly more than 9 hours. The results are comparable to those obtained in studies done nearly 30 years earlier.

Very high levels of methylephedrine have been observed in Japanese polydrug abusers taking a cough medication called BRON. Concentrations of methylephedrine less than 0.3 mg/L, the range generally observed in individuals taking BRON for therapeutic rather than recreational purposes, appear to be nontoxic and devoid of measurable effects. Methylephedrine is a minor component of most ephedra plants, but in Japan (where, unlike in the United States, methylephedrine is legally sold) it is produced synthetically, and is used in cough and cold remedies, especially BRON. In terms of catecholamine stimulation, methylephedrine appears comparable to ephedrine; however, it does not react with most standard urine screening tests for ephedrine. This can be a cause of some forensic confusion, because 10–15% of a given dose of methylephedrine is converted to ephedrine.

Although the issue has been raised in litigation, the amounts of methylephedrine and norephedrine contained in naturally occurring ephedra are so low as to be of no clinical consequence. For example, the study by Gurley et al. found that most of the commercial products tested had no methylephedrine whatsoever, but when it was present, it was usually in quantities of less than 1 mg per serving (range 0.2 to 2.2 mg). If the volume of distriution (Vd) of methylephedrine is assumed to be 3.5, approximately the same as ephedrine, then a 70-kg man ingesting a 2-mg serving of methylephedrine would produce a blood concentration of (dose = kg weight × blood concentration × Vd) 0–0.06 mg, undoubtedly below most laboratories' minimum level of detection, and a clinically insignificant finding. Similar considerations apply to the small amounts of norephedrine found in these products.

Adverse Effects and Toxicity

Two journal articles analyzing *adverse event reporters* (AERs) have been published in the peer-reviewed literature, and both reports have received wide publicity. The reports are, however, of limited use in assessing toxicity, because they are comprised of passively collected anecdotal data, which is often incomplete and unreliably reported. For example, one of the FDA ephedrine AERs "analyzed" in an article published in the *New England Journal of Medicine* described the sudden death of a teenage girl who had been born with a lethal cardiac malformation who died while playing volleyball. Postmortem blood and tissue tested negative for ephedrine, and the article failed to mention the existence of the cardiac malformation. In other AERs, massive doses of ephedrine were consumed (as with products intended for abuse, such as "*herbal ecstasy*," now withdrawn from the market). Toxicology testing was rarely performed in any of these cases, and it is not known with any certainty whether ephedrine was even taken. Even the authors of the two papers concede that anecdotal reports cannot be used to prove causality, stating that "Our report does not prove causation, nor does it provide quantitative information with regard to risk". There is little point in reviewing material that cannot be used to prove causality, and it is not included in the summaries that follow, which are comprised only of published, peer-review case reports, epidemiological surveys, and controlled clinical trials. An additional review of the utility of spontaneously reported adverse events involving supplements and, more specifically, ephedra was published by Kingston et al.. The review discussed the limitations of spontaneously reported data in assessing supplement safety and determining causality between exposure and adverse effects.

Despite conflicting data regarding the safety of ephedra from clinical studies and conclusions drawn from spontaneously reported adverse events, FDA banned the sale of ephedra-containing supplements in 2004.

Neurological Disorders

Many strokes attributed to ephedrine have actually been caused by the ingestion of ephedrine enantiomers, pseudoephedrine, phenylpropanolamine, and even methylephedrine. Two cases of ischemic stroke have been reported, but in neither case was their any toxicological testing to confirm the use of ephedrine. A decade-old report described the autopsy findings in three individuals with intracerebral hemorrhage and positive toxicology testing for ephedrine; however, one had hypertensive cerbrovasular disease and the other had a demonstrable ruptured aneurysm.

Intracerebral hemorrhage has also been described in suicide and attempted suicide victims who took overdoses of pseudoephedrine. There is also a report describing a patient who developed described arteritis following the intravenous administration of ephedrine during a surgical procedure. On the other hand, a large study to assess risk factors for stroke in young people (age 20–49) over a 1-year period was carried out in Poland, a country where ephedra-based products are widely used. Nearly one-half the cases of stroke were associated with preexisting hypertension, another 15% had hyperlipidemia, and 6% were diabetic. None of the individuals were ephedrine users.

Sometimes, especially in Japan and the Philippines, ephedrine is taken specifically as a psychostimulant. In Japan, BRON, the OTC cough medication containing methylephedrine, dihydrocodeine, caffeine, and chlorpheniramine, is very widely abused, and transient psychosis commonly results. Reports of ephedrine-related psychosis following prolonged, heavy use are fairly common. In general, psychosis is only seen in ephedrine users ingesting more than 1000 mg/day, and it resolves rapidly once the drug is withdrawn.

Ephedrine psychosis closely resembles psychosis induced by amphetamines: paranoia with delusions of persecution and auditory and visual hallucinations, even though consciousness remains unclouded. Typically, patients with ephedrine psychosis will have ingested more than 1000 mg/day. Recovery is rapid after the drug is withdrawn. The ephedrine content per serving of most food supplements is on the order of 10–20 mg, making it extremely unlikely that, in recommended doses, use of any of the products would lead to neurological symptoms.

Renal Disorders

Reports, particularly in the European literature, have described the occurrence of renal calculi in chronic ephedrine users. A review of cases from a large commercial laboratory specializing in the analysis of kidney stones found that 200 out of 166,466, or 0.064%, of stones analyzed by that laboratory, contained either ephedrine or pseudoephedrine. Unfortunately, the analytic technique used could not distinguish ephedrine from pseudoephedrine, and because pseudoephedrine is used so much more widely than ephedrine, it seems that the risk of renal calculus associated with ephedrine use must be quite small. There have been no new reports of ephedrine-related nephrolithiasis since 1999. Direct toxicity, with altered renal function and demonstrable kidney lesions related to ephedrine use, has never been demonstrated. Urinary retention, occurring as a consequence of drug overdose, was occasionally reported, but additional cases have not been described in more than a decade. The FDA and Commission E both warn against the possibility of urinary retention in patients with prostatic enlargement, but the theoretical basis for this concern is unclear, and, in any case, retention in patients with prostate disease has not been reported.

Small amounts of ephedrine are oxidized in to norephedrine and norpseudoephedrine in the liver. In patients with diminished renal function, these drugs may accumulate and have the potential to cause serious toxicity. None of the ephedrine enantiomers are easily removed by dialysis, and treatment of overdose remains supportive, using pharmacological antagonists to counter the α- and β-adrenergic effects of these drugs. Because excretion is pH-dependent, patients with renal tubular acidosis are also at risk. The FDA reports having received a number of accounts of hematuria after use of ephedra-based products, but no such cases have ever appeared in the peer-reviewed literature, and review of the reports published by the FDA shows that all of the affected individuals were taking multiple remedies, some capable of causing interstitial nephritis.

Cardiovascular Diseases

Ephedrine and pseudoephedrine share properties with cocaine and with the amphetamines because they: (1) stimulate β-receptors directly, and (2) also cause the increased release of norepinephrine. Chronic exposure to abnormally high levels of circulating catecholamines can damage the heart. This is certainly the case with cocaine and methamphetamine, but ephedrine-related cardiomyopathy is an extremely rare occurrence, occurring only in individuals who take massive amounts of drug for prolonged periods of time. Only two papers have ever been published on the subject. The two existing reports are uninterpretable, because histological findings were not described in either report, and angiography was not performed, thereby making it impossible to actually establish the diagnosis of cardiomyopathy.

Similar considerations apply to the relationship (if any) between myocardial infarction and ephedrine use. The report by Cockings and Brown described a 25-year-old drug abuser who injected himself with an unknown amount of cocaine intravenously. The only other published reports involved a woman in labor who was receiving other vasoactive drugs; and two pseudoephedrine users, one of whom was also taking bupropion, who developed coronary artery spasm.

Three cases of ephedra-related coronary spasm in anesthetized patients have also been reported, but multiple agents were administred in all three cases, and the normal innervation of the coronary arteries was disrupted in two of the cases where a high spinal anesthetic had been administered. One case of alleged ephedrine-related hypersensitivity myocarditis has been reported, but the patient was taking many other herbal supplements, and the responsible agent is not known with certainty. Although there are no reasons why ephedra alkaloids should not cause allergic reactions, the incidence appears to be extremely low.

Although clinical trials or epidemiological studies are lacking, it has been suggested that maternal use of OTC cold medication may result in fetal arrhythmias, but linkage between ephedrine and isomers and arrhythmia has never been demonstrated. The literature contains one case report describing arrhythmias occurring in a 14-year-old who overdosed on cold medications. The child had taken a total of 3300 mg of caffeine, 825 mg of phenylpropanolamine, and 412 mg of ephedrine. Clearly, large doses of ephedrine, and its enantiomers, are capable of exerting toxicity.

The paucity of peer-reviewed studies describing cardiovascular complication with ephedra alkaloids suggests that few such cases are occurring. This notion is support by the studies of Porta et al., who performed a follow-up study of more than 100,000 persons below age 65 years who filled a total of 243,286 prescriptions for pseudoephedrine. No hospitalizations could be attributed to the drug. There were no admissions within 15 days of filling a prescription for pseudoephedrine for cerebral hemorrhage, thrombotic stroke, or hypertensive crisis. There were a small number of hospitalizations for myocardial infarction, seizures, and neuropsychiatric disorders, but the rate of such admissions among the pseudoephedrine users was close to the expected rate in the population at large.

Workplace Drug Testing

Ephedra alkaloids, even when used in the recommended amounts, can cause positive urine screening tests for methamphetamine, sometimes yielding surprisingly high concentrations.

Postmortem Toxicology

Very few fatalities have ever been reported (or studied), but it appears that the therapeutic index for ephedrine is very great. A 1997 case report described a 28-year-old woman with two prior suicide attempts, who died after ingesting amitriptyline and ephedrine. The blood ephedrine concentration was 11,000 ng/mL, and the liver concentration was twice that value (kidney, 14 mg/kg; brain, 8.9 mg/kg). The amitriptyline concentration was 0.33 mg/kg in blood and 7.8 mg/kg in liver. Values in a second case report (where methylephedrine concentrations were nearly 6000 ng/mL) may or may not be relevant to the problem of ephedrine toxicity, as the individual in question took massive quantities of a calcium channel blocker, and it is not known whether methylephedrine exerts all the same effects as ephedrine. Baselt and Cravey mention the case of a young woman who died several hours after ingesting 2.1 g of ephedrine combined with 7.0 g of caffeine, but tissue findings were not described. Her blood ephedrine level was 5 mg/L, whereas the concentration in the liver was 15 mg/kg.

A report from the European literature describes the findings in a 19- year-old woman who committed suicide by taking 40 Letigen tablets (200 mg of caffeine and 20 mg of ephedrine) amounting to 10 g of caffeine and 1 g of ephedrine. She developed severe toxic manifestations from the heart, CNS, muscles, liver, and kidneys leading to several cardiac arrests, and died subsequently of cerebral edema and incarceration on the fourth day of hospitalization. Postmortem blood concentrations were not given.

Pseudoephedrine concentrations, but not measurements for ephedrine or any of the other enantiomers, have been published by the National Association of Medical Examiners in their Annual Registry report. In 15 children diagnosed with sudden infant death syndrome, the mean blood pseudoephedrine concentration was 3.55 mg/L, the median 2.3 mg/L, with a range of 0.07–13.0 mg/L (SD = 3.36 mg/L). The authors of the study take pains to point out that "The data do not allow definitive statements about the toxicity of pseudoephedrine at a given concentration".

In the only autopsy study yet published, all autopsies in the San Francisco Medical Examiner's jurisdiction from 1994 to 2001 where ephedrine or any its isomers (E+) were detected were reviewed. Cases where ephedrine or its isomers were detected were compared with those in a control group of drug-free trauma victims. Of 127 ephedrine-positive cases identified, 33 were the result of trauma. Decedents were mostly male (80.3%) and mostly Caucasian (59%). Blood ephedrine concentrations were less than 0.49 mg/L in 50% of the cases, with a range of 0.07–11.73 mg/L in trauma victims, and 0.02–12.35 mg/L in nontrauma cases. Norephedrine was present in the blood of only 22.8% (mean concentration of 1.81 mg/L, SD=3.14 mg/L) and in the urine of 36.2% of the urine specimens, with a mean concentration of 15.6 mg/L, SD=21.50 mg/L). Pseudoephedrine (PE) was detected in the blood of 6.3%. More than 88% of the decedents who tested positive for ephedrine or one of its isomers also tested positive for other drugs, the most common being cocaine (or its metabolites) and morphine. The most frequent pathological diagnoses were hepatic steatosis and nephrosclerosis. Left ventricular hypertrophy was common, and coronary artery disease was detected in nearly one-third of the cases. The most common findings in the ephedrine-positive deaths reviwed were those generally associated with chronic stimulant abuse. There were no cases of heat stroke and no cases of rhabdomyolysis.

Methamphetamine Manufacture

Either (-)-ephedrine or (+)-pseudoephedrine can be used to make meth- amphetamine by reductive dehalogenation using red phosphorus as a catalyst. If (-)-ephedrine is used as the starting material, the process will generate (+)-methamphetamine. If psuedoephedrine is used, the result will be dextromethamphetamine. As this synthetic route has become nearly universal, both state and federal governments have enacted laws limiting the amount of pure ephedrine or pseudoephedrine that can be purchased.

Drug Interactions

The ephedra alkaloids are all sympathomimetic amines, which means that a host of drug interactions are theoretically possible. In fact, only a handful of adverse drug interactions have been reported in the peer-reviewed literature, The most important of these involve the monoamine oxidase inhibitors (MAOI). Irreversible, nonselective MAOIs have been reported to adversely interact with indirectly acting sympathomimetic amines present in many cough and cold medicine. In controlled trials with individuals taking moclobemide, ephedrine's effects on pulse and blood pressure were potentiated, but only at higher doses than those currently provided in health supplements. Ephedrine-MAOI interaction may, on occasion, be severe enough to mimic pheochromocytoma. In addition, there is decreased metabolic clearance of pseudoephedrine when MAOIs are administered concurrently. At least one case report suggests that selective serotonin reuptake inhibitor antidepressants can react with pseudoephedrine, leading to the occurrence of "*serotonin syndrome*". Bromocriptine, the ergot-derived dopamine agonist can interact with pseudoephedrine, and would presumably interact with ephedrine as well. Surgical patients being treated with clonidine have an enhanced pressor response to ephedrine, apparently a result of clonidineinduced potentiation of α_1-adrenoceptor-mediated vasoconstriction. In some clinical trials, the coadministration of ephedrine with morphine has been shown to increase analgesia, but this approach to pain relief remains somewhat controversial.

Reproduction

Use of ephedra-containing products is likely unsafe during pregnancy because of reports of psychoses and cardiovascular effects.

Regulatory Status

In 2004, the FDA issued a final rule prohibiting the sale of dietary supplements containing ephedrine alkaloids (ephedra), citing concerns over safety and potential risk of illness or injury.

The FDA reviewed evidence about ephedra' s pharmacology: peer-reviewed scientific literature on ephedra' s safety and effectiveness, adverse event reports, and a seminal report by the RAND Corporation, an independent scientific institute. Spontaneously reported adverse effects with high-profile sports figures and others raised public awareness and fueled the debate over safety. Subsequent to the ban, various trade groups and supplement companies have criticized the ban, and an appeal of the decision with temporary suspension of sanctions in some jurisdictions, pending further review, has occurred. Regardless of the regulatory outcome, reintroduction of OTC ephedra-containing supplements is not likely to occur. Although banned in the United States, use of ephedra in other countries is likely to continue.

7

Evening Primrose

Evening primrose is a botanical plant that has the following National Oceanographic Data Center Taxonomic Code (Kingdom: *Plantae*; Phylum: *Tracheobionta*; Class: *Magnoliopsida*; Order: *Myrtales*; Family: *Onagraceae*; Genus: *Oenothera* L.; Species: *Oenothera biennis* L.). A fragrant wildflower and biennial herb native to North America, the evening primrose reaches a height of 4 to 5 ft with flowers 2 to 3 cm long, and blossoms in the evening during June through September. A flower blooms only for one evening, thus the name "*evening primrose*". The evening primrose can be found in North America east of the Rocky Mountains, and was naturalized into Europe and Asia from North America in the early 17th century. Its leaves are alternate, rough, hairy, lanceolate, 3 to 6 in. long, and lemon-scented. The fruit is a 1-in., oblong capsule that is approx 4 cm long, containing many tiny reddish seeds; seeds are 1.5 mm long, dark gray to black in color, and have irregular sharp edges. The entire plant can be eaten (e.g., roots, leaves, flowers, buds, seedpods); leaves are cooked and eaten like spinach and the roots are boiled and taste sweet. Evening primrose was a staple food for many Native American tribes and a famine food for Chinese farmers. European settlers and Native Americans used the whole plant to ameliorate ailments such as bruising, stomachaches, and shortness of breath.

Evening primrose oil (OEP) is derived from the plant's small, dark seeds. China is now the major grower of evening primrose seed in the world, supplying an estimated 90% of the world's crop. A total of approx 400 t of seeds are processed each year in the United States and Canada. One major supplier of OEP derives the oil from specially selected and hybridized forms of *Oenothera* species. Today, the oil is used medicinally to treat a myriad of conditions related to *essential fatty acid* (EFA) deficiencies, low dietary intake of linoleic acid, and a variety of reproductive, cardiovascular, inflammatory, and neurological disorders. It is added to foods as a source of essential fatty acids and used in topical products such as soaps and cosmetics.

Current Promoted Uses

Currently promoted uses of OEP include: EFA deficiency mastalgia, fibrocystic breast disease, endometriosis, menopause, *premenstrual syndrome* (PMS), and the prevention of preeclampsia, diabetic neuropathy, psoriasis, eczema/dermatitis, rheumatoid arthritis, cardiovascular disease, gastrointestinal disorders, attention deficit disorder in children, and hypercholesterolemia. OEP is used topically as an ingredient in some soaps, cosmetics and medicinals.

Sources and Chemical Composition

The seeds of *O. biennis* contain approx 14–26% OEP, which is a fixed oil. Within this oil, several important fatty acids are present:

- 50–85% of *cis*-linoleic acid
- 2–16% of *cis*-γ-linolenic acid
- 6–11% of *cis* 6,9,12-octadecatrienoic acid; oleic acid
- 7–10% of palmitic acid
- Miscellaneous components: stearic acids, steroids, campesterol, vitamin E, and β-sitosterol.

A descriptive report of OEP produced in China states the following information about OEP: refractive index (20°C) of 1.48, specific gravity (20°C) of 0.93, iodine value of 140, saponification value of 188, thiocyanogen value of 84, and unsaponifiable matter of 1%.

In other parts of the plant, mucilage and tannin are present. OEP contains the highest amount of γ-linolenic acid (an EFA) of any food substance.

Products Available

A total of approx 400 t of seeds are processed each year in the United States and Canada. One major supplier of OEP derives the oil from specially selected and hybridized forms of *Oenothera* species. OEP in oral tablets or capsules usually range from 500 to 1300 mg. Most commercial products are standardized for a γ-linoleic acid content of 9%. Dosage forms include oral formulations (capsules, tablets, oil swallowed directly or mixed with another liquid/food) and topical.

Examples of products containing OEP include Efamol Pure Evening Primrose Oil, Efamol PMS Control, Efamol Fortify, Efalex capsules, Efalex liquid, and Efanatal. Efamol Pure Evening Primrose Oil is a natural colored, oval, soft gelatin capsule and a 500-mg capsule contains Efamol Pure Evening Primrose Oil 500 mg (linoleic acid 165 mg and γ-linolenic acid 40 mg). Efamol PMS Control is an opaque, pink, oval, soft gelatin capsule and a 695-mg capsule contains Efamol Pure Evening Primrose Oil 250 mg (linoleic acid 320 mg and γ-linolenic acid 20 mg), vitamin C (as ascorbic acid) 30 mg, magnesium (as heavy magnesium oxide) 20 mg, vitamin B6 (as pyridoxine HCl) 20 mg, niacin (as niacinamide) 6 mg, zinc (as zinc sulfate monohydrate) 2 mg, vitamin E (as *d*-α-tocopheryl acetate) 15 IU, and *d*-biotin 40 μg. Efamol Fortify is a white, oblong, soft gelatin capsule and a 750-mg capsule contains calcium (as calcium carbonate) 100 mg, Efamol Pure Evening Primrose Oil 400 mg (255 mg linoleic acid and 32 mg γ-linolenic acid), marine fish oil 44 mg with an eicosapentaenoic acid content of 7 mg, and vitamin E (as *d*-α-tocopheryl acetate) 15 IU. Efalex is a clear, oblong, soft gelatin capsule and a 450-mg capsule contains a docosahexaenoic acid-rich fish oil 294 mg with a docosahexaenoic acid content of 60 mg, Efamol Pure Evening Primrose Oil 140 mg (γ-linolenic acid 12 mg and arachidonic acid 5.25 mg), vitamin E (as *d*-α-tocopheryl acetate) 15 IU, and thyme oil 1 mg. Efalex Liquid is a pale yellow-green, lemon-lime flavored, free-flowing oil. One teaspoon (5 mL) contains sunflower oil 3584 mg, docosahexaenoic acid-rich fish oil 520 mg with a docosahexaenoic acid content of 120 mg, Efamol Pure Evening Primrose Oil 300 mg (γ-linolenic acid 24 mg and arachidonic acid content of 10.5 mg), vitamin E (as *d*-α-tocopheryl acetate) 3.7 IU, and thyme oil 2 mg. Efanatal is a pink, oval, soft gelatin capsule and a 517-mg capsule contains Efamol Pure Evening Primrose Oil 140 mg (linoleic acid 162 mg, γ-linolenic acid 20 mg, and arachidonic acid 4.3 mg), fish oil 250 mg, docosahexaenoic acid 62.5 mg, and vitamin E (as *d*-α-tocopheryl acetate) 7.5 IU. Other products containing OEP are available from manufacturers such as Jamieson, Holista, and Nutrilite. Some OEP products on the market may contain other oils in their formulations including borage oil and black current oil.

Dosage

Use of more than 4 g OEP daily (300–600 mg γ-linolenic acid) is not recommended. However, adult doses of 3–8 g/day have been used for various conditions. For a OEP product with a standardized γ-linolenic acid content of 8%, the following dosages are recommended for the following conditions: atopic eczema, 4 to 8 g daily for adults, 2 to 4 g daily for children; cyclical and noncyclical mastalgia, 3 to 4 g daily; PMS, 3 g daily.

Pharmacological/Toxicological Effects

Dermatological Effects

Clinical evidence of nutritional supplementation with OEP to correct dermal conditions is mixed. One theory for the mixed results is that in some persons, once sensitized, immunological factors may override what help OEP can offer. Very high doses of OEP or linoleic acid, or modest doses of γ-linolenic acid, with corresponding correction of plasma EFA levels, produce some clinical improvement.

A defect in the capability of the enzyme δ-6-desaturase to convert linoleic acid to γ-linolenic acid is known to occur in patients with atopic dermatitis. Patients with atopic eczema have a dietary deficiency in metabolites of linoleic: γ-linolenic acid, dihomo-γ-linolenic acid, arachidonic acid, adrenic acid, and docosapentaenoic acid caused by a reduced rate of activity in the δ-6-desturase enzyme. Galli et al. compared blood samples from babies born to parents who suffered from atopic eczema. Results showed that dihomo-γ-linolenic acid and arachidonic acid were consistently and significantly lower in children who later had atopic eczema.

Some studies have shown that OEP administration can improve the percentage of body surface involvement, itch, dryness, scaling, and inflammation associated with atopic eczema. A meta-analysis of nine controlled trials involving OEP in the treatment of atopic eczema showed a highly significant improvement in the symptom of itch over placebo ($p < 0.0001$). In 1993, Berth-Jones et al. conducted a randomized, double-blind, parallel-group–designed study to investigate whether supplementation with OEP alone or a combination of OEP and fish oil helped with clinical symptoms of atopic dermatitis. A total of 133 patients (adults and children were evenly distributed) with chronic hand dermatitis enrolled and were randomized to receive either Epogam (per 500 mg capsule of OEP [321 mg linoleic acid and 40 mg γ-linolenic acid]), Efamol Marine (per 430 mg capsule of OEP/fish oil [17 mg eicosapentaenoic acid and 11 mg docosahexaenoic acid]), or placebo (paraffin/olive oil). No improvement with OEP was found.

In 1996, Whitaker et al. conducted a clinical trial to test if OEP supplementation affected the changes in lamellar bodies and lipid layers of the stratum corneum in patients with chronic (longer than 12 months) hand dermatitis. This parallel, double-blind, placebo-controlled trial had 39 patients with chronic hand dermatitis or eczema and 10 age- and sex-matched healthy controls for statistical comparison. Treatment lasted for 16 weeks, with the active group taking OEP (twelve 500-mg Epogam capsules daily for a total dose of 600 mg γ-linolenic acid) and the placebo group taking placebo (twelve 500-mg sunflower capsules daily), after which there was an 8-week washout period. Although the Epogam group improved in the clinical impressions of dermatitis, there was no statistical difference between groups and no structural change in skin specimens was seen.

Anti-Inflammatory Effects

Increased concentrations of eicosanoids (leukotriene B_4, prostaglandin E_2 [PGE_2] and thromboxane A_2) have been reported to exist in the colon mucosa and rectal areas of patients with ulcerative colitis. In 1993, a randomized, placebo-controlled study was conducted by Greenfield et al. examining the effect of OEP and fish oil supplementation on cell membranes and symptom control in 43 patients diagnosed with stable ulcerative colitis. Treatment with OEP increased red-cell membrane concentrations of dihomo-γ-linolenic acid by 40% at 6 months ($p < 0.05$), and compared to MaxEPA and placebo, OEP significantly improved stool consistency at 6 months, with this difference being maintained 3 months after OEP treatment was discontinued ($p < 0.05$). There was no difference in stool frequency, rectal bleeding, relapse rates, sigmoidoscopic findings between the three groups. OEP appeared to be of minimum benefit over placebo and fish oils.

Autoimmune

In a randomized, double-blind, placebo-controlled, three-arm, parallel study that used OEP treatment, 49 adult participants with a diagnosis of rheumatoid arthritis that required nonsteroidal anti-inflammatory medication (NSAID) but not second-line therapy were included. Treatment groups consisted of the control group (liquid paraffin placebo), OEP group (OEP daily dose containing 540 mg γ-linolenic acid), and OEP/fish oil group (dose not recorded). At 12 months, both active treatment groups reported significant subjective improvement compared to the placebo group and had significantly reduced their NSAID use. However, at 15 months, both treatment groups had relapsed. There was no evidence that OEP or OEP with fish oil had modified the disease process in any way.

Researchers conducted a 6-month, double-blind, placebo-controlled study involving 40 patients (male and female) with rheumatoid arthritis and upper gastrointestinal lesions caused by NSAIDs. For 6 months, 19 patients (17 females and 2 males) received 6 g of OEP daily (total daily dose of γ-linolenic acid 540 mg) and 21 patients (15 females and 6 males) received 6 g of olive oil daily. The results of this study found that there was a significant reduction in morning stiffness after 3 months. No patient was able to stop NSAID medication after completing OEP treatment and only 23 percent of patients could reduce their dose. These results were similar to that of the placebo (olive oil) group. Jäntti et al. examined the effect of OEP on clinical symptoms and plasma prostaglandin levels of patients with rheumatoid arthritis. Study results showed that plasma concentrations of PGE_2 decreased and thromboxane B_2 increased in both groups in addition to no clinical benefits reported. Other experimental studies have also concluded that oral OEP has no general therapeutic effect in patients with rheumatoid arthritis.

Manthorpe et al. examined the effect of OEP supplementation on lacrimal gland function in patients with primary Sjogren's syndrome using a double-blind, crossover design. The active treatment group received the following twice daily: Efamol (1500 mg [9% γ-linolenic acid, 73% *cis*-linoleic acid]), Efavit (375 mg vitamin C, 75 mg pyridoxine, 75 mg niacin, 15 mg zinc sulfate), and vitamin E (40.8 IU). The control group received the same number of placebo capsules and directions. Study results were mixed, with benefit seen in the lacrimal film function (Schirmer's I-test, $p < 0.03$) and nonsignificant findings for the remaining outcome measures. Because of the vitamins given with the OEP, it is difficult to say whether the OEP was of any benefit. In a randomized, placebo-controlled trial by Theander et al., 90 patients diagnosed with primary Sjogren's syndrome (with or without signs of autoimmunity) were given either OEP or corn oil (placebo) for 6 months and their symptom levels recorded. Patients were evaluated at baseline, 3, and 6 months. No significant improvements were found for any of the outcomes with OEP supplementation.

Increased levels of arachidonic acid and 4-series leukotriene have been reported in the skin plaques of patients with psoriasis. OEP is rich in three fatty acids (eicosapentaenoic, γ-linolenic, and docosahexaenoic acid), and eicosapentaenoic acid may help improve psoriasis by inhibiting the formation of 4-series leukotrienes by forming the 5-series leukotrienes, which are considered biologically less active than the 4-series.

In a double-blind, placebo-controlled trial by Veale et al., the effect of OEP supplementation on the improvement of psoriatic arthritis was examined in 38 patients with chronic stable plaque psoriasis and inflammatory arthritis. Results reported no changes in outcome measurements except a decrease in leukotriene B_4 production during the active phase in the Efamol Marine group compared to baseline ($p < 0.03$) and a rebounding increase in thromboxane B_2 during the group's placebo phase run-out phase. The authors suggest that the dose used in this study was sufficient to show some competition with arachidonic acid in its metabolic pathways but not high enough to show improvement in clinical outcomes.

Neurological System Effects

In diabetes, the δ-6-desaturation of linoleic acid into γ-linolenic acid is impaired. With evidence that a high intake of linoleic acid may have some benefit in cardiovascular problems in diabetics, there are hypotheses that supplementation with products high in γ-linolenic acid might benefit diabetic neuropathy. The 1993 study by the Gamma-Linolenic Acid Multicenter Trial Group specifically investigated the effects of OEP (12 capsules daily of a product identical to Epogam, 480 mg total daily dose of γ-linolenic acid) on the clinical outcomes of 111 patients with mild diabetic neuropathy over 1 year using a randomized, double-blind, placebo-controlled, parallel design. Participants were evaluated at baseline, 3, 6, and 12 months. Compared to placebo, OEP supplementation improved 8 out of 10 neurophysiological measures and 5 out of 6 neurological assessments ($p < 0.05$). The authors noted that the changes seen were of a magnitude that was clinically meaningful and consistent among the clinical, thermal, and neurophysical assessments.

Using a double-blind, placebo-controlled study design, Jamal and Carmichael investigated the effect of 6-month OEP supplementation in clinical improvement in 22 patients with either type I or II diabetes mellitus with distal diabetic polyneuropathy. OEP (a total daily dose of 4 g containing 360 mg γ-linolenic acid) was given to 12 patients, and placebo was given to 10. Compared with the placebo group, the OEP group showed statistically significant improvement ($p < 0.05$) in neuropathy symptom scores, median nerve motor conduction velocity/compound muscle action/potential amplitude, peroneal nerve motor conduction velocity/compound muscle action/ potential amplitude, median sensory nerve action potential amplitude, ankle heat threshold, and cold threshold.

Two major controlled trials have examined supplementation of OEP and its effect on attention-deficit/hyperactivity disorder (ADHD) with mixed results. In a double-blind, placebo-controlled, crossover study, Aman et al. examined the effect of OEP supplementation on ADHD in 31 children with ADHD (4 girls, 27 boys). A total of 26 children (mean age of 9 years) fulfilled the following inclusion criteria: 90th percentile or greater scores on both the Attention Problem subscale III of the Revised Behavior Problem Checklist and the Inattention subscale II of the Teacher Questionnaire. Each child received either OEP supplementation (6 Efamol capsules daily containing a total daily content of 2.16 g linoleic acid and 270 mg γ-linolenic acid) or placebo (500 mg liquid paraffin) for 4 weeks each, then switched to the other treatment with a 1-week washout period between crossovers. When the experiment-wise probability level was set at 0.05, the authors concluded that OEP supplementation showed no effect in hyperactive children. In the second trial, Arnold et al. compared *d*-amphetamine to OEP treatments using a double-blind, placebo-controlled, crossover treatment of 18 boys suffering from ADHD. Outcomes were parent and teacher ratings using standardized hyperactivity scales at screening, baseline, and every 2 weeks during the 3-month study period. Parent ratings showed no effect regarding OEP treatment. Teachers' ratings showed a trend of OEP effect between placebo and *d*-amphetamine with the only statistically significance ($p < 0.05$) demonstrated on the Conners Hyperactivity Factor.

Only one double-blind, crossover study has been conducted to examine the effect of OEP supplementation in 13 patients (8 men, 5 women) diagnosed with schizophrenia. Active treatment (4 g OEP, 40 mg vitamin E, 1000 mg vitamin C, 200 mg vitamin B_6, 300 mg vitamin B_3, and 40 mg zinc sulfate) lasted 4 months, with a 2-month washout period before crossing over to placebo treatment (content not described) for 4 months. Nonsignificant results were obtained when comparing mean scores during the active and placebo treatment periods.

Endocrine System Effects

Because levels of γ-linolenic acid are lower in women with PMS compared to non-PMS women, it is thought that a defect in converting linoleic acid to γ-linolenic acid may contribute to the sensitivity to normal changes in prolactin that happen during the menstrual cycle. Unfortunately, most studies of OEP in treatment of PMS have been open-label, nonplacebo-controlled studies. Only two small studies are considered well-designed and are summarized below. Khoo et al.

examined the effect of OEP on PMS symptoms of 38 women, aged 20 to 40 years, using a randomized, double-blind, placebo-controlled, crossover study design. Treatment duration for the first phase lasted 3 cycles, after which women crossed over into the other group for the next 3 months. Active treatment was OEP supplementation (8 Efamol Vita-Glow capsules daily, each capsule containing 72% linoleic acid, 9% γ-linolenic acid, and 12% oleic acid). Content of placebo capsule was not stated. Results reported showed that over 6 months, there were no significant differences in the symptom scoring between the active and placebo groups. The authors determined that the slight improvements noted by women with moderate PMS were caused by a placebo effect. Collins et al. conducted a 10-month randomized, double-blind crossover trial to determine the effect of OEP supplementation in 27 women diagnosed with PMS using *Diagnostic Manual of Mental Disorders*, criteria. All women were given placebo in the first month, which was considered the baseline month. All women with PMS received placebo in the second cycle to reduce placebo effects. For the OEP phase, total daily dose was 12 Efamol capsules (each capsule contained 4.32 g linoleic acid, 540 mg γ-linolenic acid). For the placebo phase, the same number of capsules was given and contained paraffin. After starting the treatment in the third cycle, women in one group crossed over to the other group in the seventh cycle. Of the 68 women who participated, 38 completed the study. Analyses of all outcome measures showed that OEP did not improve PMS symptoms or their cyclic nature. All women had improvements in their PMS symptoms over time. The study investigators stated that this result came from a placebo or study participation effect.

Chenoy et al. conducted a randomized, double-blind, placebo-controlled study of 56 women that examined the effects of OEP on menopausal flushing (hot flashes). Inclusion criteria were that women had suffered hot flashes at least 3 times a day, and had increased follicle-stimulating hormone and luteinizing hormone levels and/or amenorrhea for at least 6 months. Baseline levels were taken for 1 month when no treatment was given. At the beginning of the second month, 6 months of treatment began with the OEP group taking 4 g of OEP daily (4 capsules twice a day, each capsule containing 500 mg of OEP with 10 mg of vitamin E) and the control group taking the same regimen of placebo capsules. Women recorded the number and severity of flushing and sweating episodes in daily diaries. Assessments were conducted at baseline, 1,4, and 7 months. Of the 35 women who finished the study, improvements between control cycle and last treatment cycle were statistically significant for the placebo group but not for the OEP group, showing that OEP offered no benefit over placebo in treating menopausal flushing.

Although there has been no direct evidence, hormone imbalances (e.g., progesterone deficiency in the luteal phase, high estrogen levels or increased sensitivity to estrogen, higher-than-normal basal prolactin levels) have been associated with mastalgia. It is suggested that women with breast pain have low levels of γ-linolenic acid, possibly caused by the competition from high levels of saturated fatty acids that make the woman less able to convert linoleic acid to γ-linolenic acid. Another proposed mechanism suggests that OEP may help reduce pain through decreased peripheral prolactin via 1-series prostaglandins that is made from an OEP constituent, dihomo-L-linolenic acid.

OEP was found to have a favorable response in 45% of patients treated at the Cardiff Mastalgia Clinic for cyclical mastalgia. In this study, results from clinical trials (ranging in design from randomized and placebo-controlled to open-label) of drug treatment for mastalgia were grouped and descriptively analyzed. Four drugs were compared: bromocriptine, danazole, OEP, and progestins (dydrogesterone and norethisterone). Typical doses and durations were different for each drug. The usual dose of OEP used was six capsules daily for 3 to 6 months; milligram, product name, or percent of fatty acids was not disclosed. Study results report that of the 291 women who received medications, 45% of those with cyclical mastalgia reported good responses using OEP compared to 70% using danazol. Women with noncyclical mastalgia had less impressive good responses from all the drugs (31% danazol vs 27% OEP).

No statistical analyses were performed to control for study biases, so study results are suspect. In a later study by Wetzig, 170 women with severe mastalgia who were treated at a single clinic were followed for 3 years, with assessments performed on their responses to various medications. Sequence of drugs given depended on previous responses: vitamin B_6 (50–100 mg twice daily), OEP (1 g two to three times daily), danazol (100 mg twice daily tapering to 100 mg daily when pain was controlled). In some cases, progesterone, tamoxifen, or NSAIDs were also prescribed. Results regarding the effect of OEP supplementation on mastalgia were similar to placebo. A more recent study by Blommers et al. examined the effect of OEP and fish oil supplementation on severe mastalgia using a randomized, double-blind, controlled design. A total of 120 women were randomly placed into four groups. Group 1 took fish oil and one control oil, group 2 took OEP and a control oil, group 3 took fish oil and OEP, and group 4 took two control oils. Duration of therapy was 6 months. Results showed that neither OEP or fish oil were better than placebo in decreasing the number of days with pain.

Prostaglandins may be an important factor in the cervical ripening process of labor. Topical or oral OEP is promoted as an agent to speed cervical ripening. For this particular condition, continuing OEP use is typically re-evaluated after 1 week. If no cervical change is noted, the woman may choose to continue for another week or change to another ripening agent. A 1999 retrospective cohort study investigated the effect of oral OEP on pregnancy length, duration of labor, incidence of postdates induction, incidence of prolonged rupture of membranes, occurrence of abnormal labor patterns, and cesarean delivery in low-risk nulliparous women. The sample (54 subjects receiving OEP and 54 random controls) was drawn from records of all nulliparous women registered for care at one birth center in the northeastern region of the United States from 1991 to 1998. Results of this study showed that there were no apparent benefits from taking oral OEP with regards to reducing the incidence of adverse labor outcomes or decreasing the overall length of labor. In fact, the study reported a trend of increased incidence of birthing problems such as prolonged rupture of membranes and the need for oxytocin augmentation or vacuum extraction.

Cardiovascular System Effects

Low levels of linoleic acid and dihomo-γ-linolenic acid may predispose coronary heart disease. For this benefit, linoleic acid needs to be converted by the enzyme δ-6-desaturase to other highly unsaturated, long-change fatty acids, such as γ-linolenic acid. OEP contains both linoleic and γ-linolenic acid, and OEP has been reported to reduce elevated serum cholesterol levels, with y-linolenic acid having a more dramatic effect of the two.

In 1986, Boberg et al. examined the effects of n-3 and n-6 long-chain polyunsaturated fatty acid supplementation on serum lipoproteins and platelet function in 28 adults with high triglyceride levels. Using a placebo-controlled, double-blind, crossover design, 14 adults were randomized to either Efamol supplement group (total daily dose of 4 g had a content of 2.88 g of linoleic acid and 0.36 g of γ-linolenic acid) or the placebo group for 8 weeks, then switched to the other group for another 8 weeks. Another 14 adults were randomized to either MaxEPA supplement group (total daily dose of 10 g had a content of 1.8 g of eicosapentaenoic acid and 1.2 g of docosahexaenoic acid) or the placebo group for 8 weeks, with the same group switching noted previously. Results showed that although OEP supplementation increased γ-linolenic and dihomogammalinolenic acid content in plasma triglycerides and cholesterol esters, compared to placebo, no statistically significant changes were demonstrated in serum lipoprotein lipids or apolipoproteins, triglyceride levels, platelet aggregation, or plasma β-thromboglobulin levels. In a randomized, placebo-controlled study of healthy men aged 35 to 54 years who had low levels of dihomo-γ-linolenic acid, the effect of OEP on the fatty acid composition of their adipose tissue and serum lipids was investigated. A total of 35 subjects were enrolled in the study and randomized into four groups. Group 1 ($n = 9$) received 10 mL OEP daily, Group 2 ($n = 8$) received 20 mL OEP daily, Group 3 ($n = 9$) received 30 mL OEP daily, and Group 4 ($n = 9$) received 20 mL of safflower oil daily for 4 months. Results showed that whereas 20 mL daily OEP supplementation increased adipose dihomo-γ-linolenic acid levels ($p < 0.01$), no effects were seen on serum cholesterol, low-density lipoprotein (LDL) cholesterol, or high-density lipoprotein (HDL) cholesterol. OEP was deemed to be an ineffective cholesterol-lowering agent.

In a randomized, blinded, crossover study, 12 males with hyperlipidemia took 3 g of OEP daily (containing linoleic acid 2200 mg and γ-linolenic acid 240 mg). After a receiving a placebo for 4 weeks, participants were randomly divided into the treatment or placebo group. For 4 months, the treatment group received OEP (total daily dose of 3 g containing 2.2 g linoleic acid and 240 mg γ-linolenic acid) and placebo group received liquid paraffin. After 4 months, each group received 4 weeks of placebo (washout period) then crossed over to the alternate group for 4 more months of supplementation. Comparing blood samples taken at placebo phase and after 4 months of OEP use, serum triglyceride levels, serum cholesterol, and LDL cholesterol had decreased 48, 32, and 49%, respectively, and HDL cholesterol had increased by 22% ($p < 0.01$). Adenosine diphosphate- and adrenaline-induced platelet aggregation were reduced 50 and 60%, respectively, after 2 and 4 months of OEP use (p-values not reported), and platelet production of thromboxane B_2 went from 26 ± 1.8 to 11.8 ± 3.8 ng/mL plasma ($p < 0.001$) after OEP use. Compared with placebo, after 3 or 4 months of OEP use, bleeding time increased 40% (from 6.8 ± 0.3 minutes to 12.0 ± 0.8 percent [$p < 0.001$]).

Using a randomized, placebo-controlled design, Leng et al. examined the effect of γ-linolenic acid on cholesterol and lipoprotein levels in patients with lower limb atherosclerosis. A total of 120 adults with stable intermittent claudication (ankle brachial pressure index of ≤ 0.9 in at least one limb) were given either active treatment or placebo for 2 years. Active treatment was three capsules twice daily of polyunsaturated fatty acid (one capsule contained 280 mg γ-linolenic acid and 45 mg eicosapentaenoic acid) or the same doses of placebo capsules (one capsule contained 500 mg sunflower oil) for 2 years. Of the 120 participants, 39 (65%) taking active treatment and 36 (60%) taking placebo completed the trial. Lipid concentrations and walking distance were not different between groups. However, hematocrit was higher ($p < 0.01$) and systolic blood pressure lower ($p < 0.05$) in the γ-linolenic acid groups.

Dietary supplementation with OEP, which contains the fatty acid prostaglandin precursors linoleic and γ-linolenic acid, may enhance the synthesis of prostaglandins, which might help lower vascular sensitivity to increased levels of angiotensin II in pregnancy. To examine the effect that OEP supplementation has in hypertension during pregnancy, randomized, placebo-controlled studies have investigated its use in women diagnosed with preeclampsia. Unfortunately, OEP did not lower blood pressure in women suffering from hypertension in pregnancy.

Cytotoxic Effects

Mansel et al. conducted a randomized, double-blind, placebo-controlled clinical trial in 200 women with proven recurrent breast cysts that could be aspirated and were determined to be noncancerous by mammography and biopsy. For 1 year, one group took six Efamol capsules per day (total daily OEP dose of 3 g containing 9% γ-linolenic acid) and the other group took placebo. After 1 year, only 15 women had dropped out of the study (eight from the placebo group, seven from the OEP group). The overall cyst recurrence rate was 44% (46% for the placebo group, and 43% for the OEP group) and statistically nonsignificant. Cyst fluid electrolyte ratio was unremarkable. Fatty acid analysis results were not stated.

Miscellaneous

Chronic fatigue syndrome (CFS) is a condition in which the etiology is unclear. The illness is characterized by persistent and relapsing fatigue, and other varying symptoms throughout the body. In 2000, a critique of the literature on all *randomized controlled trials* (RCTs) regarding treatment for CFS reported mixed results for OEP therapy. The reviewers reported two RCTs comparing OEP with placebo in patients with either a diagnosis of postviral fatigue syndrome or CFS.

In the first double-blind, randomized, placebo-controlled study, Behan et al. examined the physical and psychological effects of high doses of OEP/ fish oil supplementation on 63 adults (27 men, 36 women) with postviral fatigue syndrome. Participants were randomly assigned to placebo group (liquid paraffin containing a total daily dose of 400 mg linoleic acid and 80 IU of vitamin E) or treatment group (total daily OEP/fish oil preparation containing 288 mg γ-linolenic acid, 136 mg eicosapentaenoic acid, 88 mg docosahexaenoic acid, 2.04 g linoleic acid, and 80 IU of vitamin E) for 3 months and were evaluated at baseline, 1, and 3 months. At 3 months, 85% of the OEP group showed improvement compared to 17% of the placebo group (scale of better, worse, unchanged; $p < 0.0001$). The EFA levels were abnormal at the baseline and were corrected in the OEP group by study end ($p < 0.05$). The second study was a double-blind, placebo-controlled, randomized design in which Warren et al. looked at the effect of 3 months of OEP supplementation on physical and psychological outcome measures of 50 patients (21 men, 29 women) who were diagnosed with CFS using the Oxford Criteria. Patients were randomized into the placebo group (sunflower oil) or treatment group (eight Efamol Marine 500 mg daily, which contained, in the OEP and fish oil components, a total daily dose of 288 mg γ-linolenic acid, 136 mg eicosapentanoic acid, 88 mg of docosahexanoic acid, and 2.04 g of linoleic acid) or placebo group (sunflower oil). At the end of the 3 months, seven participants from the treatment group and five from the placebo group had quit the study because of lack of clinical response. Results showed that although both physical and psychological symptoms improved with time, the differences before and after treatment between groups were not statistically significant.

Khan et al. examined the effects of n-3 and n-6 fatty acid supplements (two of which contained OEP) on the microvascular blood flow and endothelial function in 173 healthy men and women aged 40 to 65 years in an 8-month, double-blind, randomized, placebo-controlled study. For the single OEP supplementation, the group received a total daily OEP of 5 g (which contained 400 mg/day of γ-linolenic acid). For the tuna oil/OEP supplementation, the group received a total daily tuna oil of 5 g (which contained 6% of eicosapentaenoic acid and 27% of docosahexaenoic acid per day) and OEP of 5 g. Results showed that there although there were significant improvements in the tuna oil supplementation group, there were no significant changes in any of the outcome measures with either single OEP or tuna oil/OEP supplementation group.

Pharmacokinetics

The pharmacokinetic parameters of γ-linolenic acid and its metabolic products were studied in six healthy volunteers (three males, three females) following the administration of OEP. Serum level-time courses of eight fatty acids (γ-linolenic, palmitic, linoleic, linolenic, oleic stearic, arachidonic, dihomo-γ-linolenic acids) were profiled twice over a 24-hour period after receiving six capsules of Epogam (total dose being 240 mg of γ-linolenic acid) at 7:00 AM and 7:00 PM (γ-linolenic acid total daily dose being 480 mg). The following mean pharmacokinetic parameters were obtained for γ-linolenic acid: t_{max}^{am} (hour) = 4.4 (significantly higher than t_{max}^{pm} [$p < 0.05$]); C_{max}^{am} (μg/mL) = 22.6; t_{max}^{pm} (hour) = 2.7; C_{max}^{pm} (μg/mL) = 20.7; area under the curve $(AUC)_{12h}^{am}$ ([μg · hour]/mL) = 119.0; AUC_{12h}^{pm} ([mg · hour]/mL) = 155.1; and AUC_{24h} ([mg · hour]/mL) = 274.1 (significantly higher than AUC_{24h} at baseline). This study found that the absorption of γ-linolenic acid from the gastrointestinal tract is much lower than in the morning than in the evening. The concentrations of the metabolites of γ-linolenic acid, arachidonic acid, and dihomo-γ-linolenic acid could not be established in these volunteers.

Adverse Effects and Toxicity

When taken within the recommended dosage range, the γ-linolenic acid content of OEP is equivalent to that present in a normal diet. Thus, although adverse effects are rare at recommended doses, occasionally, mild gastrointestinal effects and headache may occur with oral use of OEP. The World Health Organization Programme for International Drug Monitoring reported that, in the period between 1968 and 1997, there were 193 adverse reactions reported mentioning OEP. The most critical of these OEP reports mentioned convulsions, aggravated convulsion, face edema, and asthma. The most noncritical OEP adverse effects included headache, nausea, itching, abdominal pain, and diarrhea. In the study by Guivernau et al. reported that OEP inhibited platelet aggregation and prolonged bleeding time in 12 males with hyperlipidemia taking 3 g of OEP daily (containing linoleic acid 2200 mg and γ-linolenic acid 240 mg). Compared to placebo, bleeding time at 3 and 4 months increased 40%, with the group's mean rising from 6 to 12 minutes ($p < 0.001$).

Interactions

Current references advise caution with concurrent use of OEP and several classes of medications (anticoagulants, antipsychotics/anticonvulsants) because of possible serious side effects.

The use of anticonvuls ants and OEP may result in a delayed reduction in the effectiveness of the anticonvulsant because OEP may lower the seizure threshold. In 1981, three patients on phenothiazine therapy for schizophrenia were given OEP (around this time, OEP was being considered a possible adjunct to therapy for this mental illness). The patients suffered seizures, OEP was discontinued, and electroencephalograms were performed. The tests showed temporal lobe epileptic disorders and phenothiazine therapy was discontinued or reduced in the patients and carbamazepine started. The authors suggested that OEP supplementation be used with caution in patients taking phenothiazines. In 1983, Holman et al. reported an incident involving a 43-year old man with schizophrenia on fluphenazine decanoate therapy who suffered a grand mal seizure after using 4 g of OEP daily for 3 months. Once the OEP was discontinued, no seizures occurred in the next 7 months.

The use of OEP with antiplatelets, thrombolytics, low-molecular-weight heparins, or anticoagulants may result in a delayed but increased risk of bleeding, and concomitant use is not advised. The mechanism of action is theorized to be decreased thromboxane B_2 synthesis and increased prostacyclin production caused by γ-linolenic acid, resulting in inhibition of platelet aggregation and prolonged bleeding time.

In vitro experiments by Zou et al. in 2002 examined the effect of the *cis*-linoleic acid component of OEP on the catalytic activity of cDNA-expressed cytochrome P450 isoforms (CYP1A2, CYP2C9, CYP2C19, CYP2D6, and CYP3A4). The highest concentration of *cis*-linoleic acid tested was 179 μM. In these assays, inhibitory concentration of 50% (IC_{50}) values no greater than 10 μM were considered potent inhibitors and IC_{50} values between 10 and 50 μM were labeled moderate inhibitors. *cis*-Linoleic acid tested as a moderate inhibitor of all the cDNA-derived enzymes except CYP3A4 (resorufin benzyl ether substrate). However, there have been no case reports of toxicity or adverse reactions with OEP and drugs metabolized by this enzyme.

Reproduction

There are no known reports of OEP causing teratogenicity in humans. No effects of OEP administration on reproduction were found in 2-year teratological investigations. Specifically, reproductive investigations with OEP supplementation have been performed in mice and rats, mink, and the blue fox. In a study examining the teratogenicity of OEP, mice and rats were fed a diet containing 10% of oxidized linoleic acid. The rats, but not the mice, had babies with an increase in urogenital anomalies. Tauson et al. conducted reproduction studies in the male and female mink. The results of these studies suggested there was a tendency (nonsignificant) for a decreased rate of stillbirths and deaths during the first 21 days of life when the male was administered OEP. OEP administration did not affect reproductive performance.

Regulatory Status

OEP is regulated as a dietary supplement in the United States. It is approved in Canada as an over-the-counter product for use in EFA-deficiency conditions and as a dietary supplement to increase EFA intake. In Germany, OEP is approved for use as food and is approved there in the treatment and symptomatic relief of atopic eczema. In Sweden, OEP is classified as a natural product. OEP has a Class 1 Safety Rating with the American Herbal Product Association.

8

FEVERFEW

Feverfew is a short perennial bush that grows along fields and roadsides. It reaches heights of 15–60 cm. With its yellow-green leaves and yellow flowers, it can be mistaken for chamomile (*Matricaria chamomilla*). The flowers bloom from July to October. Since the time of Dioscorides in the first century CE, feverfew has been used for the treatment of headache, menstrual irregularities, and fever. The common name is in fact a corruption of the Latin word *febrifugia*. Other traditional uses include treatment of menstrual pain, asthma, arthritis, psoriasis, threatened miscarriage, toothache, opium abuse, vertigo, tinnitus, anemia, the common cold, and gastrointestinal disturbances. It was also used to aid in expulsion of the placenta and stillbirths, and in difficult labor. Feverfew has been planted around houses to act as an insect repellant, as well as for use as a topical remedy for insect bites.

CURRENT PROMOTED USES

In the 1970s, use of feverfew as an alternative to traditional medicines for relief from arthritis and migraine headache began gaining popularity. Prevention of migraine headache and nausea and vomiting associated with migraine headache is the most commonly promoted indication for feverfew.

SOURCES AND CHEMICAL COMPOSITION

Tanacetum parthenium Schulz-Bip, formerly *Chrysanthemum parthenium* (L.) Bernh, *Leucanthemum parthenium* (L.) Gren and Gordon, *Pyrethum parthenium* (L.) Sm; also described as a member of the genus *Matricaria*; featherfew, altamisa, bachelor's button, featherfoil, febrifuge plant, midsummer daisy, nosebleed, Santa Maria, wild chamomile, wild quinine, amargosa, flirtwort, manzanilla, mutterkraut, varadika.

Products Available

Feverfew is available as a fresh leaf; dried, powdered leaf; capsules; tablets; fluid extract; dry standardized extract; crystals; and oral drops. Brand names include Migracare (600 μg of parthenolide per capsule), Migracin (feverfew extract 1:4 and white willow bark), MigraSpray, MygraFew, Lomigran, 125-mg Migrelief (light green round tablet containing 600 μg of parthenolide), Partenelle, Phytofeverfew, and 125-mg Tanacet (not $<0.2\%$ parthenolide). Feverfew contains flavonoid glycosides and sesquiterpene lactones. Parthenolide can constitute up to 85% of the sesquiterpene lactones in feverfew grown in Europe, but is present in lesser amounts or is even totally absent from North American feverfew.

Parthenolide is concentrated in the flowers and leaves, as opposed to stems and roots, and parthenolide content of the leaves may decrease during storage. The vegetative cycle also influences parthenolide content. Although parthenolide is thought to be the active ingredient in feverfew, and preparations are often standardized based on parthenolide content, there may be other active compounds, including the lipophilic flavonol tanetin, other methyl monoterpene ethers, and chrysanthenyl acetate, monoterpene.

Most tablet and capsule formulations contain 300 mg of feverfew, and the recommended dose is usually two to six tablets or capsules per day. A dose of 250 μg of parthenolide is considered an adequate daily dose, and 0.2% parthnolide is considered the acceptable minimum parthenolide concentration; therefore, the manufacturer's recommended dose is probably in excess of what is considered therapeutic. In the prevention of migraine headache, doses used in studies have been 50–100 mg of dried feverfew leaves daily (60 mg of dried feverfew leaves = 2.5 leaves). However, the parthenolide content of the North American plant is low, and parthenolide content in feverfew products varies widely, and may be lower than stated on the label or even absent from some preparations. For example, no parthenolide could be detected in two-thirds of feverfew products purchased in Louisiana health food stores. The parthenolide content of powdered feverfew leaves falls during storage. Given that the active ingredients of feverfew have yet to be definitively determined, it is difficult to designate a therapeutic or toxic dosage range.

Pharmacological/Toxicological Effects

Neurological Effects

Feverfew's mechanism of action in the prevention of migraine headaches is not known. It is speculated that feverfew affects platelet activity or inhibits vascular smooth-muscle contraction, perhaps by inhibiting prostaglandin synthesis. Results of in vitro studies suggest that rather than acting as a cyclooxygenase inhibitor, feverfew inhibits phospholipase A2, thus inhibiting release of arachidonic acid from the cell membrane phospholipid bilayer.

Drugs that are serotonin antagonists are used in migraine prevention (e.g., methysergide). During a migraine, serotonin is released from platelets, and in vitro studies using a bovine platelet bioassay have shown that parthenolide, as well as other sesquiterpene lactones, inhibits platelet serotonin release. Both parthenolide and a chloroform extract of dried, powdered leaves were also able to inhibit serotonin release and platelet aggregation in an in vitro study using human platelets and a variety of platelet-activating agents. The effect of these substances on platelet aggregation caused by a variety of chemicals was tested, and was similar except that inhibition of platelet aggregation induced by the calcium ionophore A23187 by chloroform extract leveled off at a relatively low concentration and was not complete, whereas parthenolide inhibited aggregation in a dose-dependent manner, suggesting a different mechanism of action.

Similarly discrepant results were reported in a study comparing chloroform extracts of fresh and dried feverfew and parthenolide. In this in vitro study, both the fresh extract and parthenolide were able to irreversibly inhibit contraction of rabbit aortic ring and rat anococcygeus muscle in a dose-dependent manner. In contrast, the extract from dried powdered feverfew leaves was spasmogenic, causing a slow, maintained, reversible contraction. The differences in pharmacological effect were explained by the differences in composition of the extracts; unlike the extract of fresh leaves, the extract of dried powdered leaves did not contain parthenolide or other sesquiterpene lactones. The specific functional group responsible for inhibition of smooth muscle contraction has been identified as the α-methylene moiety present on parthenolide and other sesquiterpene lactones. It has been hypothesized that the irreversible inhibition of platelet aggregation and inhibition of smooth muscle contraction are caused by covalent binding of parthenolide and other lactones to sulfhydryl (SH-) groups on proteins.

Another study using chloroform extract of fresh feverfew leaves demonstrated reversible blockade of open voltage-dependent potassium channels, but not of calcium-dependent potassium channels, in smooth muscle cells in vitro. Inhibition of potassium channels would be expected to increase the excitability of smooth muscle cells, potentiate the effects of depolarizing stimuli, and open voltage-dependent calcium channels, thus leading to muscle contraction. In the study described previously, the extract of dried, powdered feverfew had this very effect, which could be explained by potassium channel blockade; however, the fresh extract had the opposite effect (i.e., it irreversibly inhibited contractility). In addition, parthenolide, which was present in fresh but not dried extracts, did not appear to inhibit potassium channels. The substances in feverfew that cause potassium channel blockade and muscle contraction have not been identified, but because voltage-dependent potassium channels present in smooth muscle cells are similar to those present in neurons, it is possible that feverfew interferes with the neurogenic response in migraine.

One of the first studies to attempt to objectively evaluate the efficacy of feverfew for migraine prophylaxis enrolled 17 patients with common or classical migraine who had been self-medicating with raw feverfew leaves (average 2.44 leaves [60 mg]) daily for at least 3 months. Patients were randomized to receive either 50 mg of freeze-dried feverfew powder or placebo for 6 months. One patient in each group was taking conjugated equine estrogens and one patient in the feverfew group was taking Orlest 21, an oral contraceptive. Efficacy was assessed using patient diaries in which patients recorded the duration and severity of headache pain, severity and duration of nausea and vomiting, and analgesic use on an ordinal scale. The frequency of migraine, nausea, and vomiting, was significantly ($p < 0.02$) lower in the feverfew group, but analgesic use was similar. Two patients taking placebo withdrew from the study because of recurrent severe migraine. Patients taking feverfew reported a similar number of migraine attacks during the study compared to before the study, when they were self-medicating with feverfew. Conversely, placebo patients reported a frequency of headache that was greater than when they were self-medicating, and similar to the frequency of headache before beginning feverfew self-treatment. At the end of the study, the patients assessed the overall efficacy of the treatment; feverfew had a more favorable rating than placebo ($p < 0.01$). Because there was underreporting of headache in the placebo group, the difference between feverfew and placebo may have been even greater. Adverse events were not reported in the feverfew group, but patients did complain of the product's taste. A potential problem with this study was blinding; most patients guessed correctly which treatment they were receiving. Another criticism of this study is that because the participants were recruited from a population already taking feverfew and who presumably felt they were benefiting from feverfew, the investigators were in effect selecting known "*feverfew responders*" for their study. Such a selection process limits the extent to which these study results can be extrapolated to the general population.

In a subsequent study, efficacy of feverfew in migraine prophylaxis was further assessed in a double-blind, randomized, crossover design. One capsule of dried feverfew leaves (70–114 mg, average 82 mg) was compared to placebo in 72 adult volunteers with classical or common migraine. All subjects had migraine of at least a 2-year duration, and suffered at least one attack per month. Patients were excluded if they were being treated for any other disease, but women taking oral contraceptives were eligible for the study if they had been on the same contraceptive for at least 3 months. Females of child-bearing potential were excluded unless they were using adequate contraception. All migraine-related drugs were stopped at the beginning of the trial, which commenced with a 1-month single-blind placebo run-in period. Patients were then randomized to placebo or feverfew for 4 months each. Efficacy was assessed based on a patient diary in which patients recorded the number, severity, and duration of any migraine attacks, as well as the presence of nausea and vomiting, on a scale from 0 to 3. In addition, every 2 months, the patient's overall impression of migraine control was assessed using a 10-cm visual analog scale. There was a significant difference ($p < 0.05$) between placebo and feverfew in number of attacks only after month 4, but there wasa significant difference between the two groups in overall impression after month 4 ($p < 0.05$) and after month 6 ($p < 0.01$) when assessed via the visual analog scale. Feverfew decreased the number of classical migraine attacks by 32% (95% confidence interval [CI] 11–53%, $p < 0.05$), but the effect on the number of common migraine attacks was not statistically significant ($p = 0.06$). When assessing the responses of patients who had never used feverfew before study enrollment (n = 42/59), the number of attacks was reduced by 23% (95% CI 10–33%, $p = 0.06$). This nonsignificant result gives credence to the concerns about selection bias in the study by Johnson and colleagues. The overall impression of both patients with common and classical migraines was favorable based on the visual analog scale ($p < 0.01$). Vomiting associated with attacks was also decreased with feverfew, and there was a trend toward reduction in migraine severity. Duration of attacks was unchanged. Incidence of adverse effects, including mouth ulceration, indigestion, heartburn, dizziness, lightheadedness, rash, and diarrhea was low and comparable to placebo.

Another randomized, double-blind, crossover study assessed the efficacy of 100 mg of feverfew (0.2% parthenolide) daily compared to placebo in 57 patients. Efficacy was assessed using a questionnaire. Feverfew was superior to placebo in reducing intensity of migraine pain and other symptoms. Unfortunately, no results were reported for the actual number of headache attacks occurring during the study. An alcoholic extract of feverfew providing 0.5 mg of parthenolide daily for 4 months was not superior to placebo in the number of migraine attacks in a randomized, double-blind, crossover study in 44 evaluable patients.

Surprisingly, melatonin, a human pineal hormone, has been identified in fresh green feverfew leaves at a concentration of 2.45 μg/g, and in a commercially available feverfew tablet at a concentration of 0.143 μg/g. Each Tanacet tablet contains 70–80 ng of melatonin, and the recommended dose is one or two tablets daily. Freeze-dried green leaf contains 2.19 μg/g of melatonin, fresh golden feverfew leaf contains 1.92 μg/g, oven-dried green leaf contains 1.69 μg/g, freeze-dried golden leaf conatins 1.61 μg/g, and oven-dried golden leaf contains 1.37 μg/g. Because chronic migraine headaches are associated with lower circulating melatonin levels, it is possible that melatonin plays a role in feverfew's purported efficacy in preventing migraine headache. This finding underscores the need to fully characterize the ingredients in herbs and medicinal preparations made from them.

A concentrated CO_2 extract of *T. parthenium* (feverfew) indentified as MIG-99 was evaluated in a 12-week, double-blind, multicenter, randomized, placebo-controlled, dose-response study involving 147 patients. The clinical effectiveness of three dosage levels of MIG-99 (2.08, 6.25, and 18.75 mg) administered three times daily was studied. In general, the compound failed to demonstrate a significant prophylactic effect in any treatment group. Only the maximum migraine intensity, severity, and the number of attacks with confinement to bed were reduced by MIG-99. In the intent-to-treat analysis, MIG-99 was shown to be effective only in a small, predefined subgroup of patients receiving the 6.25-mg dose. These patients were noted to have a total of four attacks reported in a baseline period. Regarding toxicity and safety, the incidence of adverse events was similar between all treatment groups as compared to placebo, and the incidence of patients reporting at least one adverse effect was lowest in the patients receiving the highest dose. Additionally there were no negative laboratory investigations or changes in vital signs during the treatment regimen in any patient group.

A randomized, double-blind, placebo-controlled trial comparing the effects of a compound containing a combination of riboflavin (4000 mg daily), magnesium (300 mg daily), and feverfew (100 mg standardized to 0.7 mg parthenolide daily) to placebo (25 mg riboflavin) showed a placebo effect comparable to the combination compound. In this particular study, the placebo effect exceeded that reported for any other placebo in migraine prophylaxis trials. The trial was undertaken to study patient response to a "natural" multicombination product containing ingredients with previously demonstrated efficacy in at least one double-blind, placebo-controlled trial. Although there was no statistical difference between groups during the 3-month trial, both groups were superior to baseline in reduction of number of migraines, migraine days, and migraine index, but not superior to previously reported positive results for any of the agents alone. Possible reasons for the high placebo response (44%) included a potential therapeutic effect of the small dose of riboflavin in the placebo group, adverse interaction between the three agents used in the combination product, and a short duration of study (3 months).

In a study designed to evaluate the pharmacokinetics and toxicity of parthenolide, the active component of feverfew, doses of 1,2,3, and 4 mg were studied in a dose escalation fashion. Administration of feverfew in escalating doses up to 4 mg showed no toxicity and a maximum tolerated dose was not reached. Despite a parthenolide detection level of 0.5 ng/mL, no measurable concentrations of this component could be measured at any of the administered doses levels.

Larger studies are needed to definitively determine the efficacy of feverfew in the prevention of migraine and to identify the component or components responsible for its pharmacologic effects. Although parthenolide is considered the active constituent of feverfew, the pharmacokinetics of this constituent have not been characterized, and challenges remain in detecting this component analytically to allow evaluation of its metabolic fate.

Anti-Inflammatory Effects

Organic and aqueous feverfew powdered leaf extracts were found to inhibit IL-1-induced prostaglandin E2 release from synovial cells, IL-2- induced thymidine uptake by lymphoblasts, and mitogen-induced uptake of thymidine by peripheral blood mononuclear cells (PBMCs). Parthenolide also inhibited thymidine uptake by PBMCs. Both parthenolide and the extracts were cytotoxic to the PBMCs and synovial cells; thus, the anti-inflammatory effects of feverfew may be secondary to cytotoxicity. These results reflect those of previous researchers who found parthenolide and other sesquiterpene lactones to be cytotoxic to cultures of human fibroblasts, human laryngeal carcinoma cells, and human cells transformed with simian virus 40.

The anti-inflammatory effect of dried powdered feverfew leaf was compared to placebo in the treatment of *rheumatoid arthritis* (RA). This double-blind, randomized study used dried powdered feverfew leaf 70–86 mg (mean 76 mg), equivalent to 2–3 μmol of parthenolide. A total of 41 female patients with RA from a rheumatology clinic participated. Patients were allowed to continue their usual doses of nonsteroidal anti-inflammatory drugs and other analgesics. If a patient deteriorated acutely during the study, a single intraarticular dose of 20 mg of triamcinolone hexacetonide was allowed at week 3. Efficacy was determined by clinical assessments at weeks 3 and 6, and included duration of early morning stiffness in minutes, inactivity stiffness (present/absent), pain (10 cm visual analog scale), grip strength, and Richie articular index. Patients were also questioned about adverse effects. At weeks 0 and 6, hemoglobin, white blood cell count, platelet count, urea, creatinine, erythrocyte sedimentation rate, C reactive protein, immunoglobulin G (IgG), IgM, IgA, latex fixation test, Rose-Waaler titer, C3 degradation products, and Steinbrocker functional capacity were determined. At week 6, a global impression from both the patient and the clinician were recorded as better, same, or worse. One patient in the placebo group dropped out after the third day because of lightheadedness, but complete data were obtained for the remaining 40 patients. One patient receiving feverfew reported minor ulceration and soreness of the tongue. At baseline, hemoglobin and serum creatinine levels were lower in the placebo group than in the feverfew group. By week 3, urea levels had significantly increased ($p = 0.04$) in the feverfew group, but this was not apparent at week 6. At week 6, grip strength and IgG were increased in the feverfew group compared with baseline ($p = 0.47$ and 0.025, respectively). Overall, the results of this study do not support the efficacy of 76 mg of dried feverfew leaf in the treatment of RA.

Mutagenicity/Carcinogenicity/Teratogenicity

In 30 patients with migraine who had been taking feverfew leaves, tablets, or capsules for at least 11 months, there was no increase in chromosomal aberrations or sister chromatid exchange in circulating lymphocytes compared to patients with migraine not taking feverfew matched for age and sex. The Ames salmonella mutagenicity test was also performed on urine samples from 10 patients using feverfew and 10 matched nonusers, with no indication of mutagenicity.

No problems have been reported in offspring of pregnant women who used feverfew, but feverfew has purportedly been associated with spontaneous abortion in cattle and uterine contractions in term human pregnancies.

Adverse Effects and Toxicity

Case Reports of Toxicity Caused by Commercially Available Products

Adverse effects associated with feverfew use include dizziness, lightheadedness, nausea, heartburn, indigestion, bloating, gas, constipation, diarrhea, inflammation, and ulceration of the oral mucosa, weight gain, palpitations, heavier menstrual flow, contact dermatitis, and rash. Feverfew belongs to the *Compositae* family, and persons allergic to other members of this family such as chamomile, ragweed, asters, chrysanthemums, and echinacea could also be allergic to feverfew. Out of 300 feverfew users, 18% of those questioned reported adverse effects, with mouth ulceration reported in 11.3%. Feverfew-induced mouth ulceration is not a manifestation of contact dermatitis; it is a systemic reaction. In contrast, inflammation of the tongue and oral mucosa accompanied by lip swelling and loss of taste is probably caused by direct contact with feverfew and is not associated with use of feverfew capsules or tablets.

In the study by Johnson and colleagues, in which 10 patients who had been taking fresh feverfew leaves were switched to placebo, patients experienced recurrence of migraine, tension headaches, joint pain and stiffness, nervousness, insomnia and disrupted sleep, and tiredness. The investigators dubbed these symptoms the "*postfeverfew syndrome.*" Dr. Johnson had documented this syndrome in a previous publication when approx 10% of 164 patients who discontinued feverfew reported anxiety, poor sleep, joint and muscle aches, pains, and stiffness.

Drug Interactions

In vitro studies suggest that feverfew may inhibit platelet aggregation, leading to recommendations that patients avoid use of feverfew with anticoagulants and medications with antiplatelet activity. Platelets from 10 patients who had taken feverfew for at least 3.5 years responded normally to aggregation induced by adenosine diphosphate and thrombin compared to platelets from four control patients who had stopped taking feverfew at least 6 months earlier. In patients who had been taking feverfew for at least 4 years, the threshold for platelet aggregation in response to 11α, 9α; -epoxymethanoprostaglandin H2 (U46619) and serotonin was elevated. Whether these results translate into the potential for drug interactions and bleeding diatheses remains to be documented.

Regulation

In the United States, feverfew may be marketed as a dietary supplement, but is not approved as a drug. A United States Pharmacopeia advisory panel, although recognizing that feverfew has a long history of use and lack of documented adverse effects, does not recommend its use owing to the paucity of scientific evidence of safety and efficacy. The panel encourages further research, including at least one properly designed clinical trial.

In Canada, the Health Protection branch allows sale of tablets and capsules made from feverfew crude dried leaves for decreasing the frequency and severity of migraine headaches. The products should be standardized to contain no less than 0.2% parthenolide. In France, feverfew has traditional use in the treatment of heavy menstrual flow and prevention of migraine headache.

9

Garlic

Garlic use dates back to Old Testament times, when it was a favored food. Drawings of garlic from 3700 BCE were uncovered in Egyptian tombs. Over the centuries, garlic has been used to ward off vampires, demons, witches, and evil beings and was thought to have magical properties. Medicinal uses date back to 1550 BCE, when it was used as a remedy for heart disease, headaches, and tumors. It has also been used as an aphrodisiac to improve sexual performance and desire, and as a cure-all for everything from hemorrhoids to snake bites.

Current Promoted Uses

In 1997, garlic was the most widely used natural supplement in US house-holds. Garlic was shown to be used more than twice as much as any other natural supplement. Garlic is promoted to lower cholesterol and blood pressure, delay the progression of atherosclerosis, prevent heart disease, improve circulation, prevent cancer, and is used topically for tinea infections.

Sources and Chemical Composition

Allium sativum, *Allii sativi bulbus*, knoblauch, ail, ajo, allium, Camphor of the Poor, Garlic Clove, Nectar of the Gods, Poor Man's Treacle, Rust Treacle, Stinking Rose.

Products Available

Four types of garlic preparations are currently available on the US market: garlic essential oils, garlic oil macerate, garlic powder, and *aged garlic extract* (AGE). Most garlic preparations report allicin yield potentials, whereas AGE products standardize to S-allylcysteine (SAC) amounts. Some products have been shown to release differing amounts of active components depending on when the product was made.

Product Names

- Garlic-Gold, extract 600 mg (*A. sativum*), (7200-μg allicin yield)
- Garlic-Go!, 1000 mg AGE
- Garlic HP — Physiologics, 400-mg garlic bulb (1000 μg allicin/g yield)
- Garlic HP 650 — Physiologics, bulb powder (allicin yield 6500 μg, total thiosulfinates 6500 μg, alliin yield 14,500 μg, γ-glutamyl-cysteines 5200 μg)
- Garlife — Life Extension, 900-mg pure garlic extract (odor suppressed)
- Garlinase 4000 — Enzymatic Therapy, extract equivalent to 4 g fresh garlic (3.4% allicin)
- Garlique — Chattem, 400-mg bulb powder (500 μg allicin yield)
- GNC Garlic Oil — Basic Nutrition, 0.65 mg
- Herbscience Garlic, 600-mg caplets
- Kwai Odor-Free Garlic, 150-mg tablets (900 μg allicin yield)
- Kyo-Chrome AGE Cholesterol Formula, 400-mg extract powder, niacin 20 mg, chromium 200 μg
- Kyolic Aged Garlic Extract Kyolic HI-PO, 600-mg tablets AGE powder
- Kyolic Liquid Aged Garlic Extract, 1-mL AGE
- Kyolic Reserve Aged Garlic Extract, 600-mg capsules AGE powder
- Natrol GarliPure Daily Formula, 600-mg powdered bulb extract (1200 μg allicin yield, 1200 μg thiosulfinates)
- Natrol GarliPure Formula 500, 1000-mg powdered bulb extract (1500 μg allicin yield, 1600 μg thiosulfinates)
- Natrol GarliPure Maximum Allicin Formula, 600-mg powdered bulb extract (3600 μg allicin yield, 3800 μg thiosulfinates)
- Natrol GarliPure Once Daily Potency, 600-mg powdered bulb extract (6000 μg allicin yield, 6060 μg thiosulfinates)
- Natrol GarliPure Organic Formula, 1000-mg organically grown powdered bulb extract (1500 μg allicin yield, 1600 μg thiosulfinates)
- Nature's Plus Garlite, 500-mg odorless Vegicap
- Nature's Plus Ultra Garlite, 1000-mg deodorized sustained-release tablet
- Nature's Way Garlicin, 300-mg allinaise-rich garlic powder

- Nature's Resource Garlic Cloves, 400-mg capsules garlic bulb (0.8 mg allicin)
- Nature's Resource Odor-Controlled, 180-mg enteric-coated tablets garlic bulb (1.8 mg allicin)
- One-a-Day Garlic, 600-mg odor-free soft-gel, concentrated oil macerate
- Sundown Herbals Garlic Oil, 3-mg oil (1500-mg garlic clove equivalent)
- Sundown Herbals Garlic Whole Herb, 400-mg tablets garlic clove concentrate
- Sundown Herbals Garlic, 400-mg tablets garlic clove concentrate (1200-mg garlic clove equivalent)
- Sundown Herbals Odorless Garlic, 400-mg tablets garlic clove concentrate (1200- mg garlic clove equivalent)
- Sun Source Garlique, 400-mg enteric-coated, odor-free tablets, garlic powder (5000 μg allicin yield)
- Wellness GarlicCell, 650-mg enteric-coated tablets, garlic clove (6000 μg allicin yield, 6000 μg thiosulfinates)

Recommended Daily Doses in Humans

- 4 g of fresh garlic, approx 1 clove (4–12 mg of allicin or 2–5 mg of allicin)
- Dehydrated garlic powder, 600–1200 mg in divided doses
- AGE, 1–7.2 g/day
- Fresh air-dried bulb, 2–5 g
- Garlic oil, 2–5 mg
- Dried bulb, 2–4 g times daily
- Tincture (1:5 in 45% alcohol), 2–4 mL three times daily

Garlic Compounds

Raw, intact garlic contains various chemical compounds, all of which are converted to other sulfur-containing compounds when processed. All of these compounds are derived from the compound allicin. Allicin is formed from alliin, by the action of allinase, which is released when garlic is chopped or chewed. Allicin is extremely unstable and further breaks down to produce hundreds of organosulfur compounds such as diallyl sulfide (DAS), diallyl disulfide (DADS), diallyl trisulfide, ajoenes, methyl allyl di- and trisulfides, vinyl dithiins, and other sulfur compounds, depending on how the garlic is prepared. By the formation of these compounds, allicin is responsible for most of the biological activity of garlic; however, it is also a major contributor in garlic's characteristic odor.

Different methods of processing garlic, resulting in products containing different sulfur-containing thiosulfinate derivatives, have been discussed. A bulb of raw garlic, on average will contain up to 1.8% alliin, a small amount of SAC, which is a less-odorous biologically active compound, but no allicin. When garlic is chopped or crushed, 1 mg of alliin is converted to 0.48 mg of allicin. Cooking whole or coarsely chopped garlic destroys allinase, the enzyme necessary for production of allicin, ajoene, diallyl sulfide, diallyl disulfide, and vinyl dithiins; only cysteine sulfoxides such as alliin remain.

Crushing or finely chopping garlic followed by boiling in an open container leads to volatilization and loss of many chemically unstable, but potentially medicinal thiosulfinates. Steam distillation produces an oily mass of active compounds including diallyl, methyl allyl, dimethyl, and allyl 1-propenyl oligosulfides that originate from the thiosulfinates. Maceration of garlic in vegetable oil or soybean oil produces vinyl dithiins, ajoenes, and diallyl and methyl allyl trisulfides. These latter two methods are used to prepare some commercially available garlic capsules. When garlic is allowed to ferment (cold aging, AGE products), water-soluble SAC, *S*-allyl-mercaptocysteine, and other biologically active compounds are produced.

Garlic powder is produced by drying and pulverizing sliced or crushed garlic. The drying process is thought to cause powders to lose approximately one-half the amount of alliin found in whole garlic cloves. If dried at low temperatures, the garlic powder will remain odor-free until the product reaches the gastrointestinal (GI) tract after ingestion. In contrast to common belief, odorless garlic products still produce the same adverse drug reactions as those nonodorless products. Kwai brand coated odorless garlic powder tablets contain dried garlic powder prepared by freeze-drying fresh garlic. After the tablets are ingested, the alliin is converted to allicin in the GI tract by the enzyme allinase, which can come into contact with alliin once the coated tablets disintegrate and mix with intestinal water. Kwai is one of the most common garlic preparations used in studies.

Regardless of the processing procedure used, no garlic preparation available contains allicin, because of its high volatility. Many products report an "allicin yield" potential when consumed. However, studies have shown that allicin is not produced in significant amounts after ingestion of garlic products, which may be owing to inactivation of alliinase in the acidic stomach. Therefore, allicin is likely not an appropriate marker of the potential activity of the product. Enteric-coated products may preserve the activity of allinase, by delaying dissolution of the product. AGE products are standardized to SAC, which is found in detectable levels in the body and may therefore be a better standardization marker for garlic products than allicin yield.

PHARMACOLOGICAL/TOXICOLOGICAL EFFECTS

Cardiovascular Effects

Antioxidant and antiatherosclerotic effects

Garlic has been shown to have significant effects on the cardiovascular system. Such areas include improvement in lipids, modest effects on blood pressure, platelet inhibition, antioxidant effects, and a decrease in fibrinolytic activity. In vitro studies have shown garlic possesses specific antiatherosclerotic effects such as reducing inducible nitric oxide synthase (iNOS) mRNA expression, inhibition of oxidized low-density lipoprotein (LDL)-induced lactate dehydrogenase (LDH) release and inhibition of oxidized LDL-induced depletion of glutathione.

Results from a study in nine subjects found that supplementation with AGE at a dose of 2.4g/day significantly inhibited the oxidation of LDL, but ingesting 6 g/day of crushed raw garlic did not have a significant effect. The authors believe that this difference in response may be owing to the fact that the active ingredient in raw garlic is allicin, whereas SAC is believed to be the active component of AGE in preventing atherosclerosis. However, when compared to á-tocopherol (Vitamin E), which is well documented at preventing lipid oxidation, both AGE and raw garlic were less effective at inhibiting oxidation ($p < 0.05$). In addition, it has been shown that 900 mg/day of garlic powder vs placebo for 4 years caused a significant decrease in arteriosclerotic plaque volume in both men and women with advanced atherosclerotic plaques and at least one cardiovascular risk factor.

The effects of garlic as an antioxidant and its ability to alter the atherosclerotic process require additional study. To date, no trials evaluating patient outcomes have been completed.

Antihyperlipidemic effects

Garlic as a lipid-lowering agent is perhaps the most studied topic related to its use in cardiovascular health. The mechanism by which garlic lowers lipoprotein levels is not well understood. Animal data shows that garlic significantly decreases hydroxymethylglutaryl coenzyme A (HMG-CoA) reductase activity, and may have some effects on cholesterol α-hydroxylase, fatty acid synthetase, and pentose-phosphate pathway enzyme activity.

A recent meta-analysis using multiple databases, from inception until November 1998, compiled all randomized, double-blind, placebo-controlled trials using monopreparations of garlic, to test the effectiveness of garlic in lowering total cholesterol (TC). Inclusion criteria included trials in which participants had elevated TC, defined as 5.17 mmol/L (200 mg/dL) at baseline, and reported TC levels as an end point. Studies were excluded if they did not contain enough data to compute effect size. Of the 39 garlic-in-hyperlipidemia studies identified, 21 were excluded because they were not placebo- controlled, randomized, double-blinded, did not use a monopreparation of garlic, did not report TC, or have a baseline TC meeting inclusion criteria. An additional five trials did not include enough data to perform statistical pooling. Of the 13 studies cited in the meta-analysis, 10 used Kwai powder tablets in doses of 600, 800, and 900 mg/day. One study used 700 mg of spray-dried powder per day, another used 0.25 mg/kg body mass of essential oil, and the other study used 10 mg/day of steam-distilled oil. Study duration ranged from 8 to 24 weeks. Of the 13 trials, 10 required a diagnosis of hypercholesterolemia or hyperlipoproteinemia, whereas the other trials required diagnosis of coronary heart disease, hypertension, or healthy participants. A total of 796 participants were involved, and all trials excluded participants using hypolipidemic drugs. Results showed that TC levels decreased by a modest 5.8% (0.41 mmol/L; 15.7 mg/dL) in participants taking garlic compared to placebo ($p < 0.01$). Of the five methodologically similar trials using Kwai 900 mg/day, no significant difference was seen in reducing total cholesterol with garlic. Additionally, in an analysis of the six trials that controlled for diet, no significant difference was seen in reducing total cholesterol with garlic. The authors also looked at data presented in these studies regarding changes in LDL and high-density lipoprotein (HDL) levels. No significant difference was seen in reducing or increasing these values, respectively.

Several more recent studies have confirmed the TC-lowering effect seen in this meta-analysis. A randomized, double-blind, placebo-controlled study in 50 subjects with hypercholesterolemia and LDL levels between 150 and 200 mg/dL, triglycerides less than 300 mg/dL, an average age of 53 years, and who were not using lipid-lowering drugs, evaluated the effect of 300 mg three times daily of garlic powder for 12 weeks. Patients were classified by their LDL pattern A or B.

Pattern B LDL has been shown to be more atherogenic than pattern A This study was designed to not only look at the effect of garlic on lipoprotein levels, but also LDL particle size, LDL and HDL subclass distribution, and the effect on lipoprotein(a) [Lp(a)]. The only significant difference found was a significant decrease in LDL peak particle diameter in LDL pattern A. It is unclear what the implications of this decrease in diameter are. Results showed no significant difference in plasma lipid levels, overall LDL peak particle diameter, LDL or HDL subclass distribution, apolipoprotein B, or Lp(a) in the garlic vs placebo groups.

Another double-blind, placebo-controlled, randomized study of 34 men, average age of 48 years, with total cholesterol levels between 220 mg/dL and 285 mg/dL evaluated the effects of 7.2 g of AGE daily for 5 months. At 2 and 4 months after beginning the study, no significant difference was seen in TC or LDL cholesterol levels. At 5 months, a significant drop (7% in TC, 10% in LDL) was seen in the garlic group vs placebo. Plasma HDL and triglyceride levels did not change.

Overall, there is conflicting data regarding the effects of garlic on serum lipid levels. The diverse nature in the design of these studies makes it difficult to pool data. In addition, the use of various garlic preparations may have differing effects on lipids because of the diverse activity of organosulfide compounds present in each product. However, a larger number of studies have found garlic to provide a significant but small decrease in LDL and total cholesterol when garlic is used for up to 4 months. Further study is needed to determine whether garlic has a prolonged affect on lipids and if the effects are sustainable. Compared to the available lipid-lowering prescription drugs, garlic provides a small-percent decrease in lipid values and has not been shown to have morbidity and mortality benefits in these patients.

Platelet inhibitory and fibrinolytic effects

Platelet inhibition is another widely studied effect of garlic use. Platelet inhibition has been demonstrated in several in vitro and animal studies with fresh garlic cloves, ajoene, garlic oil, and AGE. Mechanisms proven by in vitro studies include a dose-dependent, irreversible inhibition of platelet aggregation through almost complete suppression of thromboxane production, a dose-dependent inhibition of collagen-induced platelet aggregation, and inhibition of adenosine diphosphate (ADP) and epinephrine-induced platelet aggregation. Multiple mechanisms may be responsible for the platelet inhibitory affects of garlic. It is thought that the inhibition of thromboxane production is caused by inhibition of cyclooxygenase, but not lipoxygenase; however, some studies question whether garlic inhibits cyclooxygenase. There may be a direct inhibition of thromboxane. β-Thromboglobulin release is decreased, which suggests that the effect may be more on the platelet activation phase. The specific components of garlic may also have different effects on the various mechanisms of antiplatelet activity. Some forms of garlic may include adenosine, which increases *cyclic adenosine monophosphate* (CAMP) levels and thus decreases thromboxane formation.

The antiplatelet effects of garlic are thought to be caused by allicin, SAC, adenosine, *methyl allyl trisulfide* (MATS), diallyl disulfide, and diallyl trisulfide. It has been demonstrated that raw garlic extract is more effective than boiled garlic extract in inhibiting platelets ($p < 0.001$). However, a double-blind, randomized, placebo-controlled study found no significant difference in platelet aggregation when subjects took the equivalent of 15 g raw garlic in capsule form. The garlic preparation consisted of garlic cloves homogenized in water and further processed into an oil extract. Higher doses of garlic may be needed for inhibition of thromboxane synthesis, whereas lower doses may have other mechanisms. A randomized, placebo-controlled, double-blinded crossover study showed that AGE increased the threshold concentrations needed for ADP-, epinephrine-, and collagen-induced platelet aggregation in human blood. Doses of 7.2 g AGE per day significantly increased the threshold of ADP-induced platelet aggregation ($p < 0.05$), whereas lower doses of 2.4 and 4.6 g AGE per day significantly increased the collagen- and epinephrine-induced threshold. Higher doses of 7.2 g AGE per day did not show a significant difference than the lower doses for the latter two substances. Platelet adhesion to collagen-coated surfaces, fibrinogen, and von Willebrand factor were measured. At a dosage of 4.8–7.2 g AGE per day, adhesion to collagen-coated surfaces was significantly reduced ($p < 0.05$). All doses significantly decreased adhesion to fibrinogen ($p < 0.01$) and only the highest dosage of 7.2 g AGE per day significantly reduced adhesion to von Willebrand factor ($p < 0.05$). Similar results were seen in an earlier study of 15 men with hypercholesterolemia.

A double-blind, randomized, matching placebo-controlled parallel group investigation was done to evaluate the effect of 800 mg dried garlic powder for 4 weeks (Kwai/Sapec; 300-mg tablets; contains 1.3% alliin, which corresponds to an Allicin release of 0.6%) in patients with an increased risk of juvenile ischemic attack owing to increased circulating platelet aggregates. The ratio of circulating platelet aggregates decreased by 10.3%, and spontaneous platelet aggregation decreased by 56.3% during the treatment period compared to baseline ($p < 0.01$) and placebo ($p < 0.01$). Plasma viscosity also significantly decreased in the garlic group after 4 weeks of treatment compared with baseline and placebo ($p < 0.0001$). These levels returned to pretreatment levels 4 weeks after treatment was stopped.

In another study, 800 mg of dried garlic powder daily for 15 weeks significantly improved pain-free walking distance in patients with arterial occlusive disease. In this randomized, placebo-controlled, double-blind study, 60 patients underwent 15 weeks of physical therapy, 30 of the subjects received garlic, and 30 baseline-matching patients received an identical placebo. After 6 weeks of treatment, pain-free walking distance was significantly farther in the garlic group ($p < 0.038$). Cholesterol levels ($p < 0.011$), plasma viscosity ($p < 0.0013$), and spontaneous thrombocyte aggregation ($p < 0.013$) were significantly lower in the garlic group. This is the only published study addressing a clinically relevant outcome associated with platelet inhibition caused by garlic supplements.

Fibrinolytic effects of garlic have also been evaluated. Garlic oil was shown to increase fibrinolytic activity by 55% ($p < 0.01$) after 3 months of treatment, with 2 g twice daily for 3 months. Fibrinogen was not affected. A dried garlic preparation (Sapec) was shown to significantly increase tissue plasminogen activator activity compared to placebo after 1 day and 14 days of treatment.

The antiplatelet and antifibrinolytic activity of garlic is of great interest to researchers. Many studies have confirmed these effects as a result of garlic consumption. As with the lipid-lowering effects of garlic, more clinical outcome trials are needed to justify its use in patients with cardiovascular risk factors. In addition, comparative studies with aspirin would be needed to show if there are any benefits to using garlic instead. Because of the demonstrated antiplatelet effect of garlic, its use should be avoided in patients with bleeding disorders and discontinued 1–2 weeks prior to surgery.

Antihypertensive effect

In addition to its effects on lipids and platelet inhibition, garlic has been studied for its effects on lowering blood pressure. A meta-analysis of the effects of garlic on blood pressure was conducted by Silagy and Neil in 1994. Each of the eight randomized studies identified within the analysis used the dried garlic preparation Kwai, 600–900 mg daily (1.8–2.7 g/day fresh garlic), for at least 4 weeks in 415 subjects. Overall, there was an average decrease in *systolic blood pressure* (SBP) of 7.7 mmHg (95% confidence interval [CI] 4.3–11), and a decrease in *diastolic blood pressure* (DBP) of 5 mmHg (95% CI 2.9–7.1) in those subjects taking garlic. However, only two of the placebo-controlled trials were limited to hypertensive patients. These studies showed an average decrease in SBP of 11.1 mmHg (95% CI 5–17.2) and a decrease in DBP of 6.5 mmHg (95% CI 3.4–9.6) in those subjects taking the garlic preparation. In a pilot study, 2400 mg dried garlic powder (Kwai) containing 1.3% allicin, was administered to nine patients with persistent severe hypertension (DBP ≥ 115 mmHg). A statistically significant decrease was seen in the DBP at 5–14 hours ($p < 0.05$), with a maximum decrease at 5 hours after the dose (16 ± 2 mmHg). No significant difference was seen in SBP at any time-point; however, a trend was present. Other studies, which had primary outcomes other than blood pressure, have also shown similar findings.

GI Effects

Garlic was effective against castor oil-induced diarrhea, and relieved abdominal distension/discomfort, belching, and flatulence in 30 patients. Small doses of garlic are purported to increase the tone of smooth muscle in the GI tract, whereas large doses decrease such actions. An ethanol-chloroform extract of fresh bulb-antagonized acetylcholine and prostaglandin E induced rat fundus smooth muscle contraction at a concentration of 0.002 mg/mL; however, an ethanol extract of fresh garlic bulb caused rat fundus smooth muscle stimulation at a concentration of 0.016 mg/mL.

In vitro data shows an antibacterial effect of garlic against *Helicobacter pylori*; however, studies in humans with documented *H. pylori* infection showed no in vivo effect on *H. pylori* with dried garlic powder, oil, or freshly sliced cloves and no effect of garlic oil on symptoms or grade of gastritis. This demonstrates the importance of in vivo data with garlic, rather than extrapolating from in vitro studies.

Animal studies in rats show a protective effect of garlic from intestinal damage from methotrexate and 5-fluorouracil, but human data is not available.

Antimicrobial Activity

Antibacterial activity

Garlic has in vitro activity against many Gram-negative and Gram-positive bacteria, including species of *Escherichia*, *Salmonella*,

Staphylococcus, *Streptococcus*, *Klebsiella*, *Proteus*, *Bacillus*, *Clostridium*, and *Mycobacterium tuberculosis*. Even some bacteria resistant to antibiotics, including methicillin-resistant *Staphylococcus aureus*, multidrug-resistant strains of *Escherichia coli*, *Enterococcus* spp., and *Shigella* spp. were sensitive to garlic. Activity against *H. pylori* is discussed in the GI effects section. A study in 30 subjects was done to determine activity of garlic against oral microorganisms. After using both garlic and chlorhexidine, antimicrobial activity from the subject's saliva was shown against *Streptococcus mutans* and no other oral microorganisms, but adverse effects were significantly higher for garlic. Antibacterial activity is thought to be caused by the allicin component of garlic. A characteristic unique to allicin is the low likelihood of most bacteria to develop resistance to it. However, more investigation should be done regarding this issue. Data is insufficient for the use of garlic to treat bacterial infections. In vitro data does not always correlate with in vivo clinical data, and such studies are not currently available.

Antifungal activity

Garlic has in vitro antifungal effects against *Cryptococcus neoformans*, *Candida* spp., *Trichophyton*, *Epidermophyton*, *Microsporum*, *Aspergillus* spp., and *Mucor pusillus*. When five volunteers consumed 10–25 mL of fresh garlic extract, urine samples had antifungal activity, but susceptibility from serum samples dropped significantly.

Data is also available suggesting efficacy of topical garlic on fungal infections. For tinea pedis, 1-week topical treatment with ajoene 1% twice daily resulted in mycological cure 60 days later in 100% of patients, compared to 94% for 1% topical terbinafine and 72% for 0.6% topical ajoene. Another study showed that 0.6% topical ajoene was as effective as 1% terbinafine cream, both applied twice daily for 1 week, for the treatment of tinea cruris and corposis. After 60 days, effectiveness (clinical plus mycological cure) was 73 vs 71%, respectively. In addition, a 0.4% cream was also shown to be effective. Although a topical preparation is not available commercially, it could likely be compounded.

Antiviral effects

Garlic has been shown in in vitro studies to have antiviral activity against several viruses including cytomegalovirus, influenza B, *Herpes simplex* virus types 1 and 2, parainfluenza virus type 3, and human rhinovirus type 2. Antiviral activity is thought to be caused more by the ajoene component than the allicin component of garlic.

Antiparasitic effects

Garlic has in vitro activity against *Entamoeba histolytica*, *Giardia lamblia*, *Leishmania major*, *Leptomonas colsoma*, and *Crithidia fasciculate*. In vivo and clinical data is needed before garlic can be used for treatment of infections with these organisms.

Antineoplastic Effects

In vitro and animal studies show that the organosulfur components of garlic suppress tumor incidence in breast, blood, bladder, colon, skin, uterine, esophagus, and lung cancers. Potential mechanisms include decreasing nitrosamine formation, decreased bioactivation of carcinogens, improved DNA repair, immune stimulation, and antiproliferative effects (regulation of cell cycle progression, modification of pathways of signal transduction, and induction of apoptosis). Other factors that may play a role in cancer prevention are cytochrome P450 enzyme stimulation, sulfur compound binding, or antioxidant activity. The chemical components of garlic that have shown these effects are ajoene, allicin, diallyl sulfide, diallyl disulfide, diallyl trisulfide, SAC, and S-allylmercaptocysteine. Heating garlic (microwave or oven) destroys the active allyl sulfur compound formation; however, if crushed garlic is allowed to stand for 10 minutes before heating, the total loss of anti-cancer activity is prevented. Although much of the anticancer data is from in vitro and animal studies, epidemiological studies are available.

Colorectal cancer

Several case–control studies and cohort studies were done evaluating dietary raw and cooked garlic consumption and association with colorectal cancer. The results were mixed but generally positive. One study showed an association of garlic with a reduction in the incidence of colon cancer. Another study showed an inverse relationship with rectal cancer in women for garlic consumers but no association in men. The third case-control study showed weak evidence of garlic consumption associated with a lower risk of colon cancer for men, although this was not significant, and no effect for women was shown. Two cohort studies showed a nonsignificant inverse association with colon cancer, although one showed a significant inverse association when limited to just the distal colon (relative risk [RR] 0.52 [95% CI 0.3-0.93])). These studies evaluating dietary garlic consumption cannot be extrapolated to garlic supplements. Only one study evaluated the effects of garlic *supplements* on colon and rectal cancer. This cohort study did not show an association between garlic supplement use and colon and rectal cancers. A meta-analysis showed that issues with the studies, including publication bias, heterogeneity of effect estimates, differences in doses, and confounding factors such as total vegetable consumption may not allow for definite conclusions. Overall, dietary garlic may have some efficacy in prevention of colorectal cancer, but there is not enough evidence for garlic supplements.

Gastric cancer

Two epidemiological studies show an inverse association between dietary raw and cooked garlic and gastric cancer and one showed a slight protective effect. These results cannot be extrapolated to garlic supplements. One cohort study was done to examine the effects of garlic supplement use on gastric cancer. This study did not show a protective effect of garlic supplements on gastric cancer. In fact, there was a small, nonsignificant increase in risk. A meta-analysis showed that issues with the studies, including publication bias, heterogeneity of effect estimates, differences in doses, and confounding factors such as total vegetable consumption may not allow for definite conclusions. Dietary garlic may have some efficacy in the prevention of gastric cancer, but insufficient evidence exists for garlic supplements.

Prostate cancer

High dietary intake of garlic (approximately 1 clove per day) is associated with a 50% reduction in the risk of developing prostate cancer. Another study showed that a reduced risk of prostate cancer was associated with both dietary garlic (odds ratio 0.64; 95% CI 0.38–1.09) and garlic supplements (OR 0.68; 95% CI 0.41–1.1), although both just fell short of statistical significance.

Other cancers

Garlic supplements have been associated with an *increased* risk of lung carcinoma (RR 1.78; 95% CI 1.08–2.92) in a cohort study. However, this was not seen in those using garlic together with any other supplement (RR 0.93; 95% CI 0.46–1.86). A case-control study showed an inverse relationship between dietary garlic consumption and the development of breast cancer; however, a cohort study evaluating the effects of garlic supplements did not show a protective effect. Insufficient epidemiological evidence exists for the effects of dietary garlic on head and neck cancers.

In summary, although the data is encouraging, more studies are needed before definitive conclusions can be made about the effect of garlic on the prevention or the cause (in the case of lung cancer) of cancer, especially with garlic supplements.

Immunostimulant Effects

Immunostimulant effects of garlic include an increase in proliferation of lymphocyte and macrophage phagocytosis, induction of the infiltration of lymphocytes and macrophages in transplanted tumors, induction of splenic hypertrophy, increased release of interleukin (IL)-2, interferon-γ, and tumor necrosis factor-α, and enhancement of natural killer cell activity. It is thought that these effects may be mechanisms of cancer prevention. Lau and colleagues tested an aqueous garlic extract from Japan, the protein fraction isolated from this same extract, and three additional extracts obtained from health food stores in Loma Linda, CA, for ability to stimulate murine T-lymphocyte function and macrophage activity in vitro.

Both Japanese extracts were shown to stimulate macrophage activity, and the protein fraction from the Japanese protein extract stimulated lymphocyte activity. Of the three extracts sold in American health food stores, only one stimulated macrophage activity. Aged garlic extract was shown in an in vitro study to enhance the proliferation of spleen cells, augment IL-2–induced proliferation, and enhance natural killer cell activity.

Other Effects

AGE, but not fresh garlic, has been shown to have antioxidant effects. The compounds with the highest activity are SAC and *S*-allylmercaptocysteine. Garlic exerts antioxidant effects by scavenging free radicals, enhancing superoxide dismutase, catalase and glutathione peroxidase, and increasing cellular glutathione. These effects of garlic may play a role in the cardiovascular, antineoplastic, and cognitive effects of garlic.

Aged garlic extract has been shown in in vitro and animal studies to protect against liver toxicity from environmental substances, such as bromobenzene, protect against cardiotoxicity from doxorubicin, and improve age-related spatial memory deficits. A placebo-controlled human study showed that garlic may also be useful as a tick repellent. In addition, a double-blind, randomized, placebo-controlled human study showed that garlic supplements taken over a 12-week period in the winter significantly reduced the incidence of the common cold ($p < 0.001$), and reduced the duration of symptoms when they occurred ($p < 0.001$).

Pharmacokinetics

Absorption

The bioavailability of the garlic component SAC was found to be 64.1, 76.6, and 98.2% in rats after oral administration of 12.5, 25, and 50 mg/kg, respectively. The bioavailability was 103% in mice and 87.2% in dogs. SAC is rapidly absorbed from the GI tract, with a peak plasma concentration occurring at 15 minutes in dogs, 30 minutes at doses of 12.5 mg/kg and 25 mg/kg in rats, and at 1 hour in rats administered 50 mg/kg.

Distribution

Egen-Schwind et al. found that 1,2-vinyl dithiin, a component of oily preparations of garlic, accumulates in fatty tissues, whereas 1,3-vinyl dithiin is more hydrophilic and is rapidly eliminated from serum, kidney, and fat tissue. The latter compound was detected in rat liver over the first 24 hours after administration, whereas 1,2-vinyl dithiin was not. Both 1,3-vinyl dithiin and 1,2-vinyl dithiin were detected in the serum, kidney, and fat. In rats, mice, and dogs, SAC is distributed mainly in the liver, kidney, and plasma. In rats, SAC levels are highest in the kidney, and plasma and tissue levels peak 15–30 minutes after oral administration.

Garlic apparently distributes into human amniotic fluid and breast milk. Placebo or garlic oil capsules were given to 10 women 45 minutes prior to routine amniotic fluid sampling. Four of the five amniotic fluid samples from the women who had ingested garlic were judged by a blinded panel to have a stronger and more garlic-like odor than a paired amniotic fluid sample from a woman in the placebo group. The ingestion of garlic by nursing mothers was shown to significantly change the perceived odor of milk, as well as significantly increase the amount of time the infant spent attached to the nipple while feeding and the number of sucks during feeding. The total amount of milk ingested by the infants was not significantly affected, however. In contrast, these authors later found that the ingestion of garlic for 3 days by nursing women decreased the infants' feeding time compared to infants of mothers who had taken placebo.

Metabolism/Elimination

De Rooij et al. conducted a study to evaluate the urinary excretion of *N*-acetyl-*S*-allyl-L-cysteine (allylmercapturic acid, ALMA). The importance of this study lies in the use of ALMA as a biomarker for occupational exposure to alkyl halides; if garlic produces detectable urine concentrations of ALMA, garlic consumption could interfere with toxicological studies. Six human volunteers were administered 200 mg of garlic extract in tablet form (Kwai). The volunteers ranged from 20 to 27 years of age, with body weights ranging from 60 to 90 kg. Urine samples were collected prior to administration of the garlic and up to 24 hours postadministration. Gas chromatography-mass spectrometry (GC-MS) was used to evaluate the excretion of ALMA. γ-Glutamyl-*S*-allyl-L-cysteine (GAC) is ALMA's most likely precursor. γ-Glutamine is hydrolyzed from GAC by glutamine-transpeptidase, resulting in *S*-allyl-L-cysteine. This compound then undergoes acetylation via *N*-acetyl transferase to form ALMA. It is difficult to calculate to what extent GAC is excreted as ALMA in the urine because GAC content of garlic varies depending on the product. By assuming that GAC represents 1% of the dry weight of garlic bulbs, and that the tablets represented 100% dry garlic, the researchers approximated that 10% of GAC is excreted as ALMA within the first 24 hours of garlic ingestion. The average elimination half-life of ALMA was 6.0 ± 1.3 hours.

N-acetyl-*S*-(2-carboxypropyl) cysteine, *N*-acetyl-*S*-allyl-L-cysteine (ALMA), and hexahydrohippuric acid were identified in the urine of humans ingesting garlic or onions. It is important to note that the study participants' urine contained *N*-acetyl-*S*-(2-carboxypropyl)-cysteine at baseline in minute amounts, even before garlic ingestion, but increased after ingestion of garlic or onions. As with the study by De Rooij, the importance of these findings lies in the use of urinary excretion of mercapturic acids as a marker for industrial exposure to halogenated alkanes, such as vinyl chloride. Elimination of other garlic components has also been studied. Allicin is metabolized in rat liver homogenate more rapidly than the vinyl dithiins, the main constituents of oily preparations of garlic.

As discussed above, 1,2-vinyldithiin is lipophilic and tends to accumulate in fat, whereas 1,3-vinyldithiin is less lipophilic and more quickly eliminated from the serum, fat, and kidney. Both vinyldithiins can be detected in the serum, fat, and kidney using GC-MS for at least 24 hours after oral administration.

SAC is thought to undergo first-pass metabolism in rats based on nonlinear increases in AUC (area under the plasma concentration vs time curve) after oral administration. SAC is likely metabolized to ALMA by acetyltransferase in the liver and kidney. The high concentration of SAC in rat kidney has been attributed to conversion of ALMA back into SAC by kidney acylase. Of the full SAC dose,

30–50% is excreted in the urine of rats as ALMA, and less than 1% of the dose is excreted as unchanged SAC in the urine and bile. In mice, both SAC (16.5%) and the *N*-acetylated metabolite (7.2%) are excreted in the urine, whereas in dogs, less than 1% of the dose was found in the urine as either SAC or ALMA. The half-life of SAC in rats ranges from 1.49 hours with an intravenous dose of 12.5 mg/kg, to 2.33 hours with an oral dose of 50 mg/kg. In mice, the half-life of SAC is 0.77 hour when given orally, and 0.43 hour for intravenous administration, and in dogs approx 10 hours after either oral or intravenous administration.

ALMA is also detectable in human urine and concentrations in blood increase in response to ingesting garlic. Therefore, because SAC is found in many garlic preparations, it may be the best standardization compound and compliance marker for garlic preparations.

Adverse Effects and Toxicity

Garlic is most commonly consumed as a food, rather than as a supplement. According to the Food and Drug Administration (FDA), chopped garlic and oil mixes left at room temperature have the ability to result in fatal botulism food poisoning. Such products need to be kept refrigerated, especially those that do not contain acidifying agents such as phosphoric or citric acid. *Clostridium botulinum* bacteria are dispersed throughout the environment, but are not dangerous in the presence of oxygen. The spores produce a deadly toxin in anaerobic, low-acid conditions. The garlic-in-oil mixture provides the environment for the spores to produce their toxin, leading to botulism. At least 40 cases of this poisoning were reported in the late 1980s.

Since the effects of garlic as a medicinal agent have been studied, reports of common side effects have been reported. The most common of which is malodorous breath and body odor. This effect generally can last many hours after garlic consumption and is not removed by brushing teeth or bathing. One study attempted to reveal the mechanism behind this unpopular effect. Air from the mouth and lungs, as well as urine samples were analyzed for sulfur-containing gases (hydrogen sulfide, methanethiol, allyl mercaptan, allyl methyl sulfide, allyl methyl disulfide, and allyl disulfide) after garlic ingestion. Most of the gas levels were present in higher levels in mouth air than lung air or urine up to 3 hours after ingestion and decreased thereafter. However, allyl methyl sulfide concentrations remained high in mouth and lung air, and urine. This indicates that this gas was absorbed and released from the lungs and in the urine. The authors concluded that systemic absorption of allyl methyl sulfide was responsible for the prolonged odor caused by garlic consumption and therefore explained why oral hygiene could not abolish the smell.

Many of the cardiovascular trials reported side effects of garlic use, with the most frequently reported being GI symptoms and garlic breath. In addition, rash and prolonged oozing from a razor cut were reported in one of these studies. Other commonly described side effects associated with garlic use include GI effects such as abdominal pain, fullness, anorexia, and flatulence.

Coagulation dysfunctions have also been reported, such as postoperative bleeding and prolonged clotting time. One case of spinal epidural hematoma associated with excessive garlic ingestion has been reported. An 87-year-old man who reported to consume an average of four gloves of garlic per day to prevent heart disease, presented to the emergency room with acute onset abdominal discomfort and bilateral sensory and motor paralysis in the lower extremities. Prothrombin time was 12.7 seconds and partial thromboplastin time was 22.3 seconds. The patient had no additional risk factors for bleeding and was taking no other medications that would affect bleeding tendency. The platelet inhibition caused by garlic was determined to be the cause.

In 2001, Hoshino et al. investigated whether different garlic preparations have undesirable effects on the GI mucosa in dogs. When administered directly to the stomach, AGE did not produce any changes compared to control to the mucosa, whereas boiled garlic powder caused redness, and raw garlic powder caused redness and erosion of the mucosa. Pulverized enteric-coated tablets caused redness and a loss of epithelial cells. Although these findings were significant, further study in humans should be done to confirm the relevance of these findings.

In addition, garlic has been shown to change the odor of breast milk in lactating women, as well as alter the sucking patterns of nursing infants.

Reports of adverse effects in garlic studies are inconsistent. Studies using AGE have reported fewer side effects and toxicities than those using other garlic preparations. Therefore, the frequency and severity of effects seen with garlic may vary with the type of preparation used.

Garlic Allergy

Allergic reactions to garlic have also been reported in the literature. Garlic allergy can manifest as occupational asthma, contact dermatitis, urticaria, angioedema, rhinitis, and diarrhea. A 35-year-old woman experienced several episodes of urticaria and angioedema associated with ingestion of raw or cooked garlic, as well as urticaria from touching garlic. Two garlic extracts as well as fresh garlic produced a 4+ reaction on *skin prick tests* (SPTs) in this patient, but no other food allergens produced positive results. The patient's symptoms were immunoglobulin E (IgE)-mediated, but she also produced specific IgG, which confounded the results of IgE testing. A group of 12 garlic workers with respiratory symptoms associated with garlic exposure underwent SPTs using garlic powder in saline, commercial garlic extract, and various other possible allergens; bronchial provocation tests with garlic powder; oral challenge with garlic dust; and specific IgE testing using the CAP methodology. Patients were classified into two groups depending on the results of the bronchial provocation tests. Seven patients had positive responses (rhinitis or asthma) to the inhalation challenge test, and were designated as Group 1. Six of these patients reacted to the garlic SPT, and five had specific garlic IgE. In addition, six patients had specific IgE to onion, three to leeks, and four to asparagus. In Group 2 (patients who did not respond to the inhalation challenge), one patient had a positive response to the garlic SPT, one to the onion SPT, and two to the leek SPT. None had garlic or onion IgE. Three patients in Group 1 reported that in the past, they had experienced urticaria, asthma, angioedema, and anaphylaxis after garlic ingestion. Two of these patients were administered garlic orally in increasing doses up to 1600 mg. The patient who had reported anaphylaxis tolerated the full dose, whereas the patient who reported urticaria developed a 35% decrease in forced expiratory volume in 1 second (FEV 1) and angioedema of the eyelids at a dose of 500 mg. Using immunoblot and IgE immunoblot inhibition analysis, the investigators also attempted to elucidate the specific garlic component to which the patients reacted. Using pooled sera from Group 1, the investigators found that several garlic allergens cross-react with grass and Chenopodiaceaepollens.

A group of 50 catering workers with eczema or dermatitis of the hand or arm were studied for suspected occupational dermatitis. All workers were prick tested with foods that commonly irritated their hands at work, as well as patch tested with garlic 50% in arachis oil, onion 50% in arachis oil, and pieces of the same prick test foods. Seven workers reacted to 50% garlic in oil and one reacted to whole garlic.

Housewives were found to be more likely to experience contact dermatitis of the hand than those exposed to garlic in other job settings such as chef, agricultural, and industrial positions. A group of 93 patients were patch tested with diallyl disulfide. Of these, 22.6% tested positive for allergy, 79.5% of whom were women. Dermatological eruptions were primarily located on the hand; however, lesions were also seen on the feet, head, legs, and in widespread distribution.

Other cases of occupational allergy and asthma associated with garlic extract include an 11-year-old boy who helped with garlic harvesting on his parents' farm and a 15-year-old who helped collect and store garlic; a 49-year-old proprietor of a spice marketing and packing firm; a 30-year-old electrician working in a spice processing plant; and a 16-year-old who had helped his father load stored garlic into a van for several years. Symptoms described included wheezing; cough, dyspnea, and chest tightness; rhinitis; and conjunctivitis. Garlic allergy was confirmed using a wide variety of tests including scratch testing; SPT; IgE to garlic using *radioallegosorbent test* (RAST), polystyrene tube solid phase radioimmunoassay technique, CAP system; oral challenge; bronchial provocation; and basophil degranulation. Patients with occupational garlic allergy are often allergic to other foods as well as to airborne allergens, including peanuts, onion, ragweed pollen, asparagus, and chives.

Topical Reactions

Topically applied garlic can cause "*garlic burns*" as well as allergic garlic dermatitis. A 17-month-old infant suffered partial thickness burns when a plaster made of garlic in petroleum jelly was applied to the skin for 8 hours. Another infant, age 6 months, suffered garlic burns when his father, disappointed that no antibiotics had been prescribed for a treatment of suspected aseptic meningitis, applied crushed garlic cloves by adhesive band to the wrists for 6 hours. After 1 week, a round ulceration 1 cm in diameter surrounded by a slightly raised, erythematous border was noted on the left wrist. A similar, more superficial lesion was also seen on the right wrist. When questioned, the parents explained that these ulcerations were the residual blisters that had formed after garlic application. The author of this case report described this reaction as a second-degree chemical burn. An allergic mechanism was ruled out because the infant had not previously been exposed to garlic or onions. A patch test was not done for ethical reasons. Although Garty hypothesized that the infants' delicate skin predisposed them to garlic burns, such reactions have also been reported in older children and adults. For example, a 6-year-old child developed a necrotic ulcer on her foot after her grandmother applied crushed garlic under a bandage as a remedy for a minor sore.

A 38-year-old woman developed a garlic burn after applying a poultice made from fresh, uncooked garlic to her breast for treatment of a self-diagnosed *Candida* infection secondary to breastfeeding her 6-month-old son. Despite a burning sensation upon application, she left the poultice in place for 2 days. The infant continued to feed with no apparent adverse effects. She presented to the emergency room 2 days after removal of the poultice. Physical exam revealed that the area where the poultice had been applied appeared as a burn with skin loss, ulceration, crusting, hyperpigmentation, granulation tissue, serous discharge, minor bleeding, and erythema on the periphery. The area was tender. The patient was treated with 1% silver sulfadiazine cream.

Another adult suffered garlic burns after applying a compress of crushed garlic wrapped in cotton to her chest and abdomen for 18 hours. The erythematous, blistering rash was in a dermatomal distribution on the right side of the patient's chest and upper abdomen, approximating the dermatomal distribution of thoracic segments 8 and 9. She reported that the pain had been present for 1 week and had a stabbing quality. She was initially diagnosed with *Herpes zoster* and was prescribed acyclovir before admitting to use of topical garlic after further questioning. Biopsy revealed full thickness necrosis, many pyknotic nuclei, and focal separation of the necrotic epidermis from the dermis. The burns healed with scarring. The patient refused patch testing, and specific IgE RAST testing to garlic was negative. The nonspecific appearance of garlic burns has been exploited. Three soldiers applied fresh ground garlic to their lower legs and antecubital fossa to produce an erythematous, vesicular rash in an effort to avoid military duty.

Eight patients who developed contact dermatitis after rubbing cut fresh garlic cloves on fungal skin infections responded to a topical fluorinated steroid but had negative garlic patch tests, suggesting irritation rather than allergy. Patch testing with 1% diallyl disulfide in petrolatum has also been recommended when allergy is suspected.

Interactions

Garlic has antiplatelet properties, and can increase the risk of bleeding when used together with drugs with antiplatelet and anticoagulant effects, such as aspirin, clopidogrel, ticlopidine, dipyridamole, heparins, and warfarin. Increased international normalized ratio (INR), has been reported when garlic was added to warfarin. Garlic supplements that contain allicin can induce the cytochrome P450 3A4 (CYP 3A4) isoenzyme and can result in clinically important decreases in concentrations of drugs metabolized by this enzyme. This interaction was proven with saquinavir. However, a garlic preparation containing alliin and alliinase (which formed one-half the amount of allicin stated on the label) did not significantly inhibit CYP 3A4, which was proven by a lack of interaction with the drug alprazolam. It is not known whether the differences in the preparations and dose of allicin or some other factor in the metabolism of saquinavir, such as P-glycoprotein, are responsible for this effect. Until more data is available, it would be prudent to avoid or use caution when allicin is used together with some drugs metabolized by CYP 3A4, including protease inhibitors, cyclosporine, ketoconazole, itraconazole, glucocorticoids, oral contraceptives, verapamil, diltiazem, lovastatin, simvastatin, and atorvastatin.

Regulatory Status

The oil, extract, and oleo resin have been deemed generally recognized as safe as food substances by the FDA, and garlic is also regulated as a dietary supplement in the United States. Garlic is approved in Germany as a nonprescription drug. In Canada, garlic is approved as a food supplement; garlic is on the general sale list in the United Kingdom; in France it is accepted for the treatment of minor circulatory disorders; and in Sweden it is classified as a natural product.

10

Ginger

Ginger is a perennial plant with thick tuberous rhizomes from which an above-ground stem rises approx 3 feet. The plant produces an orchidlike flower with petals that are greenish-yellow streaked with purple. Ginger is cultivated in areas of abundant rainfall (at least 80 inches/year). Native to southern Asia, ginger is cultivated in tropical areas such as Jamaica, China, Nigeria, and Haiti. Ginger was introduced to Jamaica and the West Indies by Spaniards in the 16th century, and exports from Jamaica to the rest of the world amount to more than two million pounds per year.

Ginger is an ingredient in more than one-half of all traditional Chinese medicines, and has been used since the 4th century BCE. Marco Polo documented its use in India in the late 13th century. African and West Indies cultures have also used ginger medicinally, and the Greeks and Romans used it as a spice. The Chinese used ginger for stomach aches, diarrhea, nausea, cholera, bleeding, asthma, heart conditions, respiratory disorders, toothache, and rheumatic complaints. In China, the root and stem are used to combat aphids and fungal spores.

Ginger is purported to have use as a carminative, diaphoretic, spasmolytic, expectorant, peripheral circulatory stimulant, astringent, appetite stimulant, antiinflammatory agent, diuretic, and digestive aid. It has also been used to treat migraines, fever, flu, amenorrhea, snake bites, and baldness.

Current Promoted Uses

In the United States, ginger is promoted to relieve and prevent nausea caused by motion sickness, morning sickness, and other etiologies.

Additionally, in Germany it is promoted for use against nervousness, coughing, urinary tract conditions, and sore throat.

Sources and Chemical Composition

Zingiber officinale Roscoe, *Zingerberis rhizoma*, ingwerwurzelstok, Jamaican ginger, African ginger, cochin ginger, *Zingiber capitatum*, *Zingiber zerumbet* Smith, calicut, gengibre, gingembre, jenjibre, zenzero.

Products Available

The best quality ginger comes from Jamaica and consists of whole ginger with the epidermis completely peeled from the rhizomes and dried in the sun for 5 or 6 days, although high-quality, partially scraped ginger used pharmaceutically also comes from Bengal and Australia. Extracts are prepared from the unpeeled root, as essential oil can be lost from peeled ginger.

Ginger is commercially available in the United States as the dried powdered root, syrup, tincture, capsules, tablets, tea, oral solution, powder for oral solution, as a spice, and in candy, ice cream, and beer.

Ginger root is available from several manufacturers as a tea, liquid extract, and as 50-, 250-, 400-, 470-, 500-, 535-, and 550-mg capsules.

Examples include:

- Alvita Teas Ginger Root tea bag
- Breezy Morning Teas Jamaican Ginger tea bag
- Celestial Seasonings Ginger Ease Herb tea bag
- Aura Cacia Essential Oil Ginger
- Abunda Life Chinese Ginger powder
- Frontier Ginger — Hawaiian Root capsule
- Nature's Herbs Ginger Root, 535-mg capsule
- Nature's Way Ginger Root, 550-mg capsule
- Nature's Plus Liquid Ginger Extract, 4% volatile oils
- Health Plus Ginger Root extract, 50-mg capsule
- Nature's Answer Ginger Root Low Alcohol (Liquid)
- Nature's Answer Ginger Root Alcohol Free (Liquid)
- Nature's Herbs Ginger Root Extract (Liquid)
- Nature's Way Ginger Extract (Liquid)
- Quanterra Stomach Relief, 250-mg dried ginger root powder (Zintona) capsule

Pharmacological/Toxicological Effects

Gastrointestinal Effects

A study was conducted to evaluate the effect of ginger on the nystagmus response to vestibular or optokinetic stimuli, as measured by electronystagmographic (ENG) techniques. Study subjects were screened prior to study enrollment and were excluded if they responded abnormally to vestibular or optokinetic tests. A total of 38 subjects, 20 women and 18 men between the ages of 22 and 34, were given 1 g of ginger (Zintona), 100 mg dimenhydrinate, or placebo in a double-blind, crossover fashion 90 minutes prior to each test. Ginger had no effect on the ENG, in contrast to dimenhydrinate, which decreased nystagmus response to caloric, rotary, and optokinetic stimulations. Therefore, the authors considered a *central nervous system* (CNS) effect had been ruled out as ginger's antiemetic mechanism of action, and a direct gastrointestinal effect was proposed.

The antimotion sickness effect of ginger was also compared to that of dimenhydrinate (Dramamine) in 18 male and 18 female college students who were self-rated as having extreme or very high susceptibility to motion sickness. The subjects were given either two ginger capsules (940 mg), one dimenhydrinate capsule (100 mg), or two placebo capsules (powdered chickweed herb [*Stellaria media*]). Subjects were led blindfolded to a previously concealed rotating chair 20 to 25 minutes after consuming the capsule(s). None of the dimenhydrinate or placebo subjects were able to remain in the chair a full 6 minutes, and three patients in the placebo group vomited. One-half of the ginger subjects stayed the full 6 minutes. It was concluded that 940 mg of ginger was superior to 100 mg of dimenhydrinate in preventing motion sickness. It is important to note that none of the subjects in the dimenhydrinate group specifically asked to have the test terminated; the test was stopped by the investigator because of the magnitude of the subjects' self-reported "intensity of stomach feeling." Although the study subjects were blinded not only to the treatments used, but also to the purpose of the study, it is unclear if the investigator was also blinded.

Anesthesiologists appreciate the fact that individuals who experience motion sickness are also at risk of having postoperative nausea and vomiting that may persist for days after surgery. Application of a scopolamine transdermal patch behind the ear for 3 days beyond surgery may serve as a useful adjunct to antiemetic therapy and eradicate this problem.

The efficacy of Ginger as a single agent was compared to various drugs alone or in combination to prevent motion sickness in a double-blind, placebo-controlled study. Three doses of ginger were investigated and, in the opinion of the authors, neither dose of ginger alone was more effective than placebo. Dimenhydrinate, promethazine, scopolamine, and *d*-amphetamine were effective as single agents. The efficacy of the first three was enhanced by addition of *d*-amphetamine to the regimen. Most effective in preventing motion sickness with limited side effects in this study was a combination of scopolamine 0.6 mg and 10 mg *d*-amphetamine.

The efficacy of ginger as an antiemetic has been studied and compared to metoclopramide after major gynecologic surgery in a double-blind, placebo-controlled, randomized study. Premedication with either powdered ginger or a placebo capsule and 10 mg intravenous metoclopramide or placebo was given 60 to 90 minutes prior to the operation. Surgical time lasted between 50 and 60 minutes and the anesthesia time exceeded 1 hour in all cases. Postoperative pain was managed with papaverine or acetaminophen, and postoperative nausea or vomiting was managed with metoclopramide. The incidence of postoperative nausea or vomiting was similar (28 and 30%) in the groups that had received ginger or metoclopramide and considerably greater in those who had received the placebo (51%).

Another placebo-controlled study tested the effectiveness of ginger in preventing postoperative nausea and vomiting. This randomized, double- blind study included 108 subjects slated for elective gynecologic laparoscopy, a procedure generally shorter than that of the previous study. The number of subjects provided 80% power to detect a reduction in the incidence of nausea from 30 to 20%. All patients received 10 mg of diazepam orally and were randomized to receive two 500-mg ginger capsules, one 500-mg ginger capsule and one placebo capsule, or two placebo capsules 1 hour prior to surgery. Nausea, when present, was rated on a scale of 1 to 3 (mild, moderate, severe). Although there was a trend favoring ginger, the difference was not statistically significant ($p = 0.36$). The investigators concluded that neither dose of ginger was effective in preventing postoperative nausea and vomiting. Blinding may have been problematic in this study because of the characteristic taste and smell of ginger, which was noted by one of the patients. Adverse effects were reported by five of the ginger patients and consisted of flatulence and a bloated feeling, heartburn (two patients), nausea, and burping. One patient in the placebo group complained of "feeling windy and having the urge to burp."

A third placebo-controlled study tested the efficacy of ginger in prevention of postoperative nausea and vomiting. This randomized, double- blind study consisted of 120 subjects slated for elective gynecologic diagnostic-laparoscopy. The subjects were given either 1 g of ginger, 100 mg of metoclopramide, or a placebo (1 g of lactose) 1 hour prior to surgery. The incidence of nausea and vomiting with metoclopramide was 27%, 21% with ginger, and 41% with placebo. Ginger was similar in effectiveness to metoclopramide in preventing postoperative nausea and vomiting ($p = 0.34$) and significantly more effective than lactose ($p = 0.006$), the placebo.

Data from the previous three randomized controlled trials on postoperative nausea were appropriate for meta-analysis. The pooled absolute risk reduction for the incidence of postoperative nausea proved the difference between the groups treated with ginger and placebo to lack significance. These values indicate a point of the number-needed-to-treat of 19 and a 95% confidence interval that also includes the possibility of no benefit.

More recently, Visalyaputra and associates examined the efficacy of a 2-g dose of ginger root, compared to placebo and intravenous droperidol, and a combination of both oral ginger and intravenous droperidol to reduce post-operative nausea and vomiting. The authors concluded that neither ginger root capsules nor administration of a combination of intravenous droperidol and oral ginger lowered the incidence of postoperative nausea and vomiting in women having gynecologic diagnostic laparoscopy.

A randomized, double-blind crossover study was conducted to determine the efficacy of ginger in treating hyperemesis gravidarum. A total of 30 pregnant women at less than 20 weeks gestation previously admitted to the hospital for hyperemesis gravidarum participated in the study. The treatment included a 250-mg ginger capsule or a placebo (lactose) capsule three times a day for the first 4 days. After a 2-day washout period, the subjects received the alternate treatment for 4 days. Ginger was significantly more efficacious in reducing symptoms of hyperemesis gravidarum than placebo ($p = 0.035$).

Lastly, Vutyavanich and colleagues, conducted a randomized, double-blind, placebo-controlled trial to study 70 women with a lesser degree of nausea and vomiting who did not require hospital admission for hyperemesis gravidarum. All had registered prior to 17 weeks gestation and met the author's criteria for exclusion of other medical causes of nausea and vomiting. Subjects received capsules containing

250 mg powdered ginger 4 times daily or an identical-appearing placebo capsule. Prior to the day of entry, each subject graded the degree of nausea and vomiting she experienced on a scale of 0 to 10. Subjects were dispensed 18 capsules of powdered ginger or placebo, advised to record the number of vomiting episodes twice daily (at noon and bedtime), and to return the 5-item Likert scale with packaging and unused capsules (if any) in a week. After a 2-day washout period, they started the second 4-day course of study drug. Outcomes: of the 32 women in the ginger group, all had one or more episodes of vomiting in the 24 hours before treatment. Only two of the placebo group had no vomiting during this time frame. Of those who received powdered ginger, vomiting was significantly less than in the placebo group. By calculating the exact number of vomiting episodes in the treatment group vs the placebo group, those receiving powdered ginger had a greater reduction in vomiting than those receiving placebo. Of the ginger-treated women, 87% were symptomatically improved as compared to 29% of the placebo group. All patients in the ginger group were compliant with the treatment regimen, as compared with 85% of the placebo group. Adverse affects in this study were minimal. Of those receiving ginger, one experienced heartburn, another abdominal discomfort, and a third had diarrhea for 1 day. The incidence of cephalagia in both groups was equal.

Ginger root has been studied as prophylaxis against seasickness in a randomized, placebo-controlled trial. A group of 80 naval cadets who were inexperienced in sailing in heavy seas received either 1 g of powdered ginger root or placebo as the ship encountered heavy seas for the first time. Scorecards were kept for the next 4 hours regarding four symptoms of seasickness: nausea, vomiting, vertigo, or cold sweats. The cadets continued their assigned tasks throughout the study. All but one scorecard was valuable. Outcomes: 48 of the 79 cadets reported symptoms of seasickness (61%) and 31 (16 in the ginger group and 15 in the placebo group) reported no symptoms at all. Five subjects in the placebo group vomited more than once but none of the ginger group was so afflicted. Although all seasickness symptoms were less severe in the ginger group, the different was not statistically significant for nausea and vertigo.

A comparative study of motion sickness has been conducted in which powdered ginger was compared with scopolamine or placebo. A group of 28 subjects sat in a rotating chair to an end point of motion sickness short of vomiting. Antimotion sickness was defined as activity allowing a greater number of head motions than the placebo. Electrical activity of the stomach was monitored by positioning electrodes over the epigastric area. Outcomes: Powdered ginger provided no protection against motion sickness; however, subjects were able to perform an average of 147.5 more head movements after receiving 0.6 mg scopolamine orally than placebo. The rate of gastric emptying was significantly delayed when tested immediately, but quickly recovered. The authors concluded ginger does not posess antimotion sickness activity nor does it significantly alter gastric function during motion sickness.

The effect of powdered ginger root on gastric emptying rate has been studied in a double-blind, random, controlled, crossover trial of 16 healthy volunteers. The subjects received either 1000 mg powdered ginger root or placebo, and gastric emptying was monitored using the oral acetaminophen absorption model. Powdered ginger did not alter gastric emptying. The authors concluded the antiemetic effect of ginger was not related to its effect on gastric emptying.

However, there is lack of consensus regarding the mechanism of the antiemetic effect of ginger. Is this effect a result of vestibular input to the vomiting center of the brain via muscarinic acetylcholine receptors, or is it a direct effect on the stomach? Studies in rats have shown 6-gingerol enhances gastrointestinal transport of a charcoal meal. It has been suggested Phillips' study failed to demonstrate this effect because of inadequate dose of 6-gingerol. Additionally, both 6-gingerol, shogaol, and galanolactone have anti-5-hydroxytryptamine (5HT) activity in isolated guinea pig ileum. Lastly, available data is inadequate to clarify the significance of CNS activity.

Abrupt discontinuation or noncompliance with serotonin reuptake inhibitor (SRI) treatment regimens may result in a recently described "SRI Discontinuation Syndrome," characterized by disequilibrium, dizziness, vertigo, and ataxia. Although no randomized, placebo-controlled studies have been published regarding this entity, case reports of successful alleviation of its symptoms by ginger root have been emerging. The dose of ginger root most frequently utilized to treat this syndrome is 500 to 1000 mg three times daily.

Anti-Inflammatory Activity

Ginger components 6-gingerol, 6-dehydrogingerdione, 10-dehydrogingerdione, 6-gingerdione, and 10-gingerdione inhibit prostaglandin synthetics in vitro. The latter four components were found to have greater potency as prostaglandin inhibitors than indomethacin. In an additional study of ginger's ability to affect arachidonic acid metabolism in human platelets and rat aorta, an aqueous extract of ginger was able to inhibit production of thromboxane and prostaglandins in a dose-dependent manner. Ginger appears to act as a dual inhibitor of both cyclooxygenase and lipooxygenase to inhibit leukotriene synthesis.

Altman and Marcussen evaluated 247 patients with osteoarthritis and moderate to severe knee pain in a randomized, double-blind, placebo-controlled, multicenter, parallel-group, 6-week study. The results of their investigation revealed small but statistically insignificant benefits of ginger over placebo.

Another placebo-controlled, 3-week treatment crossover study with a 1-week washout period between treatments studied the same ginger extract compound compared to ibuprofen and placebo. Pain relief by ibuprofen was significantly greater than placebo, but a difference between ginger extract and placebo was lacking.

The antiinflammatory effects of ginger oil on arthritic rats were studied. A 0.05-mL suspension of heat-killed *Mycobacterium tuberculosis bacilli* in liquid paraffin (5 mg/mL) was injected into the knees and paws to induce arthritis in treatment rats. Rats were randomized to receive 33 mg/ kg of ingwerol (ginger oil obtained by steam distillation of dried ginger root), 33 mg/kg of eugenol (a component of clove oil purported to have antiinflammatory activity), or normal saline orally for 26 days, beginning just prior to the induction of arthritis. Compared to normal saline, both treatments were effective in decreasing both knee and paw swelling.

Migraine Prevention

A case reported the use of ginger for the prevention of migraines. A 42-year-old woman suffered migraine with aura once or twice every 2 or 3 months for 10 years. Because the frequency and duration of migraine increased, the patient was prescribed 500–600 mg of powdered ginger to be taken at the onset of aura, then every 4 hours for the next 3–4 days. The patient reported some relief within 30 minutes of the first dose. Then she added uncooked fresh ginger to her diet. In a 13-month period, she reported only six migraines. These results should be confirmed in a double-blind, controlled trial.

Cardiovascular Effects

In vitro studies of gingerol using canine cardiac tissue and rabbit skeletal muscle demonstrated Ca^{2+}-adenosine triphosphatase (ATPase) activation in the cardiac and skeletal *sarcoplasmic reticulum* (SR). Gingerol (3–30 μM) increased Ca^{2+}-ATPase pumping rate in a dose-dependent manner. A 100-fold dilution with fresh saline solution of 30 μM gingerol completely reversed Ca^{2+}-ATPase activation. The investigators concluded that gingerol may be a useful pharmacological tool in the study of regulatory mechanisms of the SR Ca^{2+} pumping systems, and their effect on muscle contractility.

Another in vitro study examined the effect of 6-, 8-, and 10-gingerol on isolated left atria of guinea pigs. The study found the gingerols had a dose-dependent positive inotropic effect that was evident at doses as low as 10^5, 10^{-6}, and 3×10^{-5} g/mL for 6-, 8-, and 10-gingerol, respectively. Thus, 8-gingerol was the most potent gingerol in regard to cardiotonic activity.

In vitro, aqueous ginger extract has dose-dependent antithromboxane synthetase activity that correlates with its ability to inhibit aggregation of human platelets in response to adenosine diphosphate, collagen, and epinephrine. However, this may not be clinically significant; inhibition of platelet aggregation has been demonstrated in humans only after consumption of 5 g of raw ginger daily for 1 week. A single 2-g dose of dried ginger did not affect platelet function.

Mutagenicity

A study showed that 6-gingerol and 6-shogaol isolated from *Z. officinale* using column chromatography were mutagenic at 700 μM in the Hs30 strain of *Escherichia coli*. 6-Gingerol was noted to be a potent mutagen whereas 6-shogaol was less mutagenic. Another study documented the antimutagenicity of zingerone, another ginger component, in addition to the mutagenicity of gingerol and shogaol in *Samonella typhimurium* strains TA 100, TA 1535, TA 1538, and TA 98. Gingerol and shogaol activated by rat liver enzymes at doses of 5-200 μg/plate mutated strains TA 100 and TA 1535, whereas zingerone was nonmutagenic in all four strains. Zingerone also suppressed the mutagenicity of gingerol and shogaol in a dose-dependent manner. Although all three compounds are similar in chemical structure, zingerone has a shorter side chain than the mutagenic compounds; thus the side chains may be responsible for the mutagenic activity of gingerol and shogaol.

Pyrolysates of cigarettes, fish, and meats have been found to have potent carcinogenic capability. Research in Japan found evidence that vegetables, such as cabbage and ginger, contain antimutagenic factors that suppress mutagenesis. Another study suggests that ginger juice contains more antimutagenic than mutagenic substance(s), and thus has the capability to suppress mutagenesis by the contained pyrosylates.

Pharmacokinetics

No human studies of the pharmacokinetics of any ginger components have been conducted. Only one study in rats has been conducted to examine the pharmacokinetics of a ginger component, 6-gingerol. This study observed that after IV administration, the plasma concentration-time curve was best described by a two-compartment model with a rapid terminal elimination half-life of 7.2 minutes and a total body clearance of 16.8 mL/minute/kg. The protein binding of 6-gingerol was approx 92%.

Adverse Effects

Case Reports of Toxicity Caused by Commercially Available Products

Consumption of Jamaica ginger, an alcoholic ginger extract that was popular as a beverage in the rural southern United States during prohibition, resulted in a peripheral polyneuritis. In reported cases, the first symptom to appear was sore calves for 1 or 2 days. After the soreness disappeared, walking became notably difficult for the case subjects. Subjects could not walk without the aid of a cane or crutches within 1 week. Bilateral weakness of the upper and lower extremities and foot drop, without sensory disturbance or pain, was a common physical finding. The skin on the feet was noted to be red and glossy, but not swollen. Deep tendon reflexes were inconsistent among patients; ankle jerks were not present in any subject, but some had normal knee reflexes. There were no cranial nerve deficits. Although the beverage contained 60–90% alcohol, alcoholic neuropathy was ruled out as an etiology of the syndrome because of the sporadic nature of Jamaica ginger consumption. Jamaica ginger was eventually exonerated as cause of the neuropathy and an adulterating agent, triorthocresyl phosphate, was identified as the putative toxin. This chemical had been added to the beverage presumably as a tasteless substitute for the oleo resin of ginger so that the product would be more palatable. Additional research with alcohol and true United States Pharmacopeia (USP) ginger fluid extract failed to produce paralysis. Subsequent reports of cases of neuropathy associated with the use of ginger in any form have not been forthcoming.

Drug Interactions

Although no drug interactions with ginger have been reported, caution should be exercised with patients taking anticoagulants and antiplatelet drugs because of its potential antiplatelet effect.

Reproduction

In addition to its mutagenic activity, concern has been raised that the receptor binding of testosterone may be affected in the fetus because of ginger's inhibition of thromboxane synthetase. Commission E contra-indicates ginger's use during pregnancy for morning sickness, although this contra-indication has been disputed by some owing to the lack of reported adverse effects despite its long history of use in pregnancy in traditional Chinese medicine.

Regulatory Status

In Austria and Switzerland, ginger is registered as an over-the-counter drug indicated for the prevention of motion sickness, nausea, and in Austria, for vomiting in febrile pediatric patients. Australia's Therapeutic Goods Administration's Listed Products category includes ginger as an acceptable active ingredient. Likewise, in the United Kingdom, ginger is on the General Sale List of the Medicines Control Agency. In Belgium, ginger rhizome is permitted as a traditional digestive aid, and the German Commission E approves ginger for dyspeptic complaints and the prevention of motion sickness. Ginger is listed as an official monograph in the USP-National Formulary. Ginger is regulated as a dietary supplement in the United States. It is also considered "generally recognized as safe as a food substance" by the FDA.

11

GINKGO BILOBA

The ginkgo tree, *Ginkgo biloba* (GB) L., is the last remaining member of the Ginkgoaceae family, which once included many species. It has survived unchanged in China for more than 200 million years, and was brought to Europe in 1730 and to America in 1784. Since then, it has become a popular ornamental tree worldwide. Individual trees may live as long as 1000 years, and grow to a height of approx 125 feet. GB fruits and seeds have been used in China for their medicinal properties since 2800 BCE. Traditional Chinese physicians used GB leaves to treat asthma and chilblains (swelling of the hands and feet from exposure to damp cold). The ancient Chinese and Japanese ate roasted GB seeds as a digestive aid and to prevent drunkenness. GB use had spread to Europe by the 1960s.

CURRENT PROMOTED USE

GB is sold as a dietary supplement in the United States. It is purported to improve blood flow to the brain and to improve peripheral circulation. It is promoted mainly to sharpen mental focus in otherwise healthy adults as well as in those with dementia. Other conditions for which it is currently used are diabetes-related circulatory disorders, impotence, and vertigo.

PRODUCTS AVAILABLE

An acetone-water mixture is used to extract the dried and milled leaves. After the solvent is removed, the *Ginkgo biloba* extract (GBE) is dried and standardized. Most commercially prepared dosage forms contain 40 mg of GBE, and are standardized to contain approx 24% flavonoids (mostly flavone glycosides, or ginkgoflavone glycosides) and

6% terpenes (ginkgolides and bilobalide). There are a more than 500 GB preparations on the market, in a number of dosage forms.

Pharmacological/Toxicological Effects

The effects of GB are attributed to several chemical constituents of the whole plant rather than to any one individual component. These chemicals include many flavonoids (also called flavonol, flavone, or flavonoid glycosides, ginkgo flavone glycosides, dimeric bioflavones), and the terpene lac- tones (also called terpenoids, diterpenes, terpenes), including the ginkgolides and bilobalide.

Nervous System Effects

The pharmacological basis of the effects of GBE on brain function has been addressed in a number of studies. One study showed that dietary GBE 761 protected striatal dopaminergic neurons of male Sprague-Dawley rats from damage caused by N-methyl-4-phenyl-1,2,3,6-tetrahydropyridine (MPTP). MPTP, which has caused Parkinsonism in young drug abusers, is thought to damage these neurons through formation of free radicals. The mechanism of GBE's protective effect was attributed to an antioxidant action, rather than to prevention of neuronal uptake of MPTP. Whether chronic GBE ingestion could prevent development of idiopathic Parkinson's disease in humans remains to be seen.

The effectiveness of GB in improving memory and cognition remains controversial, with most studies demonstrating no effect or only very modest improvement. Readers of the original papers listed below are encouraged to closely examine the reported results and conclusions in addition to the abstract, as the claims are not always justified by the results. In one study, 40-mg EGb 761 tablets taken three times daily before meals was compared to placebo in a double-blind, randomized trial in patients with mild to severe Alzheimer type or multiinfarct dementia, diagnosed according to the *Diagnostic and Statistical Manual of Mental Disorders*, and *International Statistical Classification of Diseases*, criteria. The study lasted 52 weeks, and patients were assessed at weeks 3, 26, and 52 using the cognitive subscale of the Alzheimer's Disease Assessment Scale (ADAS-Cog), the Geriatric Evaluation by Relative's Rating Instrument (GERRI), and the Clinical Global Impression of Change (CGIC), three validated rating instruments. Thus, participants' cognitive impairment, daily living and social behavior, and general psychopathology were objectively evaluated. Modest improvement was appreciated using ADAS-Cog and

GERRI, but the CGIC score did not reveal improvement compared to placebo. Adverse effects did not differ from those of placebo. The relatively large number of dropouts (only 202 of 309 patients were assessed at week 52) raises questions about the validity of the results. In addition, a metaanalysis of four double-blind, placebo-controlled studies including a total of 424 patients with Alzheimer's found a small (3%) but clinically significant improvement on the ADAS-Cog with 120–240 mg of GB administered for 3–6 months. A number of double-blind, placebo-controlled studies have been conducted recently to assess the effect of GB on cognition and memory, particularly in elderly subjects or those with dementia. Four of these studies have reported no beneficial effect of GB administration on tests of memory and cognitive function. Other studies have reported only modest beneficial effect of GB on some measures of memory and cognition, mostly related to measures of attention. Thus, it appears that GB administration has little benefit on improvement of cognition and memory.

Anxiolytic effects have been demonstrated in animal models. The effect of Zingicomb, a combination product containing 24% ginkgo flavonoids and 23.5% gingerols, administered orally to rats at a dose of 0.5–100 mg/kg was compared with the effects of placebo and diazepam administered intraperitoneally at a dose of 1 mg/kg on anxiety-associated behaviors. The rats were subjected to an elevated plus-maze consisting of enclosed and open arms. The 0.5 mg/kg dose of Zingicomb was associated with rats spending more time in the open arms and with more excursions toward the ends of the open arms as compared to placebo. At a dose of 100 mg/kg, excursions to the ends of the open arms and scanning (protruding the head over the edge of an open arm and looking around) were fewer. These results were interpreted to mean that the preparation exhibited anxiolytic effects at a dose of 0.5 mg/kg, but anxiogenic effects at 100 mg/kg. Both the herbal product at a 0.5 mg/kg dose and diazepam increased the number of entries into the open arms, but unlike diazepam, Zingicomb did not increase open-arm scanning, nor did it attenuate risk assessment (protruding the forepaws and head from an enclosed arm). These effects of the herbal preparation were attributed to blockade of 5-hydroxytryptamine 3 (5-HT3; serotonin) receptors, which has been shown in previous studies to produce similar results in the elevated plus-maze. In addition, components of both ginger and GB have been shown in several animal studies to exert 5-HT3 receptor-blocking effects.

Though early reports had suggested that vertigo and tinnitus could be successfully relieved with GB treatment at doses of 16–160 mg/day for 3 months, this effect has not been borne out in double-blind, placebo-controlled trials. Rejali and colleagues studied the effectiveness of GB administration in 66 adult subjects with tinnitus. Using the Tinnitus Handicap Inventory as the primary outcome measure, these investigators found that administration of GB was of no benefit to patients with tinnitus. They also conducted a metaanalysis of five additional studies (plus theirs) and confirmed the lack of effect of GB in treating tinnitus. In a similar study of ginkgo treatment (Vertigoheel), Issing and colleagues found that both placebo and the ginkgo preparation improved vertigo equally, suggesting no additional benefit of ginkgo treatment. It should be noted that this study was conducted in a randomized, placebo-controlled, double-blind fashion.

Acute mountain sickness can occur when unacclimatized individuals ascend to altitudes above 2000 meters. Chow and colleagues compared the efficacy of either acetazolamide or GB prophylaxis for preventing acute mountain sickness. The trial was completed by 57 subjects, with 20 receiving acetazolamide, 17 receiving GB, and 20 receiving placebo. GB had no effect on either the symptoms or incidence of acute mountain sickness. Acetazolamide reduced the symptoms of acute mountain sickness but did not reduce the incidence. A similar lack of effect on acute mountain sickness among Himalayan trekkers taking GB was noted by Gertsch et al.

Interestingly, GB treatment has been demonstrated to be effective in reversing the symptoms of sudden hearing loss. In one study of 106 patients receiving either GBE (EGb 761) or placebo and suffering from idiopathic sudden sensorineural hearing loss, the GBE treatment appeared to speed up recovery and improve the chances of complete recovery as compared to placebo. Similarly, Reisser and Weidauer observed that GBE (EGb 761) and pentoxifylline were equally effective in reversing hearing loss and reducing tinnitus. Though the study was randomized and double blinded, no placebo control was utilized.

Cardiovascular Effects

EGb 761 at a dose of 200 mg administered to 60 patients intravenously for 4 days improved skin perfusion and decreased blood viscosity without affecting plasma viscosity. Another GB extract, LI 1730, increased blood flow in nailfold capillaries and decreased erythrocyte aggregation compared to placebo in 10 volunteers at a dose of 112.5 mg. Blood pressure, heart rate, packed cell volume, and plasma viscosity were unchanged. A study in subjects with type 2 diabetes mellitus complicated with retinopathy evaluated the effects of administration of GB (EGb 761) for 3 months on erythrocyte hemorrheology. At the end of the treatment period, it was observed that blood viscosity was significantly reduced, fibrinogen levels were decreased, and erythrocytes were more deformable. Finally, retinal capillary blood flow was improved. However, in a double-blind, placebo-controlled trial of GB in the treatment of Raynaud' s disease, after 10 weeks of treatment there was no improvement in hemorrheology between the two groups. There was a significant decrease in the number of attacks per day.

Studies have been conducted to examine the effects on GB administration on blood pressure and blood flow. In one study, either GB or placebo was administered in a double-blind, placebo-controlled crossover design to healthy volunteers and forearm blood flow was measured. Forearm blood flow was significantly higher during GB therapy than with placebo and mean arterial pressure remained unchanged, thus rendering the forearm vascular resistance significantly lower during active treatment. In a related study, Jezova and colleagues studied the effect of GB (EGb 761) treatment on changes in blood pressure and cortisol release following exposure to stress stimuli. The rise in systolic blood pressure following stress stimuli was significantly lower (~20 mmHg rise in subjects receiving EGb 761 vs an ~30 mmHg rise in subjects receiving placebo) in the GB group. Differences in diastolic pressure rise were similar (~10 mmHg difference between GB and placebo) between the two groups. GB did inhibit the stress-induced increase in cortisol release in the male subjects but had no effect in the female subjects.

Because of effects noted with in vitro studies demonstrating that ginkgolides are capable of inhibiting *platelet-activating factor* (PAF), which is involved in platelet aggregation and inflammatory processes such as those seen in asthma, ulcerative colitis, and allergies, it has been suggested that bleeding parameters might be affected also. Several case reports of bleeding disorders among people receiving GB have been described. However, at least in healthy volunteers, changes in platelet function or coagulation have not been substantiated. In a double-blind, placebo-controlled study of 32 healthy male volunteers receiving EGb 761 at three doses (120, 240, and 480 mg/day) for 14 days, no changes in platelet function or coagulation were noted. Similarly, Kohler and colleagues studied the influence of the same GBE (EGb 761) on bleeding time and coagulation in healthy volunteers. This double-blind, placebo-controlled study was carried out for 7 days in 50 healthy volunteers. No differences in bleeding time, coagulation parameters, or platelet activity were noted between the placebo and GB treatment groups. In a study of patients on chronic peritoneal dialysis, Kim and colleagues randomized the 66 patients into two groups; those receiving GB (160 mg/day) and those receiving no treatment. There was no placebo control. Except for a small but statistically significant change in the plasma D-dimer concentration, the administration of GB had no effect on any bleeding parameters. Finally, Kudolo and colleagues studied the effect of GBE on platelet aggregation and urinary prostanoid excretion in healthy subjects and patients with type 2 diabetes. Administration of GB had no effect on any parameter of coagulation or prostanoid excretion in the patients with type 2 diabetes. In the healthy volunteers, a modest but statistically significant decrease in thromboxane B_2, PGI_2, and prostanoid metabolite ratio was noted following GB treatment. It is of note that a placebo control was not included for either group.

Carcinogenicity/Mutagenicity/Teratogenicity

No mutagenic, carcinogenic, or teratogenic effects have been noted in studies performed using commercially available GB products containing 22–27% flavone glycosides and 5–7% terpene lactones.

Endocrine Effects

Kudolo studied the effect of 3-month ingestion of a GBE on pancreatic β-cell function. Having taken a 3-month course of GB, 20 normal, healthy subjects were given an oral glucose tolerance test, and fasting plasma insulin and C-peptide were measured. Fasting plasma insulin area under the curve (AUC) was increased approx 20% whereas C-peptide AUC was increased approx 70%. In a follow-up study in noninsulin-dependent patients with diabetes mellitus who received the same 3-month GB therapy, following an oral glucose tolerance test, a blunted plasma insulin response was noted, leading to a reduction in insulin AUC. Conversely, C-peptide levels were increased, leading to a dissimilar insulin/C-peptide ratio. The author suggested this indicated an increased hepatic extraction of insulin relative to C-peptide, potentially resulting in reduced insulin-mediated glucose metabolism and elevated blood glucose.

Administration of GB has also been studied for the treatment of sexual dysfunction. Kang and colleagues evaluated the efficacy of GB administered for 2 months to subjects with antidepressant-induced sexual dysfunction in a placebo-controlled, double-blind design. Compared with baseline, both placebo and GB showed improvement in some aspects of sexual function, but there was no difference in effect between placebo and GB treatment. Similarly, Wheatley used a triple-blind, placebo-controlled design to again study the effect of GB on antidepressant-induced sexual dysfunction. Again, though some individual subjects experienced improvement, no statistically significant improvement in sexual function was noted.

Drug Interactions

In two of the five spontaneous bleeding episodes, medications that can affect platelet function or *prothrombin time* (PT) (i.e., aspirin and warfarin) were involved. Because GB is known to be an inhibitor of PAF, in theory GB could interact with antiplatelet drugs (e.g., aspirin, nonsteroidal anti-inflammatory drugs, clopidogrel, ticlopidine, dipyridamole) or anticoagulants (e.g., warfarin, heparin). EGb 761 was shown to potentiate the antiplatelet effect of ticlopidine in rats. However, in two studies in humans, the coadministration of GB with warfarin had no effect on either international normalized ratio or warfarin metabolism.

With respect to the effect of GB on cytochrome P450 drug metabolizing enzymes, in vitro studies have demonstrated that GBE and components have minimal effect on CYP2C9, CYP3A4, CYP1A2, and CYP2D6. This lack of effect on these particular cytochrome P450 enzymes has been confirmed by in vivo studies using probe drug substrates. However, coadministration of GB with omeprazole (a CYP2C 19 substrate) demonstrated significant induction of omeprazole metabolism, resulting in reduced AUC. Finally, GB coadministration did not have an effect on donepezil pharmacokinetics. A study in which 400 mg of EGb was administered to 24 healthy volunteers for 13 days demonstrated that GB is not an inducer of other hepatic microsomal enzymes.

Pharmacokinetics/Toxicokinetics

Absorption

In humans, absolute bioavailability is 98–100% for ginkgolide A, 79–93% for ginkgolide B, and at least 70% for bilobalide. In two healthy volunteers, flavonol glycosides administered as the product LI 1370 at doses of 50, 100, and 300 mg were absorbed in the small intestine with peak plasma concentration attained within 2–3 hours. Additional data from human experiments from the manufacturer of 80-

mg EGb 761 solution show that the absolute bioavailabilities of ginkgolides A and B were greater than 80%, whereas that of ginkgolide C was very low. Bioavailability of bilobalide was 70% after administration of 120 mg of the extract. Corroborating these results was a later pharmacokinetic study that found mean bioavailabilities of 80, 88, and 79% for ginkgolide A, ginkgolide B, and bilobalide, respectively. Food intake did increase the time to peak concentration, but did not affect bioavailability.

A study in rats using radiolabeled EGb 761 revealed a bioavailability of at least 60%. Peak blood concentrations occurred at 1.5 hours. At 3 hours, the highest radioactivity was measured in the stomach and small intestine, indicating that these are the sites of absorption.

Distribution

Rat studies using radiolabeled EGb 761 have revealed that the extract follows a two-compartment model of distribution. The radiolabeled extract was distributed into glandular and neuronal tissues, as well as the eyes. The volumes of distribution of ginkgolide A, ginkgolide B, and bilobalide are 40–60 L, 60–100 L, and 170 L, respectively.

Metabolism/Elimination

The half-life of the flavonol glycosides administered as the product LI 1370 is 2–4 hours. Similar resuits wereobtained using 80 mg of the product EGb 761; half-lives of ginkgolides A and B were 4 and 6 hours, respectively. The half-life of bilobalide was 3 hours after administration of 120 mg of this extract. Similar results were reported in another study using this same product; mean half-lives of ginkgolide A, ginkgolide B, and bilobalide were 4.5, 10.57, and 3.21 hours, respectively.

A study in rats using radiolabeled EGb 761 revealed a half-life of 4.5 hours, with elimination following first-order (linear) kinetics.

Approximately 70% of ginkgolide A, 50% of ginkgolide B, and 30% of bilobalide is excreted unchanged in the urine. Metabolites isolated from human urine after administration of EGb include a 4-hydroxybenzoic acid conjugate, 4-hydroxyhippuric acid, 3-methoxy-4-hydroxyhippuric acid, 3,4-dihydroxybenzoic acid, 4-hydroxybenzoic acid, hippuric acid, and 3-methoxy-4-hydroxybenzoic acid (vanillic acid). In accord with previous data, these metabolites accounted for less than 30% of the administered EGb dose. Metabolites were not detectable in blood samples.

Adverse Effects and Toxicity

Case Reports of Toxicity Caused By Commercially Available Products

Spontaneous intracerebral hemorrhage occurred in a 72-year-old woman who had been taking GB 50 mg three times daily for 6 months. Bilateral subdural hematomas were discovered in a 33-year-old woman who had been taking 60 mg of GB twice daily for 2 year, acetaminophen, and occasionally an ergotamine/caffeine preparation. Bleeding time was elevated, but had normalized when checked approx 1 month after discontinuation of the product.

In a similar case, a 61-year-old man presented with a subarachnoid hemorrhage after taking 40-mg GB tablets three or four times daily for more than 6 months. Bleeding time was elevated (6 minutes, normal), but normalized with discontinuation of the product.

A 78-year-old woman suffered a left parietal hemorrhage after taking a GB preparation for 2 months. Other medications included warfarin, which she had been taking for 5 years after undergoing coronary bypass. PT was unchanged.

A 70-year-old man experienced bleeding from the iris into the anterior chamber after self-medicating with 40 mg of Ginkoba twice daily for 1 week. Other medications included 325 mg of aspirin daily for 3 years post- coronary bypass. GB, but not aspirin, was discontinued, and no further bleeding problems occurred.

A 75-year-old woman had undergone outpatient surgery and developed bleeding complications on the first postoperative night. PT, activated partial thrombin time, and platelets were normal but platelet aggregation was diminished. The patient had been taking no other medications except a GB preparation (Gingium) that she had been taking for the past 2 years. The GB product was discontinued and her platelet aggregation returned to normal after 10 days.

In a similar case, a 77-year-old woman experienced persistent bleeding after total hip arthroplasty while taking GB therapy. This bleeding persisted for 4 weeks, at which time the ginkgo was discontinued. After the GB had been discontinued for 6 weeks, the bleeding stopped.

"Gin-nan" food poisoning, a toxic syndrome associated with ingestion of 50 or more GB seeds, can result in loss of consciousness, tonic/clonic seizures, and death. Between 1930 and 1960, 70 cases were reported, with a 27% mortality rate. Infants were at greatest risk. Although ginkgotox-in (4-*O*methylpyridoxine), which is found mostly in the seeds, has been implicated as the responsible neurotoxin, its concentrations in several commercially available GB products tested were deemed too low to have a toxic effect. If used as directed, the maximum daily intake of 4-*O*-methylpyridoxine would be approx 60 μg; however, the presence of this neurotoxin raises questions about the herb's ability to lower the seizure threshold in patients with seizure disorders. The authors of this study cite evidence that bilobalide present in the formulations may decrease the severity of convulsions, thus counter-acting any neurotoxic effects of 4-*O*-methylpyridoxine.

Adverse effects listed in the German Commission E GB leaf extract monograph include gastrointestinal upset, headache, and rash.

Regulatory Status

GB leaf extract is approved by the German Commission E for memory deficits, disturbances in concentration, depression, dizziness, vertigo, headache, dementia, and intermittent claudication. It is regulated as a dietary supplement in the United States.

12

HAWTHORN

Hawthorn is a spiny, small tree or bush with white flowers and red berries (haws), each containing one to three nuts, depending on the species. Hybridization is common among individual species, making them difficult to identify. Hawthorn is a member of the rose family and is found in Europe, North Africa, and western Asia. It can reach heights of 25–30 ft and is used as a hedge. The flowers grow in clusters and bloom from April to June, and the deciduous leaves are divided into three, four, or five lobes. The use of hawthorn can be dated back to Dioscorides in the first century CE.

Uses for the herb have included high and low blood pressure, tachycardia, arrhythmias, atherosclerosis, and angina pectoris. Hawthorn is also purported to have spasmolytic and sedative effects. Native Americans used it as a diuretic for kidney and bladder disorders and to treat stomach aches, stimulate appetite, and improve circulation. The flowers and berries have astringent properties and have been used to treat sore throats in the form of haw jelly or haw marmalade.

CURRENT PROMOTED USES

Hawthorn is promoted for use in heart failure, hypertension, arteriosclerosis, angina pectoris, Buerger's disease, paroxysmal tachycardia, heart valve murmurs, sore throat, skin sores, diarrhea, and abdominal distention.

SOURCES AND CHEMICAL COMPOSITION

Crataegus oxyacantha (L.), *Crataegus laevigata*, *Crataegus monogyna Jacquin*, English hawthorn, haw, maybush, whitethorn, may, mayblossom, hazels, gazels, halves, hagthorn, ladies' meat, bread and cheese tree.

Products Available

Available products include tea, 1:5 tincture in 45% alcohol, 1:1 liquid extract in 25% alcohol, and capsules of 250, 455, and 510 mg. The French Pharmacopoeia requires 45% ethanol for the fluid extract and 60% ethanol for the tincture. It is recommended that 0.5–1 mL of liquid extract or 1–2 mL of tincture be taken three times a day. The tea is made from 0.3–1 g of dried berries infused in hot water and taken three times a day. A typical therapeutic dose of extract, standardized to contain 1.8% vitexin-4 rhamnoside, is 100–250 mg three times daily. A standardized extract containing 18% procyanidolic oligomers (oligomeric procyanidns) is dosed at 250–500 mg daily.

Pharmacological/Toxicological Effects

Cardiovascular Effects

Hawthorn extracts purportedly dilate coronary blood vessels, decrease blood pressure, increase myocardial contractility, and lower serum cholesterol. Benefits have been demonstrated in patients with heart failure. In patients with stage II New York Heart Association (NYHA) heart failure, doses of 160–900 mg/day of the aqueous-alcoholic extract for up to 56 days showed an increase in exercise tolerance, decrease in rate/pressure product, and increased ejection fraction. Degenring and colleagues, in a randomized, double-blind, placebo-controlled trial, studied a standardized extract of fresh *Crataegus* berries for the treatment of patients with NYHA II heart failure.

Using an intent-to-treat analysis, these investigators found that the hawthorn preparation significantly increased exercise tolerance as compared to placebo, but subjective symptoms of heart failure were unchanged. In a meta-analysis of 13 randomized trials of hawthorn extract in the treatment of heart failure, investigators noted that hawthorn produced a statistically significant increase in exercise tolerance over placebo. In addition, symptoms such as dyspnea and fatigue improved significantly with hawthorn treatment. Adverse events were infrequent. These investigators concluded that hawthorn provides a significant benefit in the treatment of heart failure. The active principles are thought to be flavonoids, including hyperoside, vitexin, vitexin-rhamnose, rutin, and oligomeric procyanidins (dehydrocatechins, catechins, and/or epicatechins).

Two clinical trials have also been conducted to evaluate the ability of hawthorn to reduce blood pressure and treat hypertension. Asgary et al. studied the effect of Iranian *Crataegus curvisepala* hydroalcoholic extract in 92 men and women with primary mild hypertension. These investigators found that treatment with the hawthorn extract for 4 months reduced both systolic (~13 mmHg decrease) and diastolic (~8 mmHg decrease) blood pressure as compared with placebo. The effect was progressive over the 4-month treatment period. In a similar study, a hawthorn extract was investigated for its ability to treat mild, essential hypertension. Studying 36 subjects, these investigators found no difference in blood-pressure-lowering between hawthorn and placebo treatments (though both treatments did reduce blood pressure somewhat). Thus, results of hawthorn use in the treatment of hypertension are mixed.

Investigators attempted to elucidate the mechanism of action of the flavonoids hyperoside, luteolin-7-glucoside, rutin, vitexin, vitexin-rhamnoside, and monoacetyl-vitexin-rhamno side in spontaneous-beating Langenhoff preparations of guinea pig hearts. Dose-dependent effects on contractility, heart rate, and coronary blood flow similar to that of theophylline were exhibited by luteolin-7-glucoside, hyperoside, and rutin, whereas vitexin and its derivatives were less potent. These results were different from those of previous investigators, who found a decrease in coronary blood flow, contractility, and heart rate with hyperoside, whereas vitexin decreased contractility and increased heart rate and coronary blood flow.

Vitexin-rhamnoside increased coronary blood flow, heart rate, and contractility in the previous study. These differences were attributed to differences in the experimental device. The investigators concluded that the mechanism behind the cardiac effects of these flavonoids involved phosphodiesterase inhibition, causing an increase in cyclic adenosine monophosphate concentration, as well as inhibition of thromboxane synthesis and enhancement of prostacyclin synthesis, as described by previous researchers. The authors also concluded that despite previous studies showing that vitexin-rhamnoside protected cultured heart cells from oxygen and glucose deprivation, the role of antioxidant activity as a mechanism behind the anti-ischemic effect of these flavonoids requires further study, given that vitexin-rhamnoside exhibited only minor effects in their study.

Because reactive oxygen species may play a role in the pathogenesis of atherosclerosis, angina, and cerebral ischemia, the antioxidant activity of dried hawthorn flowers and flowering tops, fluid extract, tincture, freeze-dried powder, and fresh plant extracts was investigated. Antioxidant activity, determined by the ability of the preparations to scavenge hydrogen peroxide, superoxide anion, and hypochlorous acid, was provided by all preparations, but was highest with the fresh young leaf, fresh floral buds, and dried flowers. The antioxidant activity was correlated to total phenolic proanthocyanidin and flavonoid content.

The effects of hawthorn extract LI 132 standardized to 2.2% flavonoids on contractility, oxygen consumption, and effective refractory period of isolated rat cardiac myocytes were studied. In addition, the effect of partially purified oligomeric procyanidins on contractility was also studied. The concentrations used in their study were chosen for their physiological plausibility, based on the assumption that the volume of distribution of both hawthorn extract and procyanidins in humans is 5 L, and that the daily dose is 900 mg and 5 mg, respectively. At concentrations of 30–180 μg/mL, the hawthorn extract increased myocardial contractility with a more favorable effect on oxygen consumption than β-1 agonists or cardiac glycosides. Hawthorn also prolonged the effective refractory period, indicating that it might be an effective antiarrhythmic agent. Oligomeric procyanidins at concentrations of 0.1–30 μg/mL had no detectable effect on contractility, suggesting that they are not responsible for the positive inotropic effect of hawthorn.

Tincture of Crataegus (TCR), made from hawthorn berries, was shown to have a hypocholesterolemic effect on rats fed 0.5 mL/100 g body weight for 6 weeks. These findings prompted a study that examined the ability of TCR to increase *low-density lipoprotein* (LDL) binding to liver plasma membranes in rats fed an atherogenic diet. The hypocholesterolemic effect of TCR appears to be caused by a 25% increase in LDL receptor activity, resulting in greater LDL uptake by the liver. This was caused by an increased number of receptors, not an increase in receptor binding affinity.

In addition, TCR suppressed *de novo* cholesterol synthesis in the liver, and enhanced the use of liver cholesterol to make bile acids. Despite LDL receptor upregulation, the atherogenic diet fed to the rats offset the beneficial effects; LDL levels increased 104% and liver cholesterol increased by 231%. The investigators did not attempt to determine which TCR constituent was responsible for the hypocholesterolemic effect, but hypothesized that all contribute in some manner.

Neurological Effects

The flavonoids present in hawthorn purportedly have a sedative effect.

Lethal Dose for 50% of Test Population

The Lethal Dose (LD_{50}) of an alcoholic extract of hawthorn leaves and fruit called Crataegutt administered orally was 33.8 mL/kg in rats and 18.5 mL/kg in mice. This particular extract was manufactured by Schwabe and contained 2% or 10% oligomeric procyanidins. Death occurred after approx 30 minutes and was caused by sedation and apnea.

Teratogenicity/Mutagenicity/Carcinogenicity

The German Commission E reports that hawthorn effects are unknown during pregnancy and lactation. No experimental data have been reported concerning toxicity in the embryo or fetus, or the effects on fertility or postnatal development. Commission E also reports the lack of experimental data concerning carcinogenicity. Despite experiential data that hawthorn may be mutagenic, Commission E feels that the amount of mutagenic substances ingested would not be sufficient to pose a risk to humans. Available information presents no indication of carcinogenic risk.

Pharmacokinetics/Toxicokinetics

Although the investigators of one study assumed a volume of distribution of 5 L (approximately plasma volume) for purposes of calculating a concentration to use in their in vitro study, there are no pharmacokinetic data to confirm this.

Adverse Effects and Toxicity

Case Reports of Toxicity Caused by Commercially Available Products

Although several references mention that hawthorn in high doses may cause hypotension, arrhythmias, and sedation in humans, no substantiative case reports can be located.

Drug Interactions

Drug interactions with hawthorn are theoretically possible with cardioactive medications, but have not been documented. In addition, the flavonoid constituents have been shown to have inhibitory and inducible effects on the cytochrome P-450 enzyme system, making other drug interactions possible. However, an in vivo study of a potential pharmacokinetic interaction of digoxin and hawthorn demonstrated that concurrent administration had no effect on digoxin pharmacokinetics, suggesting that the two could be safely administered together from a pharmacokinetic point of view. However, one must be mindful of additive effects and a potential pharmacodynamic interaction.

Regulatory Status

Originally, all preparations of hawthorn were approved under one German Commission E monograph based on historical experience. However, in 1993, the preparations were reevaluated and it was concluded that sufficient scientific evidence was lacking to justify use of the flowers, leaves, and berries as individual compounds. As a result, there are currently four hawthorn monographs: three Unapproved monographs for the berry, flower, and leaf individually and an Approved monograph for the flower with leaves. In addition, the Approved monograph has only one approved indication: treatment of "decreasing cardiac output according to functional stage II of the NYHA." In Canada, hawthorn carries new drug status and is not approved, as self-treatment of cardiovascular conditions is deemed inappropriate. In France, the flower and flowering top are permitted for oral use, and in Switzerland, the leaf and flower are permitted as herbal teas. In Sweden, hawthorn is classified as a natural product, whereas in the United States, it is considered a dietary supplement.

13

Hypericum Perforatum

Hypericum perforatum is Greek for "over an apparition." It was believed that evil spirits disliked the plant's odor and thus could be warded away. *Hypericum* is a perennial aromatic shrub with bright yellow flowers that bloom from June to September. The flowers are said to be at their brightest and most abundant around June 24th, the day traditionally believed to be the birthday of John the Baptist. Also, the red spots on the leaves are symbolic of the blood of St. John. The plant is native to Europe, North Africa, and West Asia, and now also found in Australia, North and South America, and South Africa. It grows in the dry ground of fields, roadsides, and woods. The commercial products are prepared from the dried flowering tops and leaves that are harvested just before or during the flowering period.

St. John's wort has been described in medical literature for thousands of years, including the writings of Hippocrates. Historically, St. John's wort has been used to treat neurological and psychiatric disturbances, gastritis, gout, hemorrhage, pulmonary disorders, and rheumatism, and has been used as a diuretic. Some forms of the herb have been used topically as an astringent and to treat blisters, burns, cuts, hemorrhoids, vitiligo, neuralgias, inflammation, insect bites, itching, redness, sunburn, and wounds. Oral doses of 300 mg of *Hypericum* extract three times daily for periods of 4 to 6 weeks is a typical dosing regimen.

Current Promoted Uses

St. John's wort is used most often for the treatment of mild to moderate depression. It is also used to treat anxiety, sleep disorders, *seasonal affective disorders* (SADs), and wound healing.

Sources and Chemical Composition

The botanical name of St. John's wort is *H. perforatum*. Other common names by which it is known are goat weed, klamath weed, rosin rose, amber touch and heal, tipton weed; blutdkraut, Johnswort, qian ceng lou, Sankt Hans urt, St. Jan's kraut, St. Johnswort, toutsaine, tupfelhartheu, walpurgiskraut, zweiroboij, amber, chassediable, corazoncillo, hardhay, hartheu, herbe de millepertuis, herrgottsblut, hexenkraut, hierba de San Juan, hipericon, hypericum, iperico, Johannesort, pelatro, perforata, Johannisblut, Johanniskraut.

Products Available

Most commercially available preparations of hypericum in the United States are dried alcoholic extracts in a solid oral dosage form. Other preparations include the dried herb, teas, tinctures or liquid extracts. The following is a list of a few of the available formulations:

1. GNC Herbal Plus — 1000-mg softgel capsule concentrated St. John's Wort
2. GNC Herbal Plus — 300-mg tablet standardized St. John's Wort (0.3% hypericin, 0.9 mg)
3. GNC Herbal Plus — 500-mg capsule fingerprinted St. John's Wort
4. Nature's Resource — 450-mg capsule time released St. John's Wort (1.35 mg hypericin)
5. Nature's Way — Capsule, Mood Aid, with 5-HTP and St. John's Wort
6. Nature's Way — Tablet, Perika St. John's Wort (3% hyperforin)
7. Nature's Way — Capsule, standardized St. John's Wort (0.3% hypericin)
8. Enzymatic Therapy — Capsule, St. John's Wort (0.3% hypericin, 3% hyperforin)
9. Herbs for Kids — St. John's Wort Blend (alcohol extract, evaporated)
10. Nature's Answer — St. John's Wort (organic alcohol)
11. Natrol — 300-mg tablet (0.3% hypericin)
12. NSI — 450-mg capsule (0.3% hypericin, 3% hyperforin)
13. Only Natural — 450 mg (0.3% hypericin)
14. Smart Basic — 300 mg St. John's Wort
15. Source Naturals — 300 mg, 450-mg tablet (0.3% hypericin)
16. Karuna — 300-mg capsule (0.3% hypericin)
17. Remotiv — Tablet (1.375 g hyperciu[illegible] perforatum herb, 500 μg hypericin)

18. NOW -- 300-mg capsule St. John's Wort
19. Kira — 300-mg capsule St. John's Wort extract

Pharmacological/Toxicological Effects

The active component of St. John's wort is not known. It is composed of many different compounds. The concentrations of these chemicals vary from brand to brand and batch to batch. Hyperforin, hypericin, and pseudohypericin are considered by most to be the major active ingredients. Hypericin, pseudohypericin, isohypericin, protohypericin, protopseudohypericin, and cyclopseudohypericin are all anthraquinone derivatives (naphthodianthrones). Hyperforin and adhyperforin are both prenylated phorolucinols.

The flavonoids that are present include kaempferol, quercetin, luteolin, hyperoside, isoquercitrin, quercitrin, rutin, hyperin, hyperoside, I3-II8-biapigenin, 1,3,6,7-tetrhydroxyxanthone, and amentoflavone. The phenols consist of caffeic, chlorogenic, p-coumaric, ferulic, p-hydroxybenzoic, and vanillic acids. The volatile oils include methyl-2-octane, nnonane, methyl-2-decane and n-undecane, α- and β-pinene, α-terpineol, geraniol, myrcene, limonene, caryophyllen, and humulene. Other chemicals that are found in St. John's wort include tannins, organic acids (isovalerianic, nicotinic, myristic, palmitic, stearic), carotenoids, choline, nicotinamide, pectin, β-sitosterol, straight-chain saturated hydrocarbons, and alcohols. Most of these agents are found in other plants that do not possess antidepressant activity, which has led to most of the research being concentrated on the naphthodianthrones and hyperforin, which are only found in a few species.

Neurological Effects

There have been many clinical trials studying the effectiveness of St. John's wort in the treatment of depression. By the spring of 2002, there were 34 controlled trials including more than 3000 patients. Most of these trials included patients with mild to moderate depression and used the *Hamilton Rating Scale of Depression* (HAMD) to measure efficacy. Schulz compared the results of all of the trials since 1990. Nine of the 11 placebo-controlled trials showed a significant difference in the HAMD scores favoring hypericum, and a trend favoring hypericum was demonstrated in the other two. Linde also compared clinical trials with hypericum, and came to the conclusion that hypericum was superior to placebo in mild to moderate depression. When compared with the synthetic antidepressants, there was one trial with amitriptyline, four with imiprimine, two with fluoxetine, two with sertraline, one with bromazepam, and one with maprotiline. Of these trials, hypericum was equal to or superior to all of them except amitriptyline. In two trials comparing hypericum in major depression (participants with HAMD scores of at least 20), hypericum failed to show any improvement over placebo or other anti-depressants. One randomized, controlled, double-blind, noninferiority trial that has been published since the Schulz review compared 900 mg/day of St. John's wort vs 20 mg/day of paroxetine in adult patients with acute major depression (HAMD score ≥22). Using the HAMD to assess efficacy, it was found that St. John's wort was at least as effective as paroxetine and was better tolerated.

Although the results from trials in patients with mild to moderate depression appear encouraging in their support of St. John's wort, there are limitations. First, the longest duration of these trials was 56 days and several of the trials were as short as 28 days. Also, most of the trials used relatively low doses of synthetic antidepressants. Finally, two of the trials did not state the exact number of responders, making the results somewhat questionable.

The exact mechanism of action responsible for St. John's wort' s neurological effects is not known. Additionally, it is not known if any one chemical constituent is responsible for its activity or if it is a combination of multiple components. It is known that the extracts of *H. perforatum* appear to inhibit the synaptic uptake of several neurotransmitters including norepinephrine, serotonin (5-HT), and dopamine. Rats that were fed high doses of hypericum extracts standardized to flavonoids (50%), hypericin (0.3%), and hyperforin (4.5%) were shown to have dose-dependent enhanced 5-HT levels in all brain regions. Norepinephrine levels were increased in the diencephalon and brain stem, but not in the cortex, and higher levels of hypericum were needed.

Dopamine levels were only increased in the diencephalon region with doses similar to those required for increased levels of norepinephrine. Cott demonstrated that hypericum extracts had affinity for adenosine, γ-aminobutyric acid (GABA)-A, GABA-B, benzodiazapine, and monoamine oxidase (MAO) types A and B receptors. However, with the exception of GABA-A and GABA-B receptors, it is unlikely that the concentrations required to produce a physiological effect can be reached. Other studies have shown that hypericum extracts do not have high affinity for GABA-A and -B. Additionally, *H. perforatum* extracts downregulate 1 receptors and upregulate 5-HT2 receptors in the frontal cortex when given to rats. *Hypericum* extract standardized to flavonoids (50%), hypericin (0.3%), and hyperforin (4.5%) was shown to inhibit the release of interleukin-6 (IL-6) in vitro. IL-6 levels have been shown to be increased in patients with depression. It is thought that IL-6 induced stimulation of corticotropin-releasing hormone, adrenocorticotropic hormone, or cortisol may be responsible for increased depression. Also, using the rat forced- swimming model for depression, high doses of the extract was shown to improve depression in wild-type rats but had no effect in rats that were IL-6 knockouts (IL-$6^{-/-}$).

The wild-type mice had a significantly greater increase in 5-HT in the diencephalon portion of the brain compared to the IL-$6^{-/-}$ mice. This finding indicates that IL-6 may be necessary to have an antidepressant response to hypericum. *Hypericum* extract was shown to inhibit the enzyme dopamine-β-hydroxylase (DβH), and its inhibition is 200 times stronger than the inhibition by pure hypericin, suggesting that hypericin is not the component responsible. DβH is the enzyme that catalyzes the conversion of dopamine into norepinephrine; thus St. John's wort may increase dopamine levels in the brain while lowering norepinephrine. High concentrations of hypericum extracts inhibit catechol-O-methyltransferase (COMT) activity. Consumption of a single dose of 2700 mg of St. John's wort extract was found to significantly increase plasma growth-hormone levels and decrease prolactin levels in human males.

It was once thought that hypericin was the main active ingredient in St. John's wort. In 1994, it was reported that hypericin inhibited MAO-A. Further studies have shown that hypericin and pseudohypericin do not inhibit MAO-A, and hypericum extracts only inhibit MAO at extremely high concentrations. Furthermore, hypericin did not display a significant (>25%) inhibition of norepinephrine, dopamine, or 5-HT uptake sites, nor did it display high affinity to 5-HT, adenosine, adrenergic, benzodiazepine, dopamine, or GABA receptors. Hypericin was found to have high (>30%) levels of inhibition of nonselective muscarinic cholinergic receptors, 5-HT1A receptors and nonselective σ receptors. Butterweck also has shown that hypericin and pseudohypericin have significant activity at D3- and D4-dopamine receptors, and that hypericin has significant activity at β-adrenergic receptors.

Most evidence now implicates hyperforin as the main component responsible for the neurological activity of St. John's wort. Hyperforin has been shown to inhibit synaptic reuptake of 5-HT, dopamine, norepinephrine, GABA, l-glutamate, and acetylcholine. It is a potent uptake inhibitor of 5-HT, dopamine, norepinephrine, and GABA with 50% inhibition concentrations (IC50) of approx 0.05–2 μg/mL. It has been shown that hyperforin increases the intracellular level of sodium, which may be directly responsible for its effect on 5-HT reuptake. Hyperforin was also shown to strongly inhibit D1- and D5-dopamine receptors and weakly inhibit binding to the opioid receptor hδ. Adhyperforin exists as a component in St. John's wort in approx one-tenth the concentration of hyperforin; but it, too, was found to be a potent uptake inhibitor of 5-HT, dopamine, and norepinephrine at lower IC50 values. Another factor that supports hyperforin's role as the active ingredient is that it is the major lipophilic constituent in hypericum extract, allowing it to cross the blood–brain barrier more easily.

Pseudohypericin has been shown to be a corticotropin-releasing factor $(CRF)_1$ receptor antagonist. CRF has been implicated as a pathogenic factor in affective disorders, with elevated levels that are normalized after treatment with antidepressants found in the cerebrospinal fluid of patients with depression. CRF acts on CRF_1 receptors in the pituitary gland to stimulate the release of adrenocoticotropic hormone, which stimulates the release of glucocorticoid stress hormones from the adrenal glands. It is possible that St. John's wort' s activity comes from pseudohypericin' s ability to block the CRF_1 receptor.

Amentoflavone is a biflavonoid with some pharmacological activity that may contribute to the activity of St. John's wort. It was found to significantly inhibit binding at 5-HT1d, 5-HT2c, D3-dopamine, δ-opiate, and benzodiazepine receptors.

Along with depression, hypericum has been studied in SAD. There have been two studies in which participants received 300 mg St. John's wort three times daily with or without bright-light therapy either for 4 or 8 weeks. In both studies there were significant reductions in HAMD scores or SAD scores, but no statistically significant difference in scores between the groups that received light therapy and those that did not.

A study using rats to measure the anxiolytic activity of *Hypericum* was conducted with efficacy being measured by several means. In this study, rats were given either *Hypericum* extract 100 or 200 mg/kg or lorazepam 0.5 mg/kg. Using the open-field observation test and the maze test to measure anxiety, the *Hypericum* treatment groups showed anxiolytic efficacy and were superior to placebo, whereas the lorazepam was either equivalent to or superior to the *Hypericum* groups. With respect to social interaction, both treatment groups with *Hypericum* increased the amount of time the animals spent in social interactions with respect to control animals. Lorazepam-treated rats were comparable to the higher dose *Hypericum* group.

Obsessive-compulsive disorder (OCD) is a neurological disorder that affects 1.2–2.4% of the population. Drugs that inhibit 5-HT uptake are often used to treat OCD, with limited results. In a 12-week, open-label study, 13 people were treated with 450 mg of *Hypericum* standardized to 0.3% hypericin twice daily. Efficacy was measured by the Yale-Brown Obsessive Compulsive Scale (Y-BOCS). Of the 13 members, 12 completed the trial, with an average reduction in their Y-BOCS scores of 7.42 from baseline, which is comparable to the results in studies using antidepressants. Additionally, five out of 12 patients rated themselves as much or very much improved, six out of 12 were minimally improved, and one noted no change. Interestingly, although the patients' average HAMD scores were a subclinical 6.09 at baseline, they dropped significantly to 1.91 at the end of the study.

Hypericum has also been studied for its effect on sleep. In a small trial, 14 females were given 300 mg *Hypericum* three times daily for 4 weeks, given a 2-week washout period, then given placebo for 4 weeks. The continuity of sleep, onset of sleep, intermittent wake-up phases, and total sleep were not improved. There was, however, a significant increase in deep sleep (stage 3 and 4, slow wave) that was shown by analysis of electroencephalogram activities. Thus, *Hypericum* may be able to improve sleep quality.

Somatoform disorders are a group of diseases that include the complaint of physical pain, which lead the patient to believe they have a physical disease, though none can be found by medical investigation. A study was conducted where 151 patients received either *Hypericum* 300 mg twice daily or placebo. Efficacy was measured using the Hamilton Anxiety Scale, subfactor somatic anxiety (HAMA-SOM). After 6 weeks, the average HAMA-SOM decreased from 15.39 to 6.64 in the *Hypericum* arm and from 15.55 to 11.97 in the placebo arm, which was statistically significant, demonstrating the superiority of St. John's wort over placebo.

Antimicrobial Effects

St. John's wort has been used topically for wound healing for hundreds of years. Antibacterial properties have been reported as early as 1959, with hyperforin found to be the active component. Using multiple concentrations, it was discovered that no hyperforin dilutions had antimicrobial effects on Gram-negative bacteria or *Candida albicans*. There was, however, growth inhibition for all of the Gram-positive bacteria tested, some with the lowest dilution concentration of 0.1 μg/mL. Hyperforin was also shown to be effective at inhibiting methacillin-resistant *Staphylococcus aureus*.

Along with antibacterial properties, it has also been reported that both the hypericin and pseudohypericin components of St. John's wort have antiviral properties. In vitro studies showed antiviral activity against cytomegalovirus, *Herpes simplex*, human immunodeficiency virus (HIV) type I. Influenza virus A, moloney murine leukemia virus, and sindbis virus. Hypericin and pseudohypericin are thought to work by inhibiting viral replication via disruption of the assembling and processing of intact virions from infected cells. Mice coinjected with 150 μg of hypericin/pseudohypericin and the Friend virus had a 100% survival rate at 240 days whereas all control mice that were only injected with the virus were dead by day 23. Animals treated with lower doses (10 and 50 μg) were also protected, but not to the same degree. In an in vitro study, HeLa cells carrying HIVcat transcriptional units were incubated at concentrations of 25, 50, and 100 μg/mL of hypericin and 100 μg/mL of *Ginkgo biloba*, then exposed to ultraviolet (UV) light. It was found that hypericin inhibited the UV-induced HIV gene expression by 50, 81, and 88% correlating with the 25, 50 100 μg/mL concentrations when compared to control cells (g2). *G. biloba* inhibited the UV-induced HIV gene expression by 19%. The first study with St. John's wort in people with HIV was halted because of phototoxicity; further studies are on the way. When the first study in patients with AIDS was stopped, no significant improvements were seen in CD4 counts, HIV titer, HIV-RNA copies, or HIV p24 antigen levels. Flavonoid and catechins in St. John's wort have been shown to have some activity against influenza virus.

Mutagenicity

Quercetin, a flavonoid component of St. John's wort and several other medicinal plants, has been implicated as a mutagen. However, St. John's wort aqueous ethanolic extract showed no mutagenic effects in mammalian cells. Tests used included the HGPRT (hypoxanthine guanidine phosphoribosyl transferase) test, the UDS (unscheduled DNA synthesis) test, the cell transformation test using Syrian hamster embryo cells, the mouse-fur spot test, and the chromosome aberration test using Chinese hamster bone marrow cells.

Neuropathic Pain

Neuropathic pain is commonly treated with tricyclic antidepressants. Although generally efficacious, these drugs do have the potential to cause serious side effects. A crossover trial was conducted in which participants received St. John's wort standardized to 2700 μg of hypericin per day or placebo for 5 weeks, with a 1-week washout period between treatments. Patients rated several types of pain on a scale of 1–10. A total of 47 patients completed the trial, which showed a trend toward lower total pain with the St. John's wort treatment; however, it was not statistically significant. There was also a trend toward people reporting moderate to complete pain relief during their treatment with St. John's wort. When the study population was further broken down into patients with and without diabetes, it was found that in the 18 participants with diabetes, there was still a trend toward lower total pain and a significant reduction in lancinating pain, whereas in the 29 participants without diabetes, there was no significant differences or trends in any pain scores. Interestingly, 25 participants preferred the St. John's wort treatment arm, 16 preferred placebo, and six did not have a preference.

Inflammation/Asthma

There are many articles that address the role of St. John's wort in inflammation. As previously mentioned, St. John's wort is an inhibitor of IL-6, which is an important cytokine involved in inflammation. Additionally, hyperforin was found to inhibit cyclooxygenase (COX)-1 and 5-lipoxygenase (5-LO), key enzymes in the formation of proinflammatory eicosanoids. Moreover, it inhibited both enzymes at IC50 concentrations of 0.09 to 3 μM, which is close to the plasma concentrations achieved with standard dosing. Hyperforin was three times more potent then aspirin in its ability to inhibit COX-1 and almost equipotent to zileuton in its ability to inhibit 5-LO. Hyperforin did not significantly inhibit COX-2, 12-LO, or 15-LO enzymes. St. John's wort's ability to act as a 5-LO inhibitor could lead to a future role in asthma.

Another way that St. John's wort may reduce inflammation is by reducing inducible nitric oxide synthase (iNOS), which is increased in the early phases of inflammation. Nuclear factor-κB (NF-κB) and signal transducer and activator of transcription-1α (STAT-1α) are both implicated in inducing iNOS leading to the production of nitric oxide (NO), which is produced in large amounts near areas of inflammation. St. John's wort was found to inhibit STAT-1α, thereby reducing both iNOS and NO formation. Surprisingly, St. John's wort did not inhibit NF-κB, which was shown in earlier reports to be inhibited by quercetin, a component of St. John's wort.

Atopic Dermatitis

After it was found that St. John's wort, and more specifically hyperforin, has an inhibitory effect on epidermal langerhan cells, there was speculation that it may treat atopic dermatitis. A 4-week trial was conducted in which 21 patients with mild to moderate atopic dermatitis were treated twice daily with a cream standardized to 1.5% hyperforin on one side of their body and placebo on the other side. The primary end point of the study was severity scoring of atopic dermatitis (SCORAD) index, based on extent and intensity of erythema, papulation, crust, excoriation, lichenification, and scaling. Among the 18 participants that completed the study, the SCORAD index fell from a baseline score of 44.9 to 23.9 in the hyperforin group. The SCORAD index also fell from 43.9 to 33.6 in the placebo group.

These results show statistically significant superiority of hyperforin cream over placebo, with no difference in skin tolerance to the two treatments. Of note, a secondary end point of the study showed a reduction of skin colonization with *S. aureus* with both hyperforin and placebo, with a trend toward better antibacterial activity with hyperforin cream. Although these results are positive, further studies should be conducted comparing hyperforin to corticosteroids in the treatment of atopic dermatitis.

Antioxidant

Free radicals are highly reactive molecules that have been implicated in cardiovascular and neurodegenerative disease. Hunt et al. generated superoxide radicals in both cell-free and human placental tissue to determine if St. John's wort has antioxidant qualities. They then tested St. John's wort samples that were standardized to either hypericin or hyperforin. In cell-free studies, both samples had a prooxidant effect at a 1:1 concentration. Both showed an inverse dose-related relationship in their antioxidant effect at concentrations from 1:2.5 to 1:20, with 1:20 having the greatest antioxidant effect in both groups. St. John's wort standardized to hypericin was superior in its antioxidant properties compared with hyperforin. Both were shown to be significant antioxidants in human placental vein tissue at a 1:20 dilution, the only concentration tested owing to results in the cell-free experiments.

Premenstrual Syndrome

There are numerous accounts of anecdotal evidence supporting the use of St. John's wort for *premenstrual syndrome* (PMS). One open, uncontrolled study was conducted to determine the efficacy of St. John's wort in treating PMS. The primary outcome was measured by a daily symptom check-list of 17 symptoms rated on a scale of 0 to 4 based on the *Hospital Anxiety and Depression* (HAD) scale and modified Social Adjustment Scale (SAS-M) broken down into four subscales: mood, behavior, pain, and physical. A total of 25 women were selected to participate in the study in which they received 300 mg hypericum standardized to 900 μg hypericin daily The results from the daily symptoms survey after the first cycle show a statistically significant reduction from the baseline value of 128.42 to 70.11. After the second cycle, there was a further reduction to 42.74. Of the four subscales, St. John's wort had the greatest improvement on the mood subscale (57%) and the least improvement on the physical subscale (35%). Of the individual symptoms, crying (92%) and depression (85%) were improved the most with treatment, and food cravings and headaches were improved the least.

Tumor Growth Inhibition

Hypericin, as mentioned earlier, is a fluorescent photosensitizer. When subjected to UV light, hypericin produces singlet oxygen, a nonradical oxygen species, which is highly reactive and cytoxic. In vitro studies with hypericin have shown significant growth inhibition in various human malignant cells, and in vivo studies demonstrate that it accumulates in bladder tumor cells when injected intravesically. In vivo studies were conducted in rats with transitional cell carcinoma of the bladder. Rats who were given hypericin IV and then photo-irradiated had their tumors eliminated in 15 days. Further studies could demonstrate success in human models with lower toxicity than current therapies such as bacillus Calmette-Guerin immunotherapy. It is also thought that other agents present in St. John's wort have cytotoxic qualities. When human erythroleukemic cells (K562) (human chronic myelogenous leukemia) were incubated with purified hypericin in the dark, there was only a weak inhibitory effect on cell growth and no apoptotic effect. When K562 cells were incubated with various extracts of *Hypericum*, there was significantly more growth inhibition and apoptosis. Extracts of *Hypericum* that were high in flavonoid content and low in hyperforin content had significantly greater growth-inhibitory activity compared to extracts with similar hypericin content, but low flavonoid and high hyperforin content. This supports earlier work that flavonoids have antiproliferative effects on malignant cell lines. Additionally, when the same extracts that were incubated in the dark were incubated with 7.5 J/cm^2 light activation, the IC50 values were lowered by roughly half, further demonstrating the phototoxic effects of hypericin. The mechanism of action of hypericin appears to be a combination of inhibition of protein kinase C, free-radical induction, release of mithochondrial cytochrome-c, and the activation of procaspase-3. The flavonoids also appear to increase caspase activity and release of cytochrome-c.

PHARMACOKINETICS/TOXICOKINETICS

Two pharmacokinetic studies have examined the pharmacokinetics of hypericin and pseudohypericin. Standardized hypericum extract LI 160 was used in both trials. In Part I of the studies, subjects in both trials were administered a single dose of either 300, 900, or 1800 mg of the extract (one, three, or six coated tablets) at 10- to 14-day intervals. Each dose contained 250, 750, or 1500 μg of hypericin and 526, 1578, or 3156 μg of pseudohypericin, respectively. The doses were administered on an empty stomach in the morning after a 12-hour fast. Subjects fasted for an additional 2 hours after administration. Multiple plasma levels of hypericin and pseudohypericin were measured for up to 120 hours after administration. In addition, urine samples were collected in the study performed by Kerb and colleagues. After a 4-week washout from Part I, subjects were given one coated tablet containing 300 mg of hypericum extract three times a day (8 AM, 1 PM, and 6 PM) before meals for 14 days. Blood samples were obtained over the 2-week dosing period.

Absorption

For single doses of 300, 900, or 1800 mg of dried hypericum extract in humans, the median time between administration of the dose and detectable plasma concentration (t_{lag}) in hours were as follows:

- Hypericin: 2.6, 2.0, and 2.6
- 2.1, 1.9, and 1.9
- Pseudohypericin: 0.6, 0.4, and 0.4
- 0.5, 0.4, and 0.4

A difference was observed between the t_{lag} of hypericin compared with pseudohypericin. These differences may be a function of the dosage form given. Pseudohypericin may be released from the dosage form more quickly than hypericin. Also, hypericin and pseudohypericin may be absorbed in different locations in the gastrointestinal tract. Another explanation may be that hypericin may undergo first-pass hepatic metabolism.

The median maximum plasma concentrations (C_{max}) in g/L for the respective doses were as follows:

- Hypericin: 1.5, 7.5, and 14.2
- 1.3, 7.2, and 16.6
- Pseudohypericin: 2.7, 11.7, and 30.6
- 3.4, 12.1, and 29.7

The maximum plasma concentrations increased in a nonlinear fashion.

The median time to peak plasma concentration (T_{max}) in hours for the corresponding doses were as follows:

- Hypericin: 5.2, 4.1, and 5.9
- 5.5, 6.0, and 5.7
- Pseudohypericin: 2.7, 3.0, and 3.2
- 3.0, 3.0, and 3.0

Overall no correlation was observed between dose and T_{max}. However, hypericin took longer to reach maximum plasma concentration. This corresponds with the lag time data.

After multiple dosing of 300 mg of *Hypericum* extract three times daily, the data for median C_{max} and trough plasma concentration (C_{min}) were as follows:

- Hypericin: C_{max} 8.5 μg/L
- C_{max} 8.8 μg/L
- C_{min} 5.3 μg/L
- C_{min} 7.9 μg/L
- Pseudohypericin: C_{max} 5.8 mg/L
- C_{max} 8.5 mg/L
- C_{min} 3.7 mg/L
- C_{min} 4.8 mg/L

Distribution

For oral doses, the volume of distribution appears to be approx 162 L for hypericin and 63 L for pseudohypericum.

Metabolism/Elimination

The median half-lives in hours for single 300, 900, and 1800 mg oral doses were as follows:

- Hypericin: 24.8, 26.0, and 26.5
- 24.5, 43.1, and 48.2
- Pseudohypericin: 16.3, 36.0, and 22.8
- 18.2, 24.8, 19.5

After multiple doses of *Hypericum* extract 300 mg three times daily, median half-lives in hours were:

- Hypericin: 28.0
- 41.3
- Pseudohypericin: 23.5
- 18.8

The data in these two studies differ in regard to the elimination half-life of hypericin. It is difficult to ascertain whether the half-life for either hypericin or pseudohypericin is dose related.

Neither hypericin, pseudohypericin, their glucuronic acid conjugates, nor their sulfate conjugates were detected in the urine. The chemical structure and molecular size (>500 Da) of hypericin and pseudohypericin suggest metabolism via hepatic glucuronidization followed by biliary excretion.

Adverse Effects and Toxicity

Although St. John's wort has proven to be relatively safe, there is still risk associated with its use and the development of adverse drug reactions (ADRs) can occur. The exact percentage of patients taking St. John's wort and developing an ADR varies greatly between studies. Observational studies report an incidence of ADRs to be between 1 and 3%. A German study with 3250 patients taking St. John's wort (Jarsin, 300 mg St. John's wort extract) found that 79 (2.43%) patients reported an ADR and 48 (1.43%) patients had to be treated for withdrawal symptoms. Of these ADRs, 18 (0.55%) were gastrointestinal effects, 17 (0.5 2%) were allergic/rash reactions, 13 (0.4%) were tiredness, eight (0.26%) were anxiety, five (0.15%) were confusion, and 18 (0.55%) were others, including two cases each of dry mouth, sleep disorders, palpitations, weakness, and worsening of concurrent disease, and one case each of heart flutter, circulatory complaints, irritability, visual disorders, disorders of micturition, burning eyes, euphoria, and nervous tension. Over a period from 1991 to 1999, the German ADR recording system received 95 reports of ADRs out of an estimated 8.5 million patients taking Jarsin. Of these, skin reactions were the highest-reported ADR with 27 reports. Other reported ADRs include an increased prothrombin time (16 cases), gastrointestinal complaints (9 cases), breakthrough bleeding with oral contraception (8 cases), decreased cyclosporine plasma levels (7 cases), tingling paraesthesias (4 cases), and cardiovascular symptoms (3 cases). All other ADRs reported had two or fewer reported cases. In a meta-analysis of placebo-controlled trials, the frequency of ADRs with St. John's wort is similar to those reported with placebo. In a comparison of trials where St. John's wort was compared to antidepressants, 26.3% of patients taking St. John's wort reported an ADR, whereas 44.7% taking a synthetic antidepressant reported an ADR.

Grazing animals that have consumed large amounts of St. John's wort have been reported to develop photosensitivity reactions. There are numerous case reports linking the use of St. John's wort to the development of severe rashes, both associated with and without light exposure. In the AIDS study previously mentioned, 11 out of 23 patients who were receiving 6–12 mg of hypericin IV developed severe phototoxic reactions. A multidose study with 40 participants was performed to assess the phototoxic effect of St. John's wort. Participants took two 300-mg tablets of hypericum extract three times daily for 15 days and were irradiated with a Dermalight-2001 lamp on days 1 and 15. The results of this study concluded that taking hypericum did reduce the median time for both tanning and erythema by 21%. Another study in cows found that hypericin in the presence of light induced photo-polymerization of the lens proteins crystallins α, β, and to a lesser degree, γ. These changes could potentially lead to the development of cataracts.

St. John's wort has also been associated with numerous neurological adverse effects. An acute psychotic delirium episode in a 76 year-old female was attributed to St. John's wort. She was taken to the hospital after having visual hallucinations of people in her home. She was taking no prescription or herbal medications besides one 75-mg capsule of St. John's wort daily for three weeks. More seriously, there have been several reported cases of serotonin syndrome associated with St. John's wort. A 33-year-old female on no other medications started taking St. John's wort. She took a single dose on the first day and two doses the next day. She awoke at 1:00 AM after the second day with extreme anxiety and nausea, and after going to the emergency department it was found that she had a *blood pressure* (BP) of 195/110 mmHg and a pulse of 122 *beats per minute* (BPM). Over the next 4 weeks, she had four additional episodes, although less severe. A 41 year- old male had an episode of delirium, with a BP of 210/140 mmHg and a heart rate of 115 BPM. He was not taking any medications other than the St. John's wort, which he started 7 days prior to the episode. Ten hours before the episode, he had consumed aged cheeses and one glass of red wine, the ingestion of which have been associated with hypertensive crisis with MAO inhibitors. Although the previous cases illustrate that St. John's wort alone can cause serotonin syndrome, there are even more reports of patients developing this syndrome when they are taking a synthetic antidepressant, such as a *selective serotonin reuptake inhibitor* (SSRI), and add St. John's wort. One case report involved a female who was taking paroxetine 40 mg a day for 8 months, then discontinued the paroxetine and started taking St. John's wort 600 mg daily. On day 10, she had difficulty sleeping and took 40 mg of paroxetine. The next day she was found to be incoherent, groggy, slow-moving, and difficulty getting out of bed. There are also numerous case reports of hypomania and mania associated with St. John's wort.

There are several other case reports of different ADRs associated with St. John's wort consumption. A patient taking 1800 mg three times daily for 32 days discontinued her therapy because of a possible photosensitivity reaction. Within a day, she developed nausea, anorexia, retching, dizziness, dry mouth, chills, and extreme fatigue. Her symptoms peaked by the third day and gradually improved until they had completely resolved by the eighth day. Several patients taking St. John's wort have been reported to have elevated *thyroid-stimulating hormone* (TSH) levels. In a study where 37 patients with an elevated TSH level and 37 patients with a normal TSH were interviewed to determine if they had used St. John's wort, it was found that there was a probable association with St. John's wort and an elevated TSH, but this was not statistically significant. A man who had been taking St. John's wort for 9 months reported having a severely diminished libido, which resolved after he discontinued St. John's wort and began citalopram. Hair loss has also been associated with the use of St. John's wort is hair loss. A 24 year-old female who took 300 mg of St. John's wort three times daily began experiencing hair loss of the scalp and eyebrows after 5 months of therapy, with the hair loss continuing for 12 months.

Interactions

St. John's wort has been shown to have many interactions with other drugs. Although one study found that St. John's wort has no effect on the cytochrome P450 (CYP) enzyme system, most studies have shown it is a potent inducer of CYP3A4, and some studies have shown it induces CYP1A2 and CYP2C9. Other studies have not supported the induction of CYP1A2 and CYP2C9 by St. John's wort. Induction of CYP3A4 is of the greatest concern because it is an important enzyme involved with the metabolism of many prescription medications. Induction of CYP3A4 can lower serum concentrations of drugs taken in combination with St. John's wort, thus reducing the efficacy of the drug. In vitro studies have shown an inhibition of CYP2D6, 2C9, 3A4, 1A2, and 2C19. Hyperforin was shown to be a potent noncompetitive inhibitor of CYP2D6 and a competitive inhibitor of CYP2C9 and 3A4. Hypericum extracts and hyperforin have been shown to significantly induce activity of CYP3A4 in hepatocytes. Another study performed on human hepatocytes found that the hyperforin component in St. John's wort is responsible for the drug interactions caused by CYP450 induction, and the hypericin constituent doesn't seem to affect drug metabolism. Hyperforin has been shown to be a potent ligand for the pregnane X receptor, a nuclear receptor that regulates the expression of CYP3A4 and P-glycoprotein (Pgp). This significantly induces the activity of both systems. However, both hypericin and hyperforin can inhibit Pgp with acute treatment. Pgp is found in many tissues and actively pumps various drugs and natural products out of cells. Acute use of St. John's wort can lead to increased initial serum concentrations of drugs that use this transport pump. Chronic use of St. John's wort has the opposite effect and induces Pgp. Subjects treated with St. John's wort for 16 days had a 4.2-fold increase in Pgp expression. Induction of Pgp is important because it decreases the bioavailability of drugs that use the transporter.

There are numerous case reports where patients on a calcineurin inhibitor, such as cyclosporine or tacrolimus, began taking St. John's wort and developed significant reductions in plasma concentrations of the drugs. Both cyclosporine and tacrolimus are metabolized by the CYP3A4 enzyme system, and cyclosporine is also a substrate of Pgp. There are reports of acute graft rejections caused by low cyclosporine or tacrolimus serum concentrations in heart, liver, and kidney transplant recipients who were taking St. John's wort.

There are also reports of complications associated with the combined use of oral contraceptives and St. John's wort owing to enzyme induction. The most frequent complication is breakthrough bleeding, although there are also reports of unwanted pregnancies.

Patients with AIDS who are taking protease inhibitors and nonnucleoside reverse transcriptase inhibitors are at risk of being subtherapeutically treated because these drugs are metabolized by CYP3A4. Studies have shown that combined use of St. John's wort and indinavir reduced the area under the curve (AUC) of indinavir by 57%. The same held true for nevirapine with an increased oral clearance of 35%, thus significantly lowering the exposure to the drug.

Patients taking voriconazole to treat a fungal infection may also be at risk of being subtherapeutically treated if they are concurrently taking St. John's wort. One study found that the administration of St. John's wort caused a brief, clinically insignificant increase in voriconazole blood levels followed by a significant long-term reduction in voriconazole concentrations. The AUC of voriconazole was reduced by 59% after 15 days of 900 mg St. John's wort extract taken daily. This was assumed to be caused by voriconazole being metabolized by CYP3A4 and 2C19.

Imatinib mesylate, a drug recently approved for the treatment of *chronic myeloid leukemia* (CML), can also be affected by St. John's wort. Because imatinib is primarily metabolized by CYP3A4 and is also a Pgp substrate, the usage of St. John's wort in combination with imatinib has resulted in a significant reduction in exposure to the drug compared to imatinib alone. This is potentially significant because therapeutic outcomes for patients with CML have been shown to correlate with the dose and drug concentrations of imatinib.

Another enzyme system that St. John's wort has been found to affect is topoisomerase II (Topo II). Hypericin was found to be an inhibitor of cleavage complex stabilization by Topo II inhibitors, used in cancer chemotherapy. Hypericin seems to intercalate into or distort DNA structure, precluding Topo II binding and/or DNA cleavage. Because hypericin appears to antagonize Topo II-poisoning chemotherapy drugs, concomitant usage of these medications could inhibit the antitumor effects of these drugs.

There have also been several reports of delayed emergence from anesthesia; decreased *international normalized ratios* (INRs) in patients taking warfarin; and decreased drug levels of digoxin, buspirone, methadone, mephenytoin, chlorzoxazone, and some benzodiazepines with concomitant use of St. John's wort.

Reproduction

There have been only limited studies in humans and only rare anecdotal evidence of St. John's wort' s effects on reproduction and lactation. A study using hamster oocytes incubated in either 0.06 or

0.6 mg/mL of hypericum extract for 1 hour showed normal sperm penetration at the lower concentration, whereas no penetration occurred at the higher concentration. Sperm incubated in the same concentrations for 1 week demonstrated sperm DNA denaturation and decreased viability with both concentrations. None of these effects have been seen in vivo. In vitro testing using animal uterine tissue showed weak uterine tonus-enhancing activity, but there have been no reports of abortions in animals or humans taking St. John's wort. A study using female mice fed 180 mg/kg hypericum extract or placebo starting 2 weeks prior to pregnancy and lasting until delivery demonstrated that the birth weight of the male offspring was significantly lower in the hypericum arm compared to placebo (1.67 g vs 1.74 g), but the weights were equivalent by day 3. There was no difference in female weights. There were no differences in mice of both genders in any other areas measured, including body length, head circumference, sexual maturation, or attainment of developmental milestones.

A case report involving a 38-year-old female who was in a major depressive episode began taking St. John's wort at 24 gestational weeks and continued with the therapy until delivery. The pregnancy was generally unremarkable, with a relatively mild case of late onset thrombocytopenia and neonatal jaundice that developed at day 5 and responded to treatment. The child was 7 Ibs 8 oz, had Apgar scores of 9 at 1 and 5 minutes, normal physical and laboratory results, and normal behavioral assessments at 4 and 33 days.

Postpartum depression is a relatively common occurrence in women after childbirth. One female who started taking 300 mg of St. John's wort three times daily after meeting the *Diagnostic and Statistical Manual of Mental Disorders,* criteria for major depressive episode 5 months after delivery agreed to have milk samples tested. Hypericin was not detected in the milk samples, but hyperforin was detected at low concentrations, with higher levels in the hind-milk than the foremilk samples. The milk/plasma ratio was well below one for both hypericin and hyperforin. Both levels were undetectable in the infant's serum and the baby showed no negative side effects. A larger study that involved 30 women who were taking St. John's wort and breastfeeding compared results to women who were not taking St. John's wort. There were no differences in maternal events, including duration of breastfeeding, decreased lactation, or maternal demographics. Women taking St. John's wort did report a significantly higher level of infant side effects, such as lethargy and colic, vs one case of infant colic in

97 women not taking St. John's wort. None of these infants required medical attention.

Regulatory Status

The proposed United States Pharmacopoeia National Formulary (USP-NF) monograph for hypericum requires that products contain a minimum of 0.04% of hypericins.

The German E Commission has approved St. John's wort for internal consumption for psychogenic disturbances, depressive states, sleep disorders, and anxiety and nervous excitement, particularly that associated with menopause. Oily *Hypericum* preparations are approved for stomach and gastrointestinal complaints, including diarrhea. Oily *Hypericum* preparations are also approved by the Commission E for external use for the treatment of incised and contused wounds, muscle aches, and first degree burns. The USP advisory panel recognizes that St. John's wort has a long history of use. However, because of a lack of well-controlled clinical trials its use is not recommended.

14

KAVA

Kava is a term used to describe both *Piper methysticum* and the preparation made from its dried rhizome and root. This South Pacific plant is a robust, branching, perennial shrub with heart-shaped, green, pointed leaves that grows up to 28 cm long and flower spikes that grow up to 9 cm long. The shrub grows best in warm, humid conditions with lots of sunlight, at altitudes of 150–300 m above sea level, where it forms dense thickets. Kava reproduces vegetatively, without fruit or seeds, usually under cultivation. There are reports of up to 72 varieties of the kava plant, which differ in appearance, and chemical analysis has shown differences in their composition as well, which may lead to differences in physiological activity.

Kava has been described in the European literature since the early 1600s, when it was taken there by the Dutch explorers LeMaire and Schouten, who had acquired it while seeking new passages across the Pacific. Captain James Cook was the first to describe the use of kava during the religious and cultural ceremonies of the people of the South Sea Islands, where it was, and still is, prepared as a beverage and consumed for its intoxicating, calming effects that promote sociability. Thus, kava is used for the purposes that Western society uses alcohol, the Native American populations use peyote, and the people of the Middle or Far East use opium. Events typically accompanied by kava ceremonies included weddings, funerals, births, religious occasions, seasonal feasts, reconciliations, welcoming of royalty or other guests, and the exchange of gifts. Women and commoners seldom participated in these ceremonies because that was viewed as unacceptable; however, some cultures did permit use by commoners to relax after a hard day's work.

The beverage was traditionally made by mixing grated, crushed, or chewed fresh or dried root with cool water or coconut milk and then straining the mixture through plant fibers to isolate the liquid, which was consumed. However, all parts of the plant can be used. Today the beverage is most often prepared by crushing dried roots with a large mortar and pestle, then straining the mixture in the traditional way or through cotton cloth. Other folk uses of kava have included treatment of headaches, colds, rheumatism, sexually transmitted diseases, and inflammation of the uterus. It has also been used as a sedative, aphrodisiac, urinary antiseptic, wound healing agent, and a treatment for asthma. Several substances extracted from the roots were also used briefly in Europe as diuretics.

Current Promoted Users

Kava is currently promoted for relief of anxiety, stress, and insomnia. Stress may be prolonged and difficult to cope with and affected individuals may suffer from insomnia. Kava has been promoted as an axiolytic agent with little risk for dependence or adverse reactions. An unblinded, comparative, crossover trial of kava (120 mg) and valerian (600 mg) was conducted, each agent administered for 6 weeks with a 2-week wash-out period between. This was followed with administration of a combination of the two compounds.

Both stress and insomnia were measured regarding social, personal, and life events. Results: the severity of stress was equally relieved by each of the two compounds and there was further improvement of insomnia with combination therapy. With kava, 67% of the subjects reported no adverse events, 53% denied adverse events with valerian, and likewise with combination therapy. Vivid dreams were experienced by 21% of subjects taking combination therapy and 16% of those taking valerian alone. Dizziness or gastric discomfort was reported by 3%. The investigators concluded the results were extremely promising but recommended additional studies.

Sources and Chemical Composition

P. methysticum, kava-kava, awa, kew, tonga, kawa, yaqona, sakau, ava, ava pepper, intoxicating pepper.

Products Available

Kava is available from a variety of manufacturers in most health food stores under a variety of names. Kavatrol is a popular brand found in retail outlets in the United States. Kava is marketed in Europe under a variety of names including Laitan or Kavasporal in Germany,

Potter's Antigian Tablets in the United Kingdom, Viocava in Switzerland, and Mosaro in Austria.

PHARMACOLOGICAL/TOXICOLOGICAL EFFECTS

Neurological Effects

The neurological effects of kava are attributed to a group of substituted dihydropyrones called *kava lactones*. The main bioactive constituents include yangonin, desmethoxyyangonin, 11-methoxyyangonin, kavain (kawain), dihydrokavain, methysticin, dihydromethysticin, and 5,6-dehydromethysticin. It is believed that the components present in the lipid-soluble kava extract, or kava resin, are responsible for the *central nervous system* (CNS) activities of kava including sedation, hypnosis, analgesia, and muscle relaxation. Aqueous kava extract was not active orally in mice or rats.

A randomized, 25-week, placebo-controlled study by Volz and Kieser showed a significant benefit from the use of kava-kava extract WS 1490 over placebo in treating anxiety disorders of nonpsychotic origin. The study included 101 patients suffering from agoraphobia, specific phobia, generalized anxiety disorder, or adjustment disorder with anxiety—as per the *Diagnostic and Statistical Manual of Mental Disorders*—who were randomized to placebo or WS 1490 containing 90–100 mg dry extract per capsule three times daily. The main outcome criterion, the patients' score on the Hamilton Anxiety Scale, was significantly better ($p < 0.001$) for the WS 1490 patients compared to placebo at 24 weeks. Few adverse effects were judged to be related or possibly related to kava administration. Two patients in the WS 1490 group experienced stomach upset, two noted vertigo, and one experienced vertigo and palpitations. These results support use of kava as an alternative to antidepressants and benzodiazepines.

Pittler and Ernst conducted a review of double-blind, randomized, placebo-controlled trials of kava extract monotherapy for treatment of anxiety. They reviewed 14 such studies and three were determined suitable for metaanalysis. They concluded that kava extract was not only relatively safe but superior to placebo in the treatment of anxiety.

Another study compared the cognitive effects of this same kava extract at a dose of 200 mg three times daily for 5 days to oxazepam 15 mg, followed by 75 mg on the experimental day. The results suggest that kava is less likely to affect cognitive function than oxazepam, but the oxazepam dosing regimen used was not typical of that seen in practice. Nevertheless, kava is purported to promote relaxation and sleep without dampening alertness, causing heavy sedation, or causing a "*hangover*" effect the morning after consumption. The limbic structures of the brain might represent the site of action of kava, explaining its ability to promote relaxation and sleep without cognitive effects.

The mechanism of the anxiolytic effect of kava is unclear. Studies of kava' s effects in vitro, in vivo, and ex vivo report conflicting results in regard to kava's effects on benzodiazepine or γ-aminobutyric acid (GABA) receptors. This disparity may be explained by differences in GABA receptor subtypes among the different regions of the brain studied. It is thought that kavapyrones elicit a tranquilizing effect by enhancing GABA binding in the amygdala, but do not act directly as agonists at GABA receptors.

One study has suggested that a nonstereoselective inhibition of [^{3}H]noradrenaline uptake may be responsible for, or at least contribute to, kava' s anxiolytic effect. This investigation tested the effects of naturally occurring (+)-kavain, (+)-methysticin, and a synthetic racemic mixture of kavain on synaptosomes from the cerebral cortex and hippocampus of rat brains.

Both forms of kavain inhibited [^{3}H]noradrenaline uptake more than methysticin, but the concentrations necessary to achieve this effect were approx 10 times higher than those in mouse brains after a dose of kavain high enough to cause significant sedation. This indicates that inhibition of noradrenaline uptake is probably only part of the psychotropic effects of kava. No effects were seen on the uptake of [^{3}H]serotonin. A subsequent study in rats showed that (+)-kavain and other kavapyrones affect serotonin levels in the mesolimbic area. The authors postulated that this effect could explain kava's hypnotic action. Dopamine levels in the nucleus accumbens were decreased by yangonin and low-dose (+)-kavain, but were increased by higher doses of (+)-kavain and desmethoxyyangonin. The investigators attributed kava's anxiolytic and euphoric effects to its action on mesolimbic dopaminergic pathways.

A study conducted in Germany indicates that kava may have neuroprotective properties, primarily owing to its constituent methysticum and dihydromethysticum. The investigators studied the effects of kava extract WS 1490 and the individual pyrones kavain, dihydrokavain, methysticin, dihydromethysticin, and yangonin on the size of infarction in mouse brains. The extract as well as the individual pyrones methysticin and dihydromethysticin showed significant reductions in infarct area similar to those produced by memantine, an anticonvulsive agent known to have neuroprotective qualities.

Kava lactones are also centrally acting skeletal muscle relaxants. A study by Kretzschmar et al. compared the antagonistic effects of kavain, dihydrokavain, methysticin, and dihydromethysticin to those of mephenesin and phenobarbital in preventing convulsions and death caused by strychnine. All the kava pyrones showed an antagonistic effect, with methysticin being the most potent; however, kavain and dihydrokavain doses required to produce an effect approached the toxic range. In contrast to mephenesin and phenobarbital, all the pyrones tested protected against strychnine at doses up to 5 mg/kg without causing impairment of motor function. Gleitz et al., in their studies on the antiseizure properties of kavain, conclude that the inhibition of voltage-dependent Ca^{++} and Na^{+} channels by kavain resembles that of local anesthetics. They suggest kava pyrone accumulation in neuronal cell membranes may explain the antieleptic affects of kava.

Kava also produces analgesic effects that appear to be mediated through a nonopiate pathway. A study conducted by Jamieson and Duffield compared the activity of an aqueous and a lipid extract of kava as well as eight purified pyrones on two tests for antinociception in mice. Both the aqueous and lipid extracts were effective analgesics, as were four of the eight purified pyrones (lactones): methysticin, dihydromethysticin, kavain, and dihydrokavain. In hopes of discovering the mechanism of analgesia, the investigators attempted to antagonize the effects of kava with naloxone, a known inhibitor of opiate-mediated pathways of analgesia. Naloxone failed to inhibit kava's effects at doses high enough to inhibit the action of morphine, indicating that kava works through a nonopiate pathway to produce analgesia.

In humans, kava is reported to produce a mild euphoria characterized by happiness, fluent and lively speech, and increased sensibility to sounds. It has also been reported to cause visual changes such as reduced near-point accommodation and convergence, increase in pupil diameter, and oculomotor balance disturbances. It might even have an antipyretic effect.

Tolerance and development of physical dependence by laboratory animals has been investigated for both the aqueous kava extract and kava resin, which contains the pharmacologically active pyrones. Duffield and Jamieson reported tolerance to be evident in mice only after parenteral administration of the aqueous kava extract, but not when given orally. Likewise, tolerance was not seen after daily dosing with kava resin over a 7-week period of time. They concluded tolerance to kava resin was not readily demonstrable.

Kava's effects on the peripheral nervous system are limited to a local anesthetic effect, resulting in numbness in the mouth if kava is chewed. Lipid-soluble kava extract, or resin, is also capable of causing anesthesia of the oral mucosa, whereas the water-soluble fraction is not.

Dermatological Effects

There have been many reports of skin disturbances associated with the use of kava that date as far back as the 1700s. Chronic ingestion of kava may cause a temporary yellowing of the skin, hair, and nails. Two yellow pigments, flavokawains A and B, have been isolated from the kava plant and may be responsible for this discoloration. Chronic ingestion may also lead to a temporary condition known as *kava dermopathy* or *kawaism*, characterized by dry, flaking, discolored skin and reddened eyes, which is reversible with discontinuation. In the early 19th century, Peter Corney, a lieutenant on a fur-trading vessel, described this phenomenon in great detail as it applied to the use of this side effect in treating other skin disturbances:

"When a man first commences taking it, he begins to break out in scales about the head, and it makes the eyes very sore and red, then the neck and breasts, working downwards, till it approaches the feet, when the dose is reduced. At this time the body is covered all over with white scruff, or scale, resembling the dry scurvy. These scales drop off in the order of their formation, from the head, neck, and body, and finally leave a beautiful, smooth, clear skin, and the frame clear of all disease".

The exact mechanism for this dermopathy is unknown, but it has been speculated that kava may interfere with cholesterol metabolism, leading to a reversible, acquired ichthyosis similar to that seen with the use of lipid-lowering agents such as triparanol. Skin biopsies of two recent cases associated with use of the commercially available product have revealed lymphocytic attacks on sebaceous glands, with subsequent destruction and necrosis caused by $CD8^+$ cells. Yet another theory involves interference with B vitamin metabolism or action.

Musculoskeletal Effects

As mentioned above, kava is a centrally acting skeletal muscle relaxant. The kava lactones kavain, dihydrokavain, methysticin, and dihydromethysticin isolated from kava rootstock were shown to antagonize strychnine-induced convulsions in mice.

Antimicrobial Activity

Kava has been used traditionally as an antibacterial agent in the treatment of urinary tract infections; however, no clinical trials have established its efficacy. Locher et al. investigated antiviral, antibacterial, and antifungal activity of extracts of Kava leaves, stems, and roots. They concluded that *P. methysticum* exerted no antiviral or antibacterial activity, although weak antifungal activity against *Epidermophyton fluccosum* was demonstrated by extracts made from the stems of the plant.

Antiplatelet Effects

Racemic kavain, a component of kava, has been shown to have antiplatelet effects, presumably owing to inhibition of cyclooxygenase, and thus inhibition of thromboxane synthesis. Antiplatelet effects have not been observed in vivo.

Cancer Prevention

Following the establishment of the South Pacific Commission Cancer Registry in 1977, interest abounded regarding the apparent dichotomy of high tobacco consumption and low cancer incidence of a number of South Pacific nations. Fugi, for example, has an age-standardized incidence rate of 75 cases per 100,000 males (112.2/100,000 females) compared to 237/100,000 males and 220/100,000 females in the United States. Both tobacco and kava are indigenous crops of these island nations. Men traditionally stop by kava bars to enjoy a bowl of kava on the way home from work. On the other hand, female consumption is highly variable. Data analysis reveals an inverse relationship between cancer incidence and kava consumption. A large difference exists between the age-standardized cancer incidence of these South Pacific island nations and that of the United States.

Pharmacokinetics

Absorption

In mice and rats, the aqueous kava extract is inactive when administered orally.

Metabolism/Elimination

Several kava lactones have been identified in human urine samples after ingestion of a kava beverage prepared from a commercial 450-g sample of *P. methysticin* extracted with 3 L of room temperature water. Observed metabolic transformations include reduction of the 3,4 double bond and/or demethylation of the 4-methoxyl group on the α-pyrone ring system. Demethylation of the 12-methoxy substituent in yangonin and hydroxylation at carbon 12 of desmethoxyyangonin have also been observed.

Case Reports of Toxicity Caused by Commercial Kava Products

In addition, two cases of dermopathy have recently been associated with commercially available kava products. A 70-year-old man who had been using kava as an antidepressant for 2–3 weeks experienced itching, and later erythematous, infiltrated plaques on his chest, back, and face after several hours of sun exposure. Skin biopsy revealed CD8 lymphocytic infiltration with destruction of the sebaceous glands and lower infundibula. A 52-year-old woman presented with papules and plaques on her face, chest, back, and arms after taking a kava extract for 3 weeks. Skin biopsy revealed an infiltrate in the reticular dermis with disruption and necrosis of the sebaceous gland lobules. A kava extract patch test was strongly positive after 24 hours.

There have also been four cases of extrapyramidal effects associated with kava use. A 28-year-old man with a history of antipsychotic-induced extrapyramidal effects experienced torticollis and oculogyric crisis 90 minutes after a single 100-mg dose of Laitan (kava extract). These effects resolved spontaneously after 40 minutes. A 22-year-old woman experienced oral and lingual dyskinesia, painful twisting movements of the trunk, and torticollis 4 hours after a 100-mg dose of the same product taken by the previously described male. The symptoms did not resolve spontaneously, so after 45 minutes, a 2.5-mg intravenous dose of beperiden was given, with immediate relief. A third patient, a 63-year-old female, also presented with oral and lingual dyskinesia after taking Kavasporal Forte (150 mg of kava extract) three times a day for 4 days. A single 5-mg intravenous dose of beperiden was immediately effective.

Recently, an association of kava and Parkinsonism has been noted. A 45-year-old healthy woman, absent any signs of Parkinson's disease but with a family history of essential tremor, was prescribed fluoxetine and benzodiazepines for depression. Approximately 3 months later, she developed severe Parkinson's disease after 10 days use of kava extract.

Finally, a 76-year-old woman experienced worsening of Parkinson's disease symptoms after taking Kavasporal Forte for 10 days. Improvement was noted 2 days after discontinuation of the product. These extrapyramidal side effects suggest cautious use of kava in the elderly, in patients with Parkinson's disease, and in patients taking antipsychotics.

Toxicity Associated with Traditional Use by Native Populations

Chronic use of the kava beverage has been associated with a wide range of abnormalities. A study of an Australian Aboriginal community revealed malnutrition and weight loss associated with kava use. Red blood cell volume increased in proportion to kava use, whereas bilirubin, plasma protein, platelet volume, B-lymphocyte count, and plasma urea were inversely proportional to kava consumption. Although these values were not outside the normal range, it was hypothesized that malnutrition or reduced hemoglobin turnover might explain these observations. Other findings included hematuria and difficulty acidifying and concentrating the urine, suggesting an effect on the renal tubules; and increased serum transaminases and increased high-density lipoprotein cholesterol, suggesting some effect on the liver.

Transaminase elevations were greater in the kava-using Aboriginal community compared to those in a community where alcohol, but not kava, was consumed. This suggests that kava might be more hepatotoxic than alcohol. Shortness of breath and electrocardiograph abnormalities (tall P waves) consistent with pulmonary hypertension were seen and are interesting in that, like kava, the prescription anorexiants fenfluramine and dexfenfluramine withdrawn from the US market in 1998 were associated with pulmonary hypertension. It was also noted by the authors of this observational study that sudden death in relatively young men is more common in kava-using Aboriginal communities than in nonusing communities.

In the United States and Europe, evidence of hepatic failure following the use of kava extracts is accumulating. A 50-year-old male, who had previously been well, experienced liver failure after consuming kava extract for 2 months. The dosage of kava extracts was at or slightly exceeded the maximum three-capsule-a-day dose recommended on the label. A liver transplant was performed and the individual survived.

A healthy 14-year-old adolescent girl developed nausea, vomiting, general malaise, and weight loss. Several days later she became icteric and was admitted to hospital with acute hepatitis. Drug history revealed no alcohol use; two kava products and occasional ibuprofen had been used over the preceding 4 months.

The packaging of the kava products was unavailable for identification purposes. Liver biopsy revealed active fulminant hepatitis with extensive necrosis and tests for viral hepatitis were negative. She underwent a successful liver transplantation and was able to return to normal activity upon recovery. Unfortunately, no information was provided indicating that acetaminophen toxicity had been ruled out, and the observed toxic effect could also have been associated with a large, undiagnosed acetaminophen ingestion.

A 33-year-old woman took 210 mg of kava extract for 3 weeks and discontinued the product. After 2 months, she resumed taking the same product for an additional 3-week period. Symptoms of hepatotoxicity developed a day after ingesting 60 mL of alcohol. Tests for viral hepatitis were negative and liver biopsy revealed evidence of hepatic necrosis. Phenotyping of CYP4502D6 activity with debris oquine was consistant with deficiency of this enzyme. Her liver function returned to normal 8 weeks after kava discontinuation.

A US Food and Drug Administration (FDA) advisory letter dated March 25, 2002 warned health care providers of a total of 11 patients who had used kava products and developed liver failure requiring liver transplantation. Additionally, there have been 25 reports of severe liver toxicity in Germany, Switzerland, and the United States. The prevalence of CYP4502D6 deficiency in such cases has yet to be determined.

Interactions

Alcohol appears to at least add to the hypnotic effect of kava in mice, and was also observed to increase the lethality of kava. These findings may be of importance because some Australian Aboriginal populations now frequently consume kava with alcohol. Concomitant use of barbiturates, melatonin, and other psychopharmacological agents might potentiate the effects of kava as well. The hepatotoxic potential of kava also raises concerns about concomitant alcohol use.

Although a Web site promoting a kava product states that it is safe to use kava in combination with benzodiazepines, a case report suggests otherwise. The combination of kava and alprazolam was believed to be responsible for hospitalizing a 54-year-old man. The patient's semicomatose (lethargic and disoriented) state improved after several hours. He had been taking an undisclosed brand of kava purchased in a health food store in combination with alprazolam for 3 days. Other medications taken included cimetidine and terazosin.

In vitro evidence suggests that kava components may inhibit the metabolism of drugs by cytochrome P450 1A2, 2C9, 2C19, 2D6, 2E1, and 3A4. However, in vivo studies were not confirmatory except for the case of CYP2E1. Gurley and colleagues studied the ability of kava to inhibit in vivo metabolism by several of these enzymes and found that kava coadministration had no effect on CYP1A2, CYP2D6, or CYP3A4 activity but did significantly inhibit CYP2E1 activity. Because very few drugs are metabolized by CYP2E1, the clinical significance of this interaction is lessened. It appears that pharmacokinetic interactions with kava are unlikely and any drug interactions will likely be related to an additive pharmacodynamic effect (e.g., sedation).

Reproduction

No information is available concerning the potential effects of kava on reproduction.

Regulatory Status

Kava is currently sold as a dietary supplement in the United States, though an FDA advisory warning concerning the potential for liver toxicity was issued in 2002. Germany had banned the sale of kava in 2002 but the ban was lifted in 2005. A number of countries have either banned the sale of kava or issued warnings concerning its use.

15

PANAX GINSENG

Panax ginseng is a perennial herb that starts flowering in its fourth year. It grows in the United States, Canada, and the mountainous forests of eastern Asia. The translucent, yellowish-brown roots are harvested when plants reach between 3 and 6 years of age. This herb has been used in the Orient for 5000 years as a tonic. According to traditional Chinese medicine's "*philosphy of opposites*," American ginseng (*Panax quinquefolius* L.) is a "cool" or "yin" tonic used to treat "hot" symptoms such as stress, insomnia, palpitations, and headache, whereas Asian ginseng (*P. ginseng* L.) is "hot" or "yang" and is used to treat "cold" diseases. In the Orient, ginseng is considered a cure-all. This stems from the "*Doctrine of Signatures*," because the root is said to resemble a man's appearance and is therefore useful to treat all of man's ailments. Throughout history, the root has been used as a treatment for asthenia, atherosclerosis, blood and bleeding disorders, colitis, and relief of symptoms associated with aging, cancer, and senility. Ginseng is also widely believed to be an aphrodisiac.

CURRENT PROMOTED USES

Ginseng is promoted as a tonic capable of invigorating the user physically, mentally, and sexually. It is also said to possess antistress activity, or to serve as an "*adaptogen*," improve glycemic control and stimulate immune function. Claims that ginseng can improve athletic performance, enhance longevity, or treat toxic hepatitis are not supported by human trials.

SOURCES AND CHEMICAL COMPOSITION

Korean ginseng, Asian ginseng, Oriental ginseng, Chinese ginseng, Japanese ginseng, American ginseng. Note that the term "ginseng" can refer to the species of the genus *Panax*, as well as to *Eleutherococcus senticosus*. Unless otherwise noted, the information in this monograph refers specifically to species of the genus *Panax*. Depending on the particular botanical reference, there are three to six different species of *Panax* ginseng, and three with purported medicinal benefits: *P. ginseng*, *Panax pseudoginseng*, and *Panax quinquefolium*. In this chapter, the term "*Panax ginseng*" will be used to refer to these species, and "*Siberian ginseng*" will be used to refer to *E. senticosus*. The chemical composition of Siberian ginseng differs from that of *P. ginseng*; thus, the distinction between the two is important in a discussion of therapeutic and adverse effects.

PRODUCTS AVAILABLE

Two commercial forms of the herb are available. "White" ginseng consists of the dried root and "red" ginseng is prepared by steaming the fresh, unpeeled root before drying. Many different formulations of the herb are available including capsules, gelcaps, powders, tinctures, teas, slices to eat in salads, and whole root to chew. There are also a wide variety of products that claim to contain ginseng such as ginseng cigarettes, toothpaste, cosmetics, soaps, beverages (including beer), candy, baby food, gum, candy bars, and coffee. Prices vary widely based on the quantity and quality of the ginseng root used. Tinctures are more expensive but last for years. Powder capsules are cheaper but have a shelf-life of only 1 year.

One of the problems in the manufacture of ginseng is the lack of quality control and standardization. Although the amount of ginsenosides, the purported active ingredients, ranges widely among brands and often differs from the content stated on the label, testing by Consumer Reports revealed that the amount of ginsenosides in Ginsana, the ginseng market leader in the United States, is well standardized. The manufacturer claims that each Ginsana capsule contains 100 mg of standardized, concentrated ginseng. A study of the Swedish Ginsana product revealed consistency in ginseno side content between batches. Ginsana is available in the United States in softgel capsules and chewy squares. The capsules are green because chlorophyll is added.

Other brands of ginseng are most commonly available in capsule or tablet form and are usually brown. Dosage strengths normally range between 50 mg and 300 mg of *P. ginseng* extract per capsule or tablet. Also, several combination products are available. For example, Ginkogin is a combination of Panax ginseng, Ginkgo biloba, and garlic. There are other types of ginseng on the market including Siberian,

Brazilian, and Indian ginseng. These are not of the genus *Panax* and do not contain ginsenosides.

PHARMACOLOGICAL/TOXICOLOGICAL EFFECTS

Endocrine Effects

P. ginseng may exert hypoglycemic effects possibly by accelerating hepatic lipogenesis and increasing glycogen storage. In a study of 36 newly diagnosed patients with type II diabetes, ginseng at a dose of 200 mg daily exerted a statistically significant benefit on glycosylated hemoglobin (HbA1c) compared to 100 mg of ginseng daily or placebo after 8 weeks of therapy, and patients receiving 100 mg of ginseng had smaller mean fasting blood glucose levels than patients taking 200 mg of ginseng or placebo. The actual difference among the mean HbA1c in the three groups was small; the 200-mg ginseng group had a mean glycosylated hemoglobin of 6 vs 6.5% for the 100-mg ginseng and placebo groups. Likewise, the actual difference among mean fasting blood glucose in the three groups was small; the mean fasting blood glucose was 7.7 mmol/L for the 100-mg ginseng group, 7.4 mmol/L for the 200-mg ginseng group, and 8.3 mmol/L for the placebo group at the end of the study. The observed differences might be attributed to differences in body weight among the three groups. The small study sample limits the generalizability of these results.

Vuksan and colleagues observed that whether given concurrently or prior to glucose challenge in patients with type 2 diabetes, ginseng blunted the glycemic response by approx 20%. In nondiabetic individuals, reduction in glycemic response was only noted when ginseng was administered 40 minutes prior to the glucose challenge. In a related study, investigators demonstrated that dose of ginseng but not timing of administration resulted in a statistically significant reduction in post-prandial glycemia in patients with type 2 diabetes following a glucose challenge. At 120 minutes postchallenge, reductions in incremental glycemica as much as 60% were noted. Again, these same investigators studied 10 nondiabetic individuals who received different doses of ginseng at different times prior to glucose challenge. Compared with placebo, all doses of ginseng reduced the glycemic response up to 90 minutes in some cases.

However, time of administration had no effect. Ironically, these same investigators later reported that the effect of ginseng on postprandial glycemia in healthy individuals was time of administration-dependent but not dose-dependent, conflicting with their previous reports.

Vuksan and colleagues reported that a batch of ginseng that was lower in ginsenosides than previous batches had no effect on postprandial glycemia. Finally, it has been reported that different types of ginseng can have differing effects on postprandial glycemia (decreasing, null or increasing) and that these divergent effects may be related to the ginsenoside composition in the preparations. Thus, at the present time, it is difficult to predict the effects of ginseng administration on glycemia because varying effects may be noted depending on the composition and preparation of the ginseng.

All the ginsenosids (saponins) so tested have shown antifatigue actions in mice. This may reflect the purported "*adaptogenic*" action of ginseng, which can be defined as an increase in resistance to stresses and is thought to be secondary to normalization of body processes through regulation of the production of various hormones. In evaluating the administration of Siberian ginseng for treatment of chronic fatigue syndrome, Hartz and colleagues found no measurable positive effect in those individuals receiving ginseng as compared to subjects receiving placebo.

With respect to increasing exercise performance, Hsu and colleagues reported that ginseng attenuated the formation of creatine kinase induced by submaximal exercise in subjects undergoing a treadmill test. However, no increase in aerobic work capacity was noted. In a related study of exercise performance effects, Siberian ginseng administration had no effect on steady-state substrate utilization or any physiological measure in individuals undergoing prolonged cycling exercise. The study was conducted in a randomized, double-blind, placebo-controlled fashion and followed 7 days of treatment with either ginseng or placebo.

Ginseng appears to have a modulating effect on the hypothalamic-pituitary-adrenal axis by inducing secretion of adrenocorticotropic hormone from the anterior pituitary to increase plasma cortisol, perhaps accounting for improvement in 11 quality of life measurements in a large double-blind study using ginseng extract G115.

Although many products containing ginseng are marketed specifically for postmenopausal women, a recent review concluded that there is insufficient evidence that ginseng is effective for treatment of menopausal symptoms. In vitro, Siberian ginseng extract, but not *P. ginseng* extract, binds to estrogen receptors. Both extracts have affinity for progestin, glucocorticoid, and mineralocorticoid receptors. A recent study reported that a morning/evening formulation containing ginseng and other constituents relieved menopausal symptoms, but no placebo control was included so it is difficult to tell whether the effect was caused by the formulation or a placebo effect.

Neurological Effects

Commercially available *P. ginseng* products have been reported to have stimulant effects on the *central nervous system* (CNS) in humans. In animal models, ginseng extracts have been shown to have CNS-stimulant effects. Ginsenoside Rg1 inhibits neuronal apoptosis in vitro, and ginsenoside Rb1 reverses short-term memory loss in rats.

It has been suggested that ginseng may hold promise for the treatment of dementia in humans. To this end, a number of studies have been performed to evaluate the effects of ginseng on cognition. Wesnes and colleagues studied the memory-enhancing effects of either *P. ginseng* or *Ginkgo biloba* in healthy middle-aged volunteers. These investigators found that administration of either agent resulted in a small but statistically significant improvement in the Index of Memory Quality (~7.5%) as compared to placebo. In a similar study, another group studied the effects of either ginseng, *G. biloba*, or the combination on the modulation of cognition and mood in healthy young adults. These investigators found that all three treatments improved secondary memory performance and that ginseng administration elicited some improvement in the speed of performing memory tasks and the accuracy of attentional tasks.

Only ginkgo elicited a self-rated improvement in mood. Scholey and Kennedy again studied the effects of *P. ginseng* and *G. biloba* on several tests of cognitive demand. Increasing doses of ginseng improved accuracy but slowed responses on the Serial Sevens test and the combination product caused a sustained improvement in the number of Serial Sevens responses. This was accompanied by improved accuracy on this same test, again in a dose-dependent fashion. These same investigators later conducted a study of the effects of *P. ginseng* as compared to guarana in several cognitive performance tests. Again, ginseng administration led to an improvement the speed of attention task performance, but little evidence of increased accuracy was noted.

However, two studies have also suggested that administration of ginseng (or a combination of ginseng and *G. biloba*) has no effect on cognition (and mood). Hartley and colleagues evaluated the effects of a 6- or 12-week course of a ginkgo/ginseng combination product on the mood and cognition of postmenopausal women. Subjects were administered a battery of mood, somatic anxiety, sleepiness, and menopausal symptom tests. The Gincosan treatment had no measurable effect on any parameter. In a similar study of ginseng administration, investigators found no effect of ginseng on positive affect, negative affect, or total mood disturbance in a randomized, placebo-controlled, double-blind trial. Persson and colleagues studied the memory-enhancing effects of either ginseng or *G. biloba* taken over a sustained period of time (mean intake time of 5.3 months) in healthy community-dwelling volunteers. No improvement in memory performance evaluated by eight separate tests was noted in either the group receiving ginseng or the group receiving *G. biloba*. Thus, it appears that conflicting results still exist as to the ability of ginseng to improve memory and cognition; however, even in those studies demonstrating a positive effect, the enhancement was generally small in magnitude.

The administration of ginseng has also been studied in the treatment of *attention-deficit hyperactivity disorder* (ADHD). Lyon et al., conducted a pilot study ($n = 36$) evaluating the effects of a combination product containing ginseng and ginkgo for the treatment of ADHD. The investigators reported improvement in 31–67% of the subjects depending on the outcome measure; however, no placebo control was included, so it is difficult to ascertain if the effect was caused by the treatment or a placebo effect.

Cardiovascular Effects

In animal studies, ginsenoside Rb1 decreases blood pressure, perhaps owing to relaxation of smooth muscle. In humans, small studies suggest ginseng may decrease systolic blood pressure at a dose of 4.5 g/day, and enhance the efficacy of digoxin in class IV heart failure. In contrast, ginseno side Rg1 has been purported to have hypertensive effects. Finally, it has been reported that ginseng has no effect on blood pressure in individuals with hypertension.

An in vitro study using a crude extract of ginseng saponins and rabbit corpus-cavernosal smooth muscle suggests that some component of ginseng may be a nitric oxide donor, capable of causing relaxation of smooth muscle in the corpus carvernosum. This finding might provide a scientific basis for claims that ginseng enhances sexual potency, and for the results of a study that showed increased penile rigidity and girth compared to placebo or trazodone in patients with erectile dysfunction.

Red ginseng powder may be useful in hyperlipidemia; it was shown to decrease triglycerides as well as increase high-density lipoprotein (HDL) in a pilot study. A previous rat study lends validity to ginseng's ability to decrease triglyceride levels, but a study in patients with diabetes showed no effect on total cholesterol, low-density lipoprotein (LDL), HDL, or triglyceride levels.

Hematological Effects

P. ginseng may inhibit platelet aggregation by regulating the levels of cGMP and thromboxane A2.

Immunological Effects

Red ginseng stimulates accumulation of neutrophils in a dose-dependent manner following intraperitoneal injections in mice. Data show *P. ginseng* extracts are also able to stimulate an immune response in humans. Chemotaxis of polymorphonuclear cells was increased compared to placebo. Both the phagocytosis index and fraction were enhanced in the ginseng groups and intracellular killing was increased compared to the placebo group. Total lymphocytes and helper T-cells were increased as well. There have been other reports of increases in cell-mediated immunity as well as natural-killer cell activity.

Predy and colleagues evaluated the ability of ginseng to prevent upper respiratory infections in a randomized, placebo-controlled trial. Administration of ginseng for 4 months resulted in a reduction in both the mean number of colds experienced, the number of individuals experiencing two or more colds, and the total number of days of cold symptoms. Similarly, McElhaney et al. studied the ability of ginseng to prevent acute respiratory illness in institutionalized older adults. The incidence of confirmed influenza cases was lower in the ginseng-treated group as compared to placebo treatment.

Antineoplastic Effects

Data from in vitro studies, animal models, case-control studies, and cohort studies suggest ginseng may prevent or ameliorate various cancers. These studies have been reviewed in detail elsewhere. Suh and colleagues studied the effects of red ginseng on the recurrence of cancer after curative resection in patients with previous gastric cancer during postoperative chemotherapy. Survival rate was approximately twice that of control, but placebo treatment was not used. Prospective, placebo-controlled studies of ginseng's ability to prevent or treat cancer are lacking.

Case Reports of Toxicity Caused by Commercially Available Products

In 1979 the term "*ginseng abuse syndrome*" (GAS) was coined as the result of a study of 133 people who had been using a variety of ginseng preparations for at least 1 month. Most study subjects experienced CNS excitation and arousal. A total of 14 patients experienced GAS, defined as hypertension, nervousness, sleeplessness, skin eruptions, and morning diarrhea. Five of these subjects also exhibited edema. The effects of ginseng on mood appeared to be dose-dependent; four patients experienced depersonalization and confusion at doses of 15 g, and depression was reported following doses greater than 15 g. A total of 22 subjects experienced hypertension. All of the patients experiencing GAS or hypertension were also using caffeinated beverages. Six other subjects also experienced GAS but were considered "*atypical*" because they were either using Siberian ginseng instead of *P. ginseng*, or were injecting ginseng, and thus were not included in the study results. One subject experienced anaphylaxis followed by confusion and hallucinations after injection of 2 mL of ginseng extract. The average daily dose of the 14 patients experiencing GAS was 3 g of ginseng root, and most users reported titrating the dose to minimize nervousness and tremor. One subject experienced hypotension, weakness, and tremor when ginseng use was abruptly discontinued. The author compared ginseng's effects to those of high doses of corticosteroids. GAS seemed to be found predominantly during the first year of use, possibly because by the 18-month follow-up visit, ginseng use had declined to an average of 1.7 g daily, and by the 24-month visit, one-half of the patients with GAS had discontinued ginseng use, and 21% of the remaining subjects had stopped using it. Eight subjects were still experiencing diarrhea and nervousness at the 2-year follow-up. Because this study was not controlled, the existence of GAS has been questioned.

Hypertension, shortness of breath, dizziness, inability to concentrate, a loud palpable fourth heart sound, "*thrusting*" apical pulse, and hypertensive changes on fundal examination were reported in a 39-year-old man who had taken various ginseng products for 3 years. His blood pressure measured 140/100 mmHg on three occasions over 6 weeks, and when referred for management of his hypertension it was 154/106 mmHg. He was advised to discontinue the ginseng products, and 5 days later was normotensive at 140/85 mm Hg. At 3-month follow-up, he remained normotensive and his other symptoms had resolved. No attempt was made to confirm the identity or composition of the ginseng products.

An episode of Stevens-Johnson syndrome was reported in a 27-year-old man following ginseng administration (two pills a day for 3 days). Infiltration of the dermis by mononuclear cells was noted. The patient recovered completely within 30 days.

An association between ginseng and mastalgia has been reported. A 70-year-old woman developed swollen, tender breasts with diffuse nodularity after using a *P. ginseng* powder for 3 weeks. Symptoms ceased following discontinuation of the herb and reappeared with two additional rechallenges. Prolactin levels were within normal limits.

A 72-year-old woman experienced vaginal bleeding after taking 200 mg daily of a Swiss-Austrian geriatric formulation of ginseng for an unspecified time. In a similar case, a 62-year-old woman had undergone a total hysterectomy 14 years previously and had been taking Rumanian ginseng alternating with Gerovital every 2 weeks for 1 year. The patient derived a marked estrogenic effect from the product based on microscopy of vaginal smears as well as the gross appearance of the vaginal and cervical epithelium. The patient was dechallenged from the products for 5 weeks, rechallenged with Gerovital for 2 weeks, then rechallenged with ginseng for 2 weeks. Estrone, estradiol, and estriol levels were essentially unchanged over this time period, but the estrogenic effects on the vaginal smear coincided with ginseng use. Using gas chromatography, the investigators found no estrogen in the tablets the patient had been taking. They did discover that a crude methanolic extract of the ginseng product competed with estradiol for the estrogen and progesterone binding sites in human myometrial cytosol.

A 44-year-old woman who had experienced menopause at age 42 experienced three episodes of spotting associated with use of Fang Fang ginseng face cream. Interestingly, these episodes of bleeding were associated with a decrease in follicle-stimulating hormone levels and a disordered proliferative pattern on endometrial biopsy. The woman discontinued use of the cream and experienced no further bleeding. Whether the products used in these reports of vaginal bleeding and mastalgia contained *P. ginseng* or Siberian ginseng (*E. senticosus*) was not investigated. Whether *Panax* or Siberian ginseng causes estrogenic effects requires further study.

Maternal ingestion of 650 mg of Siberian ginseng twice daily was associated with androgenization in a neonate. The product had been taken for the previous 18 months, including the pregnancy. During pregnancy, the mother noted increased and thicker hair growth on her head, face, and pubic area, and had experienced repeated premature uterine contractions during late pregnancy. At birth, the Caucasian child weighed 3.3 kg, had thick black pubic hair, hair over the entire forehead, and swollen red nipples. The woman continued to take the ginseng product for 2 weeks after the baby's birth, during which time she breast-fed the baby. She was advised to discontinue the product when the baby was 2 weeks old, and his pubic and forehead hair began to fall out. By 7.5 weeks of age, hair was scant, but his testes were enlarged. Weight gain was 1.1 kg during the first 3.5 weeks of life, and 1.4 kg during the next 3.5 weeks. At age 7.5 weeks, his weight (5.8 kg), length (60.6 cm), and head circumference (41.5 cm) were at or above the 97th percentile. At that time, testosterone, 17-hydroxyprogesterone, and cortisol levels were normal. Subsequent information did not confirm the product's androgenic effects. A sample of the raw material used in manufacturing the preparation used by this patient was identified as *Periploca sepium*, not Siberian ginseng. No androgenic effects were noted in rats administered the manufacturer's sample. *P. sepium* was reported previously to be mislabeled as Siberian ginseng, perhaps owing to similarities in the Chinese terms for these herbs.

Drug Interactions

A probable interaction between warfarin and apanax ginseng product has been reported. A 47-year-old man with a St. Jude-type mechanical aortic valve had been controlled on warfarin with an *international normalized ratio* (INR) of 3.1 (goal 2.5–3.5). He experienced a subtherapeutic INR of 1.5 following 2 weeks of ginseng administration. Other medications included 30 mg of diltiazem three times daily, nitroglycerin as needed, and 500 mg of salsalate three times daily as needed. He had been on all of these medications for at least 3 years before the abrupt change in his INR. Discontinuation of ginseng resulted in an increase in INR to 3.3 within 2 weeks. In this regard, a randomized, double-blind, placebo-controlled trial was undertaken to study the effects of ginseng on warfarin and INR. Coadministration of ginseng statistically significantly reduced the INR by –0.19 (95% confidence interval, –0.36 to –0.07) as well as reduced the INR area under the curve (AUC) and the AUC of warfarin. It should be noted that this study involved healthy volunteers and though they received ginseng for 2 weeks, they only received warfarin for three days prior to administration of ginseng and thus, steady-state warfarin concentrations were not likely achieved. In contrast, an open-label, randomized, three-way crossover study evaluated the effects of 1 week of either ginseng or St. John's wort on the INR and pharmacokinetics of warfarin following a single dose of warfarin 25 mg. These investigators found no effect of ginseng on either the INR or the pharmacokinetics of (S)-warfarin (the more active enantiomer) or its (S)-7- hydroxywarfarin metabolite.

In a phenotypic trait measure study of effects of various herbal preparations on cytochrome P450 enzyme activity, Gurley and colleagues evaluated the effects of ginseng administration on CYP1A2, CYP2D6, CYP2E1, and CYP3A4 activity in healthy human volunteers. Metabolism of probe drugs for each of these enzymes was studied in the absence and presence of ginseng administered for 28 days. Ginseng administration had no effect on the metabolism of any of the probe drugs, suggesting that ginseng administration will not result in drug interactions with drugs metabolized by CYP1A2, CYP2D6, CYP2E1, or CYP3A4. However, the enzyme that is responsible for the metabolism of (S)-warfarin is CYP2C9 and was not evaluated in this study. These findings of lack of effect on CYP2D6 and CYP3A4 were corroborated by a similar study that found no effect of ginseng administration on the activity of either of these two enzymes.

Manic-like symptoms were reported in a patient treated with phenelzine and ginseng. The symptoms disappeared with cessation of the herbal therapy. Users should also exercise caution if ginseng is taken in combination with caffeinated beverages, hypertension and nervousness have been reported when the two are combined.

Although Siberian ginseng is not of the same genus as *P. ginseng*, it may be confused with and substituted for *P. ginseng*, and thus a discussion of drug interactions with Siberian ginseng is warranted. Siberian ginseng has been reported to inhibit the metabolism of hexobarbital in mice by 66%. Siberian ginseng ingestion was associated with elevated digoxin levels in a 74-year-old man whose digoxin levels had been maintained between 0.9 and 2.2 ng/L (normal, 0.6–2.6 ng/L) for more than 10 years. He was asymptomatic for digoxin toxicity despite a level of 5.2 ng/L. Electrocardiogram, potassium level, and serum creatinine level were normal. The level decreased on dechallenge and increased on rechallenge. The product was analyzed for digoxin or digitoxin contamination, but none was found. The product was not analyzed to determine if it did in fact contain Siberian ginseng. It was hypothesized that some component of Siberian ginseng might impair digoxin elimination or interfere with the digoxin assay. The type of digoxin assay used in this case was not specified. To this end, the effect of different types of ginseng on assays of digoxin concentration has now been studied extensively. These investigators observed that apparent digoxin-like immunoreactivity was observed when ginseng was studied with a *fluorescence polarization immunoassay* (FPIA) technique and modest immunoreactivity with *microparticle enzyme immunoassay* (MEIA) methods using serum spiked with ginseng. Interestingly, when serum from patients receiving digoxin was studied and ginseng was then spiked into the samples, falsely high digoxin concentrations were measured with FPIA but falsely lower concentrations were measured using MEIA. Using the Tina-quant assay, no interference was noted with any of the ginseng preparations.

PHARMACOKINETICS

The structures and nomenclature of the chemical constituents of Panax ginseng have been discussed elsewhere.

Absorption

β-Sitosterol is a steroid sapogenin that has been isolated from ginseng. Approximately 50-60% of a dose of β-sitosterol is absorbed from the gastrointestinal tract in rats. After oral administration of radiolabeled ginseno side Rg1, blood radioactivity peaked at 2.1 hours. Bioavailability was 49%.

Distribution

Studies of the distribution of [^{3}H]ginseno side Rg1 following intravenous injection have been performed in mice. Tissue radioactivity was greatest in the kidney, followed by the adrenal gland, liver, lungs, spleen, pancreas, heart, testes, and brain. Plasma protein binding was 24%, and tissue protein binding was 48% in the liver, 22% in testes, and 8% in the brain.

Metabolism/Elimination

The blood radioactivity decreased in a triphasic manner after intravenous injection of [^{3}H]ginsenoside Rg1 to mice. Other Chinese studies have characterized the biotransformation of ginsenoside 20(S)-Rg2, one of the main constituents of ginseng roots and leaves. Its metabolism is complex and involves multiple hydrolysis reactions in the gastrointestinal tract. Metabolites of 20(S)-Rg2 include 20(S)-Rh1 and 20(S)-protopanaxatriol. Details of the biotransformation of 20(S)-Rg2 and chemical structures of the ginsenosides are available in the cited reference.

Corroborating two rat studies suggesting that only trace amounts of ginsenosides are excreted in the urine, low levels of ginsenoside aglycones were identified using gas chromatography-mass spectroscopy to analyze urine samples of 65 athletes claiming to have ingested ginseng within the 10 days prior to urine collection. An aglycone (molecule from which the sugar moiety has been removed) of ginsenosides, 20(S)-protopanaxatriol, was found at concentrations between 2 and 35 ng/mL in approx 90% of the urine samples studied. Another aglycone, 20(S)-protopanaxadiol, was barely detectable despite the fact that the ginsenosides from which it is derived were the major ginsenosides found in the commercially available Swedish ginseng products analyzed by the investigators.

This indicates that these two ginsenosides have different pharmacokinetics. Because the actual amount of ginseng ingested and the time since ingestion were unknown, little else can be inferred from these data.

Regulatory Status

The German Commission E approves *P. ginseng* as a non-prescription drug for use as a "tonic for invigoration and fortification in times of fatigue and debility, for declining capacity for work and concentration, and also for use during convalescence. In the United States, ginseng is regulated as a dietary supplement.

16

Saw Palmetto

Saw palmetto is a dwarf palm tree that grows in Texas, Florida, Georgia, and southern South Carolina. The tree grows up to 6 feet tall and has wide leaves divided into fan-shaped lobes that are gray to blue-green in color. The plant produces purple-black berries from September to January.

The earliest known use of saw palmetto was in the 15th century BC in Egypt to treat urethral obstruction. The Native Americans also used saw palmetto to treat genitourinary conditions. In the early 20th century, it was used in conventional medicine as a mild diuretic and as a treatment for *benign prostatic hypertrophy* (BPH) and *chronic cystitis*. Historically, saw palmetto has also been used to increase sperm production, increase breast size, and increase sexual vigor. Early settlers in the United States observed that animals that ate the berries grew fat and healthy, and by the 1870s saw palmetto was purported to improve general health, reproductive health, disposition, and body weight, and to stimulate appetite.

Saw palmetto is promoted as a treatment for BPH, to improve prostate health and urinary flow, and to improve reproductive and sexual functioning, as well as stimulate hair growth.

Sources and Chemical Composition

Serenoa repens (Bartram) Small, *Sabal serrulata* (Michaux) Nichols, *Serenoa serrulatum* Schultes.

Products Available

Saw palmetto is commercially available alone and in combination products including capsules, gelcaps, and tablets. There are more than

100 commercial products containing saw palmetto as the sole ingredient or as a combination product.

PHARMACOLOGICAL/TOXICOLOGICAL EFFECTS

In Vitro/Animal Studies

Saw palmetto's benefits in treatment of BPH are hypothesized to be caused in part by antiandrogen effects. Saw palmetto is a multisite inhibitor of androgen action. In an in vitro study, a liposterolic saw palmetto extract called Permixon was shown to compete with a radiolabeled synthetic androgen for the cytosolic androgenic receptor of rat prostate tissue. Another in vitro study found that saw palmetto lipid extract inhibits 5α-reductase, the enzyme responsible for the conversion of testosterone to its active metabolite dihydrotestosterone (DHT); inhibits 3-ketosteroid reductase, the enzyme responsible for DHT metabolism to other active androgens; and blocks androgen receptors. Saw palmetto may also improve BPH signs and symptoms by inhibiting estrogen receptors in the prostate. A study of the effects of saw palmetto on cancer cell lines has demonstrated that saw palmetto can inhibit 5α-reductase activity without affecting *prostate-specific antigen* (PSA) expression, confirming that saw palmetto can be administered without interfering with this biomarker (PSA) of tumor progression. Finally, it has recently been demonstrated in vitro that saw palmetto extracts do not affect α_1-adrenoceptor subtypes, suggesting that its primary mechanism of action is on androgen metabolism.

An in vivo study in rats evaluated the effects of saw palmetto and cernitin (another natural product) and finasteride on prostate growth. In castrated rats who were given testosterone, all three treatments significantly reduced prostate size as compared to rats (castrated + testosterone) who were not given any treatment. Though finasteride produced the greatest effect on prostate size, no statistical difference was noted among any of the three treatments.

Anti-inflammatory effects of saw palmetto also have been hypothesized to improve BPH symptoms. An acidic, lipophilic saw palmetto extract was shown in vitro to inhibit both the cyclooxygenase and 5-lipoxygenase pathways, preventing the formation of inflammatory-producing prostaglandins and leukotrienes. Finally, saw palmetto has been purported to stimulate immune function.

Human Studies

Saw palmetto extract in a dose of 160 mg or placebo three times daily was administered to 35 elderly men, and prostatic tissue was collected. The investigators found that some component of the saw palmetto extract inhibits nuclear estrogen receptors in the prostates of patients with BPH patients.

Clinically, 160 mg of Permixon twice daily was superior to placebo in a double-blind trial in 110 men with BPH. A statistically significant ($p < 0.001$) benefit compared to placebo was seen in nocturia, flow rate, postvoid residual, self-rating, physician rating, and dysuria. Compared with baseline, both placebo and saw palmetto were beneficial in improving nocturia ($p < 0.001$), but only saw palmetto improved flow rate and postvoid residual compared to baseline ($p < 0.001$). Headache was the only adverse effect. A double-blind study compared Proscar (finasteride, a prescription 5α-reductase inhibitor), 5 mg daily, with Permixon, 160 mg twice daily for 6 months. Both finasteride and saw palmetto improved International Prostate Symptom Score (I-PSS) and quality of life compared to baseline, with no statistical difference between the two treatments. Finasteride improved peak urinary flow rate more than saw palmetto ($p = 0.035$), and residual volume was decreased more with finasteride than with saw palmetto ($p = 0.017$). Finasteride decreased prostate volume more than saw palmetto ($p < 0.001$), and only finasteride decreased PSA compared with baseline ($p < 0.001$). Although only one patient in each treatment group withdrew because of sexual problems, the finasteride patients experienced a statistically significant deterioration in the sexual function score compared with baseline ($p < 0.01$). Twice as many patients withdrew from the saw palmetto group because of side effects (28 vs 14), but there were no statistically significant differences noted between the two groups in regard to any adverse effect. Hypertension was the most common adverse effect, occurring in 3.1% of the saw palmetto patients and 2.2% of the finasteride patients. Other adverse effects included decreased libido, abdominal pain, impotence, back pain, diarrhea, flulike illness, urinary retention, headache, nausea, constipation, and dysuria. A drawback of this study is that no placebo group was included; more data on the efficacy of these two drugs compared to placebo are needed.

The findings of Carraro and colleagues discussed previously suggest that Permixon does not affect PSA. These results were confirmed by an in vitro study in which Permixon 10 μg/mL (calculated plasma concentration achieved with therapeutic doses), did not interfere with secretion of PSA. These findings imply that PSA can continue to be used for prostate cancer screening in men taking saw palmetto.

Another randomized, double-blind, placebo-controlled trial of saw palmetto for the treatment of lower urinary tract symptoms also demonstrated its usefulness in these types of conditions. These investigators studied 85 men, randomized to receive either saw palmetto or placebo for 6 months. Effectiveness was monitored using the I-PSS, a sexual function questionnaire and urinary flow rate. Results of these studies demonstrated that the I-PSS symptom score decreased (i.e., improved) from 16.7 to 12.3 in those subjects receiving saw palmetto, whereas the symptom score decreased from 15.8 to 13.6 in the placebo group ($p = 0.038$). No significant difference was noted in the quality of life component of the I-PSS. Also, no differences were noted in either the sexual function questionnaire score or peak urinary flow rate between the saw palmetto and placebo groups. This study demonstrated that saw palmetto administration for 6 months resulted in an improvement in symptoms associated with BPH but not in sexual function or peak flow rate.

Several well-conducted studies of saw palmetto effect on BPH symptoms have been conducted using combination products that may have additional active ingredients. Marks and colleagues evaluated the effectiveness of a saw palmetto herbal blend (saw palmetto, nettle root extract, pumpkin seed oil extract, lemon bioflavonoid extract, Vitamin A, and other minor ingredients) in subjects with symptomatic BPH. Using a double-blind, placebo-controlled trial design, 44 subjects were investigated ($n = 21$ in the saw palmetto herbal blend group and $n = 23$ in the placebo group) following treatment for 6 months. Prostate epithelial contraction was noted where percent epithelium decreased from 17.8% at baseline to 10.7% at 6 months in the saw palmetto herbal blend treatment group ($p < 0.01$). Saw palmetto treatment increased the percent of atrophic glands from 25% to 41% ($p < 0.01$). Neither treatment (saw palmetto or placebo) altered PSA or prostate volume. Another group of investigators studied the effect of saw palmetto herbal blend (same ingredients as previously mentioned) on nuclear measurements of DNA content in men with symptomatic BPH. Using nuclear morphometric descriptors (NMDs) (size, shape, DNA content, and textural features) of the nucleus of pro static tissue, 6-month treatment of saw palmetto herbal blend was compared to placebo control. After 6 months, 25 of the 60 NMDs were significantly different in the saw palmetto treatment group, whereas none were changed in the placebo group. These investigators then used four of these 25 altered NMDs to develop a multivariate model that was proposed to be predictive of treatment effect. These investigators proposed that saw palmetto herbal blend treatment alters the DNA chromatin structure and organization of prostate epithelial cells. Using a different combination formula containing saw palmetto (saw palmetto, cernitin, β-sitosterol, and Vitamin E), Preuss and colleagues conducted a 3-month randomized, placebo-controlled trial in 127 subjects of this formulation in the treatment of BPH symptoms. These investigators found that treatment with this saw palmetto-containing product results in a statistically significant decrease in nocturia severity ($p < 0.001$, daytime frequency ($p < 0.04$) and the American Urological Association symptom index was significantly improved ($p < 0.001$). No change in PSA measurements, maximal and average urinary flow rates, or residual volumes was noted. Furthermore, no adverse effects were noted in either group.

A number of studies evaluating the effects of saw palmetto on BPH and urinary symptoms have been conducted that lack placebo controls, comparing saw palmetto to another agent or looking at longitudinal effect. Kaplan and colleagues conducted a 1-year prospective trial of saw palmetto vs finasteride for the treatment of category III prostatitis/chronic pelvic pain syndrome. Finasteride significantly decreased (~25%) the National Institutes of Health Chronic Prostatitis Symptom Index score, whereas saw palmetto had no effect on this measure. Finasteride also improved quality of life and pain measures but not urination. These authors concluded that saw palmetto resulted in no appreciable long-term improvement in category III prostatitis/chronic pelvic pain syndrome. However, this study suffers from lack of placebo control. Al-Shukri et al. studied the effects of Permixon on lower urinary tract symptoms caused by benign prostatic hyperplasia. These investigators administered Permixon 160 mg twice daily for 9 weeks and compared the results to a control group who received no treatment at all. Permixon treatment increased maximum flow rate by 6% ($p < 0.001$), decreased maximum detrusor pressure by 12.8% ($p < 0.001$) and reduced residual urine volume by 12.6% ($p < 0.001$). Furthermore, the I-PSS and the quality of life score improved (26.8 and 18.2%, respectively) in treated patients. Control subjects exhibited no change in any of these parameters. Again, this study lacks a placebo treatment group to assess any possible placebo effects. Treatment with Permixon of symptoms related to BPH has also been evaluated in a 2-year study of effect on symptoms, quality of life, and sexual function. These investigators studied 150 men receiving Permixon 160 mg twice daily for 2 years. The I-PSS score improved by 41% at the end of 2 years. Approximately one-half of the subjects had improvements in obstructive and irritative symptoms, and a 40% improvement in quality of life score was noted. Again, no control group and no placebo group were used and thus any placebo effect could not be discerned.

A meta-analysis of randomized trials comparing saw palmetto to placebo or other therapy was recently published. The authors concluded that despite methodology problems, saw palmetto appears to improve urologic symptoms and urinary flow to an extent similar to that of finasteride, but with fewer adverse effects.

Interestingly, saw palmetto has also been studied in a randomized, double- blind, placebo-controlled trial for the treatment of androgenetic alopecia. Subjects received either active formulation or placebo for an average of 5 months. In the 10 subjects studied, six of the subjects (60%) were determined to have significant improvement in hair growth as assessed by both the investigators and the subject.

Adverse Effects and Toxicity

Clinical studies have reported very few adverse effects that are of a mild nature (usually gastric distress or headache) following saw palmetto administration at normal doses. One randomized, double-blind study of finasteride, tamsulosin, and saw palmetto for 3 months observed no differences among the three treatments in terms of the effectiveness measures and no change in sexual function in those individuals receiving saw palmetto, though ejaculation disorders were noted as the most common side effect in those individuals receiving either tamsulosin or finasteride.

Case Reports of Toxicity Caused by Saw Palmetto Products

A case of toxicity associated with the use of Prostata, a preparation containing saw palmetto, zinc picolinate, pyridoxine, L-alanine, glutamic acid, *Apis mellifica* pollen, silica, hydrangea extract, *Panax ginseng*, and *Pygeum africanum*, was reported in the Annals of Internal Medicine.

A 65-year-old man developed acute and protracted cholestatic hepatitis after taking Prostata. The man stopped taking the product after 2 weeks of use because he developed jaundice and severe pruritus. On physical exam, the patient's abdomen was not tender and his liver and spleen were not palpable. Lab results were as follows: bilirubin 8.2 mg/dL, aspartate aminotransferase 1238 IU/L, alanine aminotransferase 1364 IU/L, alkaline phosphatase 179 IU/L, γ-glutamyl transferase 391 IU/L, hematocrit 41%, leukocyte count $3.3 \times 10^3/$

mm^3, platelet count 153,000 cells/mm^3, serum protein 6.3 g/dL, albumin 3.6 g/dL, carcinoembryonic antigen less than 2 mg/μL. Serological testing was negative for hepatitis A virus immunoglobulin M (IgM), hepatitis B surface antigen, cytomegalovirus IgM, and hepatitis C virus antibodies. The patient was negative for antinuclear antibodies and antismooth muscle antibodies, but positive for antimitochondrial antibodies. Liver enzyme levels remained abnormal for more than 3 months. Liver biopsy was done after 2 months and showed parenchymal infiltrate of neutrophils and lymphocytes that involved the portal tracts, early bridging, and mild periportal fibrosis. There was no evidence of bile duct damage, cirrhosis, or granulomas. The authors postulated that the patient's cholestasis was an extension of saw palmetto's estrogenic or antiandrogen effect.

In another case report, a 53-year-old white male with meningioma developed intraoperative hemorrhage during surgery for resection of the tumor. During the surgery, the patient began experiencing substantial bleeding that was difficult to control. The patient was given 4 L of crystalloid fluids, 4 U of packed red blood cells, 3 U of pooled platelets, and 3 U of fresh frozen plasma. The estimated blood loss was approx 2000 mL. The patient had not received any preoperative thromboprophylaxis and all clotting tests were normal prior to the procedure. However, after surgery, the bleeding time was several times longer than normal and eventually became normal after 5 days. No medications that could have resulted in excessive bleeding were discovered as being taken; however, upon further questioning the patient disclosed that he had been taking saw palmetto for BPH, but had not mentioned it to the physician. A conclusive cause-effect relationship was not established, however.

Pharmacokinetics/Toxicokinetics

Limited pharmacokinetic data are available because saw palmetto is a mixture of various compounds. With respect to absorption of saw palmetto components, a mean peak plasma drug concentration of 2.6 mg/L of the "*second component*" with a high-performance liquid chromatography retention time of 26.4 minutes was measured in 12 healthy young men after a single oral dose of 320 mg of saw palmetto. The time to peak concentration occurred 1.5 hours after administration. A 640-mg rectal dose of saw palmetto extract produced a peak of 2.6 μg/mL occurring 3 hours after the dose. Rat studies indicate that prostate concentrations are higher than those achieved in other genitourinary tissues or in the liver suggesting selective distribution to tissues of interest. The elimination half-life of the "*second component*" discussed previously was 1.9 hours and the mean area under the concentration vs time curve (AUC) was 8.2 mg/(L·hour) after a single oral dose of 320 mg. The AUC of the "*second component*" produced by a 640-mg rectal dose of saw palmetto extract was 10 mg/(L·hour), and plasma levels were detectable up to 8 hours postdose.

Drug Interactions

A study of the in vitro ability of saw palmetto to inhibit the metabolic activity of cytochromes P450 3A4, 2D6, and 2C9 was recently studied. These investigators found that saw palmetto had no effect on the metabolism of model substrates of cytochrome P450 3A4 and 2D6. However, saw palmetto was noted to be a potent inhibitor of cytochrome P450 2C9 activity in vitro.

Two recent in vivo studies have attempted to evaluate the effect of saw palmetto administration on cytochrome P450 metabolic activity in humans. Markowitz and colleagues studied the ability of saw palmetto administration for fourteen days to inhibit the metabolism of dextromethorphan and alprazolam, probe substrates for cytochrome P450 2D6 and 3A4, respectively. This study in six male and six female healthy volunteers found no effect of chronic saw palmetto administration on the metabolism or elimination of either probe substrate and, thus, no effect on either cytochrome P450 2D6 or 3A4 activity. In a similar study, Gurley and colleagues evaluated the effect of saw palmetto on cytochrome P450 1A2, 2D6, 2E1, and 3A4 activity in vivo. A group of 12 healthy volunteers were administered saw palmetto for 28 days and phenotyped for each of the previously listed enzyme activities before and after saw palmetto administration. No significant effect of saw palmetto on any of the phenotypic ratios was noted, suggesting that saw palmetto has no effect on in vivo cytochrome P450 1A2, 2D6, 2E1, or 3A4 activity. These results of Markowitz et al. and Gurley et al. confirm the in vitro results of Yale and Glurich regarding these enzymes. However, no in vivo studies have been conducted to date to evaluate whether saw palmetto affects cytochrome P450 2C9 activity, as suggested by Yale and Glurich. This has particular clinical significance because warfarin and phenytoin (both agents with narrow therapeutic indices) are metabolized by P450 2C9. Thus, clinical studies to evaluate this potential interaction are needed.

Reproduction

Because of its potential effects on 5α-reductase enzymes, analogous to finasteride, saw palmetto should not be used during pregnancy.

Regulatory Status

The German Commission E lists saw palmetto as an approved herb. The berry is the only part of the plant approved for use. The approved uses include urination problems associated with BPH stages I and II and urination problems associated with prostate adenoma. This evaluation is based on reasonable proof of safety and efficacy.

Saw palmetto is considered a dietary supplement by the Food and Drug Administration. Saw palmetto was previously included in the National Formulary (NF) and the United States Pharmacopeia, but was deleted in 1950 and 1916, respectively. Saw palmetto was deleted because no active ingredient could be found to account for its use. Saw palmetto was again included in the NF as an official monograph in 1998.

17

Valerian

Valerian is a perennial herb comprised of grooved hollow stems and saw-toothed green leaves. White, pale pink, or reddish flowers appear from June to August. Valerian grows to heights of 3–5 feet in the temperate climates of North America, western Asia, and Europe, often in moist soil along riverbanks. The vertical rhizome and attached roots of valerian are parts used medicinally, and are best harvested in the autumn of the second year. Although the fresh drug has no distinctive odor, over time hydrolysis of compounds present in the volatile oil produces isovaleric acid, which has an offensive, somewhat putrid odor. Fortunately, the smell can be removed from the skin and utensils by washing with sodium bicarbonate. Even though valerian has a disagreeable odor, people in the 16th century considered it a fragrant perfume. Traditional uses include treatment of insomnia, migraine headache, anxiety, fatigue, and seizures. It has also been applied externally on cuts, sores, and acne. Traditional Chinese uses include treatment of headache, numbness caused by rheumatic conditions, colds, menstrual difficulties, and bruises. The pharmacological effects of valerian have been attributed to the constituents of volatile oils, monoterpenes, valepotriates, and sesquiterpenes (valerenic acid). Some of these constituents have been shown to have a direct action on the brain, and valerenic acid inhibits enzyme-induced breakdown of γ-amino butyric acid (GABA) in the brain resulting in sedation.

Current Promoted Uses

Valerian is promoted in the United States primarily as a sedative-hypnotic for treatment of insomnia, and as an anxiolytic for restlessness and sleeping disorders associated with anxiety.

Sources and Chemical Composition

Also referred to as: *Valeriana officinalis* (L.), *Valeriana wallichii* DC. (Indian valerian), *Valeriana alliariifolia Vahl*, *Valeriana sambucifolia Mik*, *Radix valerianae*, red valerian (*Centranthus ruber* [L.] DC), valerian root, *Valerianae radix*, garden heliotrope, all heal, amantilla, and setwall.

Products Available

Crude valerian root, rhizome, or stolon is dried and used either "as is" or to prepare an extract. Valerian is available as a capsule, tablet, oral solution, or tea. Valerian is also administered externally as a bath additive.

Pharmacological/Toxicological Effects

Insomnia

Several studies have examined the effects of valerian on sleep. Donath and colleagues performed a randomized, double-blind, placebo-controlled, cross-over study assessing the short-term (single dose) and long-term (14-day multiple dosage) effects of valerian extract on sleep structure and sleep quality. There were significant differences between valerian and placebo for parameters describing *slow-wave sleep* (SWS) and shorter sleep latency, with very low adverse events. Leathwood and colleagues demonstrated valerian's effect on sleep quality. A freeze-dried aqueous extract of valerian root (*Rhizoma valeriana officinalis* [L.]) 400 mg was compared to two Hova (valerian 60 mg and hop flower extract 30 mg per tablet) tablets and placebo (finely ground brown sugar) in this crossover study involving 128 volunteers. Study participants took the study medication 1 hour before retiring, and filled out a questionnaire the following morning. This was repeated on nonconsecutive nights, such that each of the three treatments, identified only by a code number, was administered in random order three times to each patient. Valerian caused a significant improvement in subjectively evaluated sleep quality and a significant decrease in perceived sleep latency. The self-reported improvement in sleep quality was especially notable in smokers, those patients who considered themselves poor or irregular sleepers, and those who reported having difficulty falling asleep on a prestudy questionnaire. Hova did not demonstrate any beneficial effect, but it was reported to cause a "*hangover effect*" the next morning. Because subjective sleep questionnaires may not correlate with sleep *electroencephalogram* (EEG) results, a parallel EEG sleep study was performed comparing valerian to placebo in 10 young men. There was not a statistically significant difference between valerian and placebo in this small study. The authors hypothesized that the results of this experiment might have differed from the questionnaire-assessed study because of small sample size and differences in study populations. The larger study involved young and older individuals, men and women, and good and poor sleepers, whereas the EEG study involved young men with no reported sleep abnormalities. Rather than place more credence on the objective study, the investigators concluded that the questionnaire provides a more sensitive means of detecting mild sedative effects.

A double-blind, placebo-controlled study was performed in eight volunteers recruited from among the research staff at Nestle Products and their families who reported that they "usually have problems getting to sleep." Sleep latency was measured using an activity monitor and questionnaire. The investigators documented a small (7 minute) but statistically significant decrease in sleep latency with 450 mg of an extract of valerian (*V. officinalis* [L.]). No further improvement was demonstrated with a 900-mg valerian dose; however, patients receiving the higher dose were more likely to feel sleepy the next morning. Sleep quality, sleep latency, and sleep depth also improved according to a nine-point subjective rating scale. However, the appropriateness of the statistical analysis used to interpret the results of the subjective portion of the study is unclear.

A more objective double-blind, placebo-controlled trial evaluated the effect of 450- and 900-mg doses of an aqueous valerian extract (*V. officinalis* [L.]) on two groups of healthy, young (21–44 years of age) volunteers at home and in a laboratory setting. The effect of valerian on sleep was measured using a questionnaire and night-time motor activity recordings in both settings. The effects of valerian on the volunteers in the sleep laboratory were also measured using polysomnography and spectral analysis of the sleep EEG. Both groups demonstrated the mild hypnotic effects of valerian; however, the benefits of valerian were statistically significant only under home conditions.

Another double-blind, placebo-controlled crossover study evaluated Valerina Natt, a preparation equivalent to 400 mg of valerian root composed mainly of sesquiterpenes from *V. officinalis* [L.], on subjective sleep quality assessed using a three-point rating scale. Study subjects were 27 consecutive patients seen in a medical clinic for evaluation of sleep difficulty and fatigue who were willing to participate in the investigation. Statistically significant improvement in sleep quality was noted with the valerian preparation. Valerian was rated as better than placebo by 21 subjects, two rated the preparations equally, and four preferred placebo. No adverse effects were reported. Although some study subjects had experienced nightmares when using conventional hypnotics, nightmares were not reported in the study.

The effects of repeated doses (three tablets three times daily) for 8 days of Valdispert Forte (135 mg of dried extract of *V. officinalis* [L.]) in 14 elderly women with sleeping difficulties was assessed using polysomnography in a particularly well-designed study. Inclusion criteria were well defined: sleep latency longer than 30 minutes, more than three nocturnal awakenings per night with inability to go back to sleep within 5 minutes, and total sleep time less than 5 hours. Subjects could not have medical, psychological, or weight-related causes of sleep difficulty, and had to have normal health status for their age. Sedatives, hypnotics, and other *central nervous system* (CNS)-active drugs were discontinued 2 weeks prior to the study, and drug screening for morphine, benzodiazepines, barbiturates, and amphetamine was done prior to study commencement. Results showed an increase in SWS, and a decrease in sleep stage 1. There was no effect on *rapid eye movement* (REM) sleep, sleep latency, time awake after sleep onset, or self-rated sleep quality.

In aggregate, the results of these clinical studies suggest that at doses of approx 450 mg of the aqueous extract, valerian has mild hypnotic effects, possibly by affecting non-REM sleep in patients with reduced SWS. Unlike benzodiazepines, valerian appears not to adversely affect SWS or REM sleep, and does not appear to cause nightmares or hangover. Further well-designed studies are needed to objectively evaluate valerian. Results of animal studies reflect the clinical data. Sedative properties of Valdispert (dried aqueous extract of *V. officinalis* [L.]) in mice were documented based on reduced spontaneous movement and an increase in thiopental-induced sleep time; however, these effects were slightly less than those of diazepam and chlorpromazine. No significant anticonvulsant effect was observed.

Hendriks and colleagues tested several components of the volatile oil, obtained by steam distillation of *V. officinalis* [L.], on mice. The essential oil, its hydrocarbon fraction, its oxygen fraction, valeranone, valerenal, valerenic acid, and isoeugenyl-isovalerate were injected intraperitoneally at various doses ranging from 50 to 1600 mg/kg, with three mice receiving each dose. The mice were observed between 15 and 30 minutes post-injection for various symptoms suggestive of CNS stimulation or depression, analgesia, sympathomimetic or sympatholytic activity, vasodilation, or vasoconstriction. It was concluded that components of the essential oil, particularly valerenic acid and valerenal, which are present in the oxygen fraction, have a sedative and/or muscle relaxant effect. The authors tested the effect of intraperitoneal valerenic acid compared to diazepam, chlorpromazine, and pentobarbital on ability to walk on a rotating rod and grip strength in mice. The effects of valerinic acid on spontaneous motor activity and on pentobarbital-induced sleeping time were also assessed. Diazepam, a muscle relaxant, affected the grip test but not the rotarod test, whereas chlorpromazine, a neuroleptic, affected the rotarod test but not the grip test. Valerenic acid, like pentobarbital, decreased performance in both the rotarod and grip tests. The authors concluded that valerenic acid, like pentobarbital, has general CNS depressant activity. Valerenic acid also decreased spontaneous motor activity and prolonged pentobarbital-induced sleeping time. Dose–response effects of valerenic acid were also observed by the investigators. At a dose of 50 mg/kg, a decrease in spontaneous motor activity occurred. At 100 mg/kg, mice exhibited ataxia, then remained motionless. Muscle spasms occurred at 150–200 mg/kg and convulsions at 400 mg/kg, followed by death in six of seven mice within 24 hours.

Sedation is mediated predominantly through the inhibitory neurotransmitter GAB A. Although the mechanism of action of valerian as a sleep aid is not fully understood, it may involve inhibition of the enzyme that breaks down GABA. Dihydrovaltrate, hydroxyvalerenic acid, a hydroalcoholic extract containing 0.8% valerenic acid; a lipid extract; an aqueous extract of the hydroalcoholic extract, and another aqueous extract of *V. officinalis* (L.) were assessed for in vitro binding to rat GABA, benzodiazepine, and barbiturate receptors. The results indicated that an interaction of some component of the hydroalcoholic extract, the aqueous extract derived from the hydroalcoholic extract, and the other aqueous extract had affinity for the $GABA_A$ receptor. Because hydroxyvalerenic acid (a volatile oil sesquiterpene) and dihydrovaltrate (a valepotriate) did not show any notable activity, the investigators could not identify the specific constituents responsible for this activity. The lipophilic extract derived from the hydroalcoholic extract, as well as dihydrovaltrate, showed affinity for barbiturate receptors, and some affinity for peripheral benzodiazepine receptors.

Other in vitro studies have also yielded results that suggest GABA-mediated activity; however, the active constituent was unidentified.

Cavadas and colleagues verified that valerenic acid (0.1 mmol/L) was not able to displace [^{3}H] muscimol from the $GABA_A$ receptor, although both an aqueous and a hydroalcoholic extract were able to do so. The investigators then attempted to identify other compounds in the extracts capable of displacing [^{3}H] muscinol. Both glutamate and glutamine, amino acids present in the aqueous extract, had little inhibitory effect on [^{3}H] muscinol binding. However, glutamine can cross the blood-brain barrier (BBB) and can be taken up by nerve terminals and converted to GABA inside GABA-nergic neurons. Thus, glutamine could be responsible for the sedative effect of the aqueous extract, but not the hydroalcoholic extract, in which it is not present. GABA is found in both extracts, but GABA itself cannot explain the sedative effects of valerian because it is unlikely to cross the BBB in amounts significant enough to cause sedation. However, the amount of GABA present in the aqueous extract is sufficient to have effects on peripheral GABA receptors, perhaps resulting in muscle relaxation. Another study suggests a different mechanism of action involving inhibition of neuronal GABA uptake and stimulation of GABA release from synaptosomes. These investigators did not attempt to elucidate which constituent of the aqueous extract was responsible for these effects.

The CNS-depressant component of valerian is still unknown. Thus far, three major constituents of valerian have been identified: the volatile or essential oil, containing sesquiterpenes and monoterpenes, nonglycosidic iridoid esters (valepotriates), and a small number of alkaloids. Valepotriates are unstable compounds and are easily hydrolyzed by heat and moisture. In addition, valepotriates are not water soluble, and aqueous extracts contain small amounts. For example, the aqueous extract used in the study by Balderer and Borbely, described previously was analyzed using thin-layer chromatography, and no valepotriates were detectable. Furthermore, valepotriates are not well absorbed orally. Therefore, the likelihood that valepotriates are a major contributor to valerian's effects is questionable. Because of the low amount of alkaloid present in preparations, their contribution is also questionable. It is postulated that a combination of volatile oils, valepotriates, and possibly certain water-soluble constituents that have not yet been identified are responsible for valerian's sedative effects.

Antidepressant effects of valerian were identified by Oshima and associates using a methanol extract of *V. fauriei* roots. They found a strong antidepressant activity in mice as measured by the forced swimming test. One active component isolated was α-kessyl alcohol, a volatile oil component. At 30 mg/kg intraperitoneally, α-kessyl alcohol exhibited an effect similar to imipramine, a commonly used antidepressant. Kessanol and cyclokessyl acetate, guaiane-type sesquiterpenoids, also exhibited antidepressant activity. Kanokonol, kessyl glycol, and kessyl glycol diacetate, valerane-type sesquiterpenoids, did not exhibit an effect.

A 30% ethanol extract of the Japanese valerian root extract (4.1 g/kg and 5.7 g/kg) and imipramine (20 mg/kg) also demonstrated statistically significant antidepressant effects compared to placebo as measured by the forced swimming test in rats. As in the Oshima study, kessyl glycol diacetate exhibited no antidepressant activity in the forced swimming test. Because the forced swimming test can be affected by stimulants, anticholinergics, and antihistamines as well as antidepressants, the effect of the valerian extract on reserpine-induced hypothermia, a test for antidepressant activity and inhibition of neuronal reuptake of monoamines, was measured. Both valerian (11.2 g/kg) and imipramine (20 mg/kg) reversed reserpine-induced hypothermia, suggesting that the antidepressant effect of valerian is caused by reuptake of monoamine neurotransmitters, as with conventional antidepressants.

More evidence is needed to evaluate the use of valerian in children. One study using a combination product of valerian root extract and lemon balm leaf extract found that symptoms of dyssomnia or pathological restlessness might decrease in children under age 12.

Anxiety

A few studies have examined the effects of valerian on anxiety. Cropley and colleagues investigated whether kava or valerian could moderate physiological stress induced under laboratory conditions in healthy volunteers. Subject (n = 18-kava, and n = 18-valerian) and comparison group (n = 36) volunteers performed a standardized mental stress task 1 week apart. Cases had their blood pressure, heart rate, and subjective ratings of pressure assessed at rest and during the mental stress task (time 1 = *T1*). The valerian subjects took a standard dose for 7 days (time 2 = *T2*). In the valerian group, heart rate reaction to mental stress was found to decline, systolic blood pressure decreased significantly, and subjects reported less pressure during mental stress test tasks at *T2* relative to *T1*. Behavioral performance on the standardized mental stress test task did not change between the groups over the two time points. There were no significant differences in blood pressure, heart rate, or subjective reports of pressure between *T1* and *T2* in the control group.

Kohnen and Oswald conducted a study on the effects of valerian, propranolol, and combinations on activation, performance, and mood of healthy volunteers under social stressor conditions. The results of this study were equivocal and published over 15 years ago; however, it is mentioned here for historical reference.

Andreatini and colleagues examined the effect of valerian extract (valepotriates) using a randomized, parallel, double-blind placebo-controlled pilot study design in patients with generalized anxiety disorder (GAD). After a 2-week wash-out period, 36 patients with GAD as defined by the *Diagnostic and Statistical Manual of Mental Disorders,* were randomized to one of the following three treatment groups for 4 weeks: valepotriates, mean daily dose of 81.3 mg; diazepam, mean daily dose of 6.5 mg; or placebo. There was a significant reduction in the psychic factor of the Hamilton anxiety scale in the valepotriates group; however, the principal study analysis using between group comparisons on total Hamilton anxiety scale scores found negative results. The conclusion of this study suggests that there may be a potential anxiolytic effect of valepotriates on the psychic symptoms of anxiety, but the total number of subjects per group ($n = 12$) was very small and results must be viewed as preliminary.

Musculoskeletal Relaxation

Isovaltrate and valtrate (valepotriates) and valeronone, an essential oil component, isolated from *V. edulis* ssp. procera Meyer (Valeriana "mexicana") caused suppression of rhythmic contractions in guinea pig ileum in vivo at a dose of 20 mg/kg administered intravenously via the jugular vein. The investigators also demonstrated that the same compounds as well as dihydrovaltrate isolated from the same valerian species produced relaxation of carbachol-stimulated guinea pig ileum preparations in vitro. They concluded that these compounds have a musculotropic action in concentrations from 10^{-5} to 10^{-4} *M*.

Pharmacokinetics

One study has evaluated the pharmacokinetics of valerian following administration to humans. Following administration of a single 600-mg dose of valerian, the pharmacokinetics of valerenic acid were measured. The T_{max} occurred between 1 and 2 hours and the C_{max} was between 0.9 and 2.3 ng/mL. Concentrations of valerenic acid were measurable for at least 5 hours following the dose. The elimination half-life was approx 1 hour. The authors suggest that based on the expected use of valerian (sedative effects), dosing 30 minutes to 2 hours prior to bedtime would be appropriate based on the previously mentioned pharmacokinetics.

Adverse Effects and Toxicity

Reproductive System

There has been a theoretical concern with regard to pregnant women taking valerian because of possible effects on uterine contractions, but no problems were noted in three cases of intentional overdose with 2–5 g of valerian during weeks 3–10 of pregnancy. A mentally retarded child was born to a woman who overdosed on valerian 3 g, phenobarbital, glutethamide, amobarbital, and promethazine at 20 weeks of gestation, but this same woman delivered a mentally retarded child 2 years later after an overdose attempt with glutethamide, amobarbital, and promethazine.

V. officinalis (L.) was tested on rats and their offspring. A mixture, containing three valepotriates (80% dihydrovaltrate, 15% valtrate, and 5% acevaltrate), was orally administered to female rats for 30 days at 6-, 12-, and 24-mg/kg doses. Each dose was given to 10 rats, and placebo was given to another 10. No changes were noted in the average length of the estrus cycle, or the number of estrus phases during the 30-day observation period. The valepotriate mixture or placebo were also administered to 40 pregnant rats in the manner described previously from the day 1 through day 19 of pregnancy. Valerian did not increase the risk of fetotoxicity or external malformation. However, internal examination revealed a significant increase in the number of fetuses with retarded ossification with the 12- and 24-mg/kg doses. No developmental changes were detected in the offspring after treatment during pregnancy.

Cardiovascular System

Pharmacological investigations using a particular valepotriate fraction called Vpt2 extracted from the roots of *V. officinalis* (L.) have shown antiarrhythmic activity and ability to dilate coronary arteries in experimental animals. Moderate positive inotropic and a negative chronotropic effect were also observed. Vpt2 contains valtratum (50%), valeridine (25%), and valechlorin (3%), with trace amounts of acevaltrate, dihydrovaltratum, and epi-7-desacetyl-isovaltrate.

Alcoholic extracts of *V. officinalis* (L.) root (labeled V103 and V115) demonstrated hypotensive effects in rats, cats, and dogs. The V115 fraction showed greater potency and was extracted by a countercurrent distribution to yield three fractions. The first two fractions demonstrated hypotensive effects in rats, with the first fraction showing a hypotensive effect at 30 mg/kg. The third fraction produced hypertensive effects at a dose of 200 mg/kg. The authors noted that, apparently, with each succeeding extraction, less of the hypotensive principle was extracted. The hypotensive effect of the V103 fraction in rats was demonstrated at a dose of 500 mg/kg, and was hypothesized to act via a parasympathomimetic effect, blockade of the carotid sinus reflex, and CNS depression.

Cytotoxicity

The valepotriates valtrate/isovaltrate and dihydrovaltrate were isolated from *V. mexicana* and *V. wallichii*, respectively. The valepotriates tested were cytotoxic to granulocyte/macrophage colony-forming units (GM-CFCUs), lymphocytes, and erythrocyte colony-forming units (E-CFCUs). Valtrate was found to be a more potent inhibitor of GM-CFCUs (ID50 $\sim 3.7 \times 10^{-6}$ *M* vs $\sim 1.7 \times 10^{-5}$ *M*) and T-lymphocytes (ID50 $\sim 2.8 \times 10^{-6}$ *M* vs $\sim 3 \times 10^{-5}$ *M*) than dihydrovaltrate. Valtrate and dihydrovaltrate were similar in their activity against E-CFCUs (ID50 $\sim 2.3 \times 10^{-8}$ *M* vs $\sim 4.2 \times 10^{-8}$ *M*). Because pharmaceutical products containing valepotriates are orally administered, their cytotoxicity to gastrointestinal mucosal cells is of concern.

The effects of valtrate, dihydrovaltrate, and deoxido-dihydrovaltrate, valepotriates extracted from *V. wallichii* (DC.), on cultured rat hepatoma cells have been studied. Valtrate killed 50% of the cell population at a concentration of 5 μM, Deoxido-dihydrovaltrate and dihydrovaltae demonstrated this same toxicity at double the dose. Valtrate was also the most potent inhibitor of DNA and protein synthesis. These results suggest a mechanism by which valerian may cause hepatotoxicity.

Case Reports of Toxicity

Four cases of women who sustained liver damage after taking valerian-containing herbal medicines to relieve stress have been described. In addition, valerian was used by a patient who exhibited hepatotoxicity attributed to Chaparral.

Hospitals admitted 23 patients for treatment of intentional overdose with Sleep-Qik (75 mg of valerian dry extract, 0.25 mg of hyoscine hydrobromide 2 mg of cyproheptadine hydrochloride) between 1988 and 1991. Of these 23, 9 were men and 14 were women, with a mean age of 23.8 years (range 15–37 years). They were previously healthy, except for two patients with histories of psychiatric illness. The mean number of Sleep-Qik tablets taken per patient history was 33 (range 6–166), for an average of 2.5 g (range 0.5–12 g) of valerian. Four patients were asymptomatic. The other 19 patients reported drowsiness (*n* = 11), dilated pupils (*n* = 11), tachycardia (*n* = 6), nausea (*n* = 4), confusion (*n* = 3), urinary retention (*n* = 3), visual hallucination (*n* = 2), flushing (*n* = 2), dry mouth (*n* = 1), and dizziness (*n* = 1). Coingestants were alcohol (*n* = 2), a pesticide (*n* = 1), and Pansedan (*n* = 1) (*Passiflora* extract, *Viscum album* extract, *Uncariarhyncophylla* extract, and *Humulus lupulus*). One patient who was drowsy had also taken Panseden, and one who was confused had ingested alcohol.

Most patients received gastric lavage (*n* = 14), and one received syrup of ipecac. The patient who took 60 tablets of Sleep-Qik required ventilatory support. Liver function tests were performed on 12 patients approx 6–12 hours after ingestion with normal results. Drowsiness and confusion resolved within 24 hours. All patients recovered completely and were discharged after an average of 1.7 days (range 1–6 days). At an average of 43 months (range 27–65 months) after presentation, 10 patients were contacted by telephone. They had all remained well after discharge and none continued taking Sleep-Qik. Delayed onset of severe liver damage was ruled out via telephone interview, but subclinical disease could not be ruled out.

Subsequently, Chan reported on 24 cases of overdose of a product containing valerian dry extract 75 mg, hyoscine hydrobromide 0.25 mg, and cyproheptadine hydrochloride 2 mg. Six patients developed vomiting, and 15 underwent gastric lavage. Co-ingestants included alcohol (*n* = 10), cold products (*n* = 3), hypnotics (*n* = 2), unknown drugs (*n* = 2), and gasoline (*n* = 1). Symptoms were mainly CNS depression and anticholinergic symptoms. One patient required ventilatory support. Liver function tests were performed in 17 cases, and all were normal. Over the next 22–48 months postingestion, none of the patients returned to the hospital or clinic for any reason, suggesting that serious hepatotoxicity did not occur. The author points out that gastric lavage and spontaneous vomiting may have limited the amount of valerian absorbed in these patients, thus decreasing the risk of any delayed adverse effects. Other adverse effects attributed to overdose or chronic use of valerian include headaches, excitability, restlessness, uneasiness, blurred vision, and cardiac disturbances.

In another reported suicide attempt, an 18-year-old female ingested between 40 and 50, 470-mg capsules (18.8–23.5 g valerian) of 100% powered valerian root. The patient complained of fatigue, crampy abdominal pain, chest tightness, tremor of the hands and feet, and lightheadedness 30 minutes after ingestion. She presented to the emergency room 3 hours postingestion. Her vital signs were: blood pressure 111/64 mmHg, pulse 72 beats/minute, respiratory rate 14 breaths/minute, and temperature 37.6°C. Physical exam was unremarkable except for mydriasis (6 mm bilaterally). Electrocardiograph, complete blood count, and chemistry profile including liver function tests were normal. Toxicology screen was positive for marijuana, which she admitted using 2 weeks previously. She denied ingesting anything else. After two doses of activated charcoal, her symptoms resolved within 24 hours.

A withdrawal syndrome was described after abrupt discontinuation of valerian root extract in a 58-year-old man who had taken 530-2000 mg/dose five times daily as an anxiolytic and hypnotic for many years. Withdrawal symptoms included sinus tachycardia of up to 150 beats/minute, tremulousness, and delirium after recovery from general anesthesia (propofol, nitrous oxide, isoflurane, and thiopental) for open biopsy of a lung nodule. Medical history included coronary artery disease, hypertension, and congestive heart failure with an ejection fraction of 30–35%. Medications included isosorbide dinitrate, digoxin, furosemide, benazepril, aspirin, lovastatin, ibuprofen, potassium, zinc supplement, and vitamins.

The biopsy was complicated by multiple episodes of oxygen desaturation, and after extubation, the patient experienced tacycardia, oliguria, and increasing oxygen requirement. Despite naloxone administration, symptoms worsened. Swan-Ganz catheterization revealed high-output heart failure. At this time, interview with family members revealed the patient's long-standing valerian use. Because valerian withdrawal was suspected, midazolam 1 mg/hour (total dose 11 mg in 17 hours) was administered.

Signs and symptoms improved, and stabilized by the third postoperative day. He was switched to lorazepam 1 mg/hour as needed (total dose 5 mg in 24 hours), and then to a tapering dose of clonazepam. He was discharged on postoperative day 7, and was stable at 5-month follow-up. Other causes of high-output heart failure were ruled out, but because of the patient's multiple medical problems, postsurgical status, and medications administered, the cause of the patient's symptoms is unclear. The authors of this case report note that valerian has been reported to attenuate benzodiazepine withdrawal in rats.

Interactions

Two alcoholic valerian extracts were found to potentiate pentobarbital sleeping time in mice, and Valdispert, an aqueous extract prepared from *V. officinalis* (L.), increased the thiopental sleeping time in a dose-dependent manner in rats. Based on these animal studies, in vitro studies of valerian's effect on GABAnergic transmission, as well as the case series reported by Chan and colleagues, valerian would be expected to have at least an additive effect with barbiturates, alcohol, benzodiazepines, and other CNS depressants.

Valerian may have the potential to increase the level of drugs metabolized by the cytochrome P-450 3A4 (CYP3A4) enzyme. In vitro studies have found that valerian may have an inhibitory effect on CYP3A4. A clinical research study suggested that low to moderate doses of valerian did not significantly inhibit CYP3A4, although taking valerian extract 1000 mg/day increased alprazolam levels by 19%. Therefore, it may be wise to use valerian cautiously in patients taking medications that are CYP3A4 substrates such as lovastatin, ketoconazole, itraconazole, fexofenadine, alprazolam, triazolam, and various chemotherapeutic agents.

Reproduction

No information is available concerning any potential effects of valerian on female reproductive function. However, Mkrtchyan and colleagues reported that valerian had no effect on human male sterility.

Regulatory Status

Valerian was included as an official drug in the US Pharmacopeia until 1936 and in the National Formulary until 1946. Currently, the USP advisory panel does not recommend valerian's use owing to lack of adequate scientific evidence and conflicting study results. They encourage further research. Valerian is generally recognized as safe as a food and beverage flavoring by the FDA. The German Commission Monograph E has approved valerian as a sleep-promoting and calmative agent to be used in the treatment of unrest and sleep disturbances caused by anxiety. In Australia, valerian is acceptable as an active ingredient in the "listed products" category of the Therapeutic Goods Administration. In Belgium, subterranean parts, powder extract, and tincture are allowed for use as traditional tranquilizers. The Health Protection Branch of Health Canada allows products containing valerian as a single agent in the form of crude dried root in tablets, capsules, powders, extracts, tinctures, drops, or tea bags intended for use as sleeping aids and sedatives.

18

VITEX AGNUS-CASTUS

Vitex agnus-castus is a botanical plant that has the following National Oceanographic Data Center Taxonomic Code: Kingdom, Plantae; Phylum, Tracheobionta; Class, Magnoliopsida; Order, Lamiales; Family, Verbenaceae; Genus, *Vitex* L.; Species, *Vitex agnus-castus* L. The genus name *Vitex* is a Latin derivation for plaiting or weaving. The species name *agnus-castus* combines two Latin word origins: "*agnus*," which means lamb, and "*castitas*," which means chastity.

V. agnus-castus is a large deciduous shrub, native to Mediterranean countries and central Asia, and is also used in America as an ornamental plant. *V. agnus-castus* has long, finger-shaped leaves and displays fragrant blue-violet flowers in midsummer. Its fruit is a very dark-purple berry that is yellowish inside, resembles a peppercorn, and has an aromatic odor. Upon ripening, the berry is picked and allowed to dry. The twigs of this shrub are very flexible and were used for furniture in ancient times.

References to *V. agnus-castus* go back more than 2000 years, describing it as a healing herb. Ancient Egyptians, Greeks, and Romans used it for a variety of health problems. In 400 BCE, Hippocrates recommended chaste tree for injuries and inflammation. Four centuries later, Greek botanist Dioscorides recommended *V. agnus-castus* specifically for inflammation of the womb and lactation. Use of *V. agnus-castus* continued into the Middle Ages, where folklore persists that medieval monks chewed *V. agnus-castus* tree parts to maintain their celibacy, used the dried berries in their food, or placed the berries in the pockets of their robes in order to reduce sexual desire; thus, the synonym of Monk's pepper. Use of *V. agnus-castus* has persisted to modern times. Though its use was initially concentrated in the Mediterranean area, its popularity has increased in England and America since the mid-1900s.

Traditional medicinal uses of *V. agnus-castus* lie predominantly around the oral ingestion of the shrub's fruit; however, other plant parts such as leaves and flowers have been used in some preparations. The dry or liquid extract of, or oils from, the berry have been used for a variety of symptoms, most commonly related to the female reproductive system. Other uses include the treatment of hangovers, flatulence, fevers, benign prostatic hyperplasia, nervousness, dementia, rheumatic conditions, colds, dyspepsia, spleen disorders, constipation, and promoting urination. Traditional topical medicinal uses of *V. agnus-castus* include acne, body inflammation, and insect bites and stings. Use of *V. agnus-castus* is not commonly employed in traditional Chinese medicine or traditional Indian medicine (Ayurveda); however, other *Vitex* species (*negundo*, *trifoliata*) are used in these therapies.

Current Promoted Uses

Current promoted uses of *V. agnus-castus* relate to treatment of disorders of the female reproductive system such as short menstrual cycles, *premenstrual syndrome* (PMS), and breast swelling and pain (mastodynia/ mastalgia). The Commission E has approved the use of *V. agnus-castus* for irregularities of the menstrual cycle, premenstrual complaints, and mastalgia. Recent randomized, placebo-controlled studies have been conducted and found *V. agnus-castus* to be effective and well-tolerated for the relief of PMS symptoms, especially the physical symptoms of breast tenderness/fullness, edema, and headache. *V. agnus-castus* is not considered effective for PMS-related symptoms of abdominal bloating, craving sweets, sweating, palpitations, or dizziness.

V. agnus-castus is not used in foods and is not recommended for use in children, adolescents, pregnant women, or women who are breast-feeding. *V. agnus-castus* should be avoided in patients receiving exogenous sex hormones, including oral contraceptives, as *V. agnus-castus* may counteract the effectiveness of birth control pills by its effect on prolactin.

Sources and Chemical Composition

V. agnus-castus (L.), Agnolyt, arbre chaste, chaste berry, chasteberry, chaste tree, chaste tree fruit, chastetree, chastetree berry, Cloister Pepper, *Fructus Agni Casti*, Fruit de Gattilier, Gattilier, Hemp

Tree, Keuschlamm, Mönchspfeffer, Monk's Pepper, *V. agnus castus*, *V. agnus castus fructus*, Vitex.

The major constituents of *V. agnus-castus* include the following. Flavonoids: flavonol (kaempferol, quercetagetin) derivatives, the major constituent being casticin. Additional flavonoids found include penduletin, orientin, chrysophanol D, and apigenin. Water-soluble flavones: vitexin and isovitexin. Alkaloids: viticin. Diterpenes: rotundifuran (labdane-type); vitexilactone; 6-β,7-β-diacetoxy-13-hydroxy-labda-8,14-diene; 8,13-dihydroxy-14-labden; X-hydroxy-y-keto-15,16-epoxy-13, 14-labdadien;X-acetonxy-13-hydroxylabda-y,14-dien; cleroda-x,14-dien-13-ol; cleroda-x,y, 14-trien- 13-ol. Iridoid glycosides: In the leaf: 0.3% aucubin, 0.6% agnuside (the *p*-hydroxybenzoyl derivative of aucubin), and 0.07% unidentified glycosides. In the flowering stem (6'-O-foliamenthoyl-mussaenosidic acid [agnucastoside A], 6'O (6,7- dihydrofoliamenthoyl) mussaenosidic acid [agnucastoside B], and 7-O-trans-*p*-coumaroyl-6'-O-trans-caffeoyl-8-epiloganic acid [agnucastoside C], aucubin, agnuside, mussaenosidic acid, 62-O-*p*-hydroxybenzoylmussaenosidic acid, and phenylbutanone glucoside [myzodendrone]. Essential oil of leaves and flowers: monoterpenes (major chemicals found: limonene, cineole, sabinene, and α-terpineol, linalool, citronellol, camphene, myrcene) and sesquiterpenes (major chemicals found: β-caryophyllene, β-gurjunene, cuparene, and globulol). Depending on the maturity of the fruits used and the distillation processes, the components of the essential oil can vary greatly. Other constituents: fatty acids (including stearic, oleic, linoleic, and palmitic acids), amino acids (glycine, alanine, valine, leucine), castine (a bitter principle), vitamin C and carotene, and trace amounts of hormones from leaves and flowers (progesterone and 17 α-hydroxyprogesterone). Main components of the volatile oil 0.5%: mixtures of monoterpenes and sesquiterpenes, cineol, and pinene.

Products Available

V. agnus-castus is available as bulk berries, bulk powder, crushed fresh or dried berry, tea (loose or in tea bags), extract, tonic, elixir, or tincture. Chasteberry products may consist of the herb alone or in combination with other herbs and vitamins. Topically, it is used primarily as the essential oil, mixed in combination with other products in cream form.

A proprietary preparation (Agnolyt) containing an alcoholic extract of *V. agnus-castus* (0.2% w/w) has been available in Germany since the 1950s. Other products using *V. agnus-castus* synonyms in their nomenclature are available by a myriad of manufacturers. Some single-entity brand names include Agnofem, Agno-Sabona, Agnucaston, Agnufemil, Agnuside, Agnumens, Agnurell, Antimast N, Antimast T, Gynocastus, Mastodynon, and Vitex Extract. Many combination products also contain *V. agnus-castus* and include, but are not limited to, the following: Herbal Premens, Herbal Support For Women Over 45, Dong Quai Complex, Emoton, Feminine Herbal Complex (FM), Menosan, Mulimen, Phytoestrin, Virilis-Gastreu SR41, Femisana, Lifesystem Herbal Formula 4 Women's Formula (FM), PMT Complex (FM), Presselin Dysmen Olin 3 N (FM), Women's Formula Herbal Formula 3 (FM), and others.

The amount of *V. agnus-castus* contained in oral tablets or capsules varies depending on whether the product contains crushed fruit or extract of the berry. For example, tablet or capsule formulations have included the following: Chaste Berry 450 mg/Chase Berry Extract 50 mg, Chastetree fruit 500 mg, Chaste Berry Dried Extract 1.6–3.0 mg corresponding to 20 mg *Vitex*, Chaste Tree Berry Extract (0.5% agnuside) 225 mg. Commercial extract forms of chasteberry are usually standardized to contain 6% agnuside constituent. Chasteberry liquid extract may or may not contain alcohol.

Dosage

Generally, the Expanded Commission E Monographs reports the following total daily dosages:

- 30 to 40 mg of dry or fluid extracts of crushed fruit
- 0.03 to 0.04 mL of fluid extract 1:1 (g/mL), 50–70% alcohol (v/v)
- 0.15 to 0.2 mL of tincture 1:5 (g/mL), 50–70% alcohol (v/v)
- 2.6 to 4.2 mg of dry native extract (9.5–11.5:1 (w/w)

Other references have reported total daily dosages ranging from 20 to 1800 mg/day of crude *V. agnus-castus* extracts. *V. agnus-castus* is considered safe when used orally and appropriately.

Pharmacological/Toxicological Effects

Prolactin Secretion

Evidence of varying levels of discrimination exists that demonstrate *V. agnus-castus* inhibits the secretion of prolactin by the pituitary gland. In a randomized, placebo-controlled, double-blind study, Milewicz et al. examined whether *V. agnus-castus* affected elevated pituitary prolactin reserve. Participants were 52 women with luteal phase defects caused by latent hyperprolactinemia. Intervention was *V. agnus-castus* 20 mg daily or placebo, for 3 months. Only 37 women (20 = placebo, 17 =

V. agnus-castus) completed the study. Outcome measures were pre- and posthormonal analysis (blood draws taken on days 5–8 and day 20 of menstrual cycle) 1 month prior to treatment and after 3 months of treatment and latent hyperprolactinemia analysis (monitoring prolactin release 15 and 30 minutes after intravenous injection of 200 μg *thyrotropin-releasing hormone* (TRH). Results from this study showed that compared to preintervention, the *V. agnu-scastus* group had statistically significant reduced prolactin release after 3 months, whereas the control group did not. The study's information came from an English abstract of a German publication. Information about inclusion/exclusion criteria, study specifics, study funding, or author disclosures were not available.

In an open and intraindividual comparison study, Merz et al. conducted a clinical study of tolerance and prolactin secretion of *V. agnus-castus* using 20 healthy male subjects between the ages of 18 and 40 years. Placebo and three doses of *V. agnus-castus* (total daily dosages of 120, 240, and 480 mg were divided into 8-hour administration times) were given in an increasing sequence. Prolactin concentration profile after TRH stimulation was assessed by determining the maximum concentrations (C_{max}) and the area under the curve over a period of one hour ($AUC_{0\text{-}1h}$). These procedures were identical in all four study phases. Results for the $AUC_{0\text{-}24h}$ showed that as daily doses increased, prolactin levels decreased ([$AUC_{0\text{-}24h}$ {μIU · hour}/$\mu\Lambda$ ± standard deviation]; placebo: 6182 ± 1827; 120 mg: 6874 ± 1790; 240 mg: 5750 ± 1594; 480 mg: 5998 ± 1664), with statistically significant findings for the 120-mg dosage only.

Wuttke reported in a 1996 abstract the results of experiments demonstrating that 3 months of *V. agnus-castus* therapy (double-blind clinical study vs placebo) significantly reduced basal prolactin levels in patients. However, details of the experiments and study subjects were not outlined or referenced.

Follicle-Stimulating Hormone, Luteinizing Hormone

There are a limited number of human studies regarding how *V. agnus-castus* directly effects *luteinizing hormone* (LH) or follicle-stimulating hormone (FSH). In a 1994 case report by Cahill et al., a 32-year-old woman undergoing unstimulated in vitro fertilization (IVF) treatment took *V. agnus-castus* for one cycle without consulting her physician. During this cycle, she had symptoms of mild ovarian hyperstimulation in the luteal phase. Her FSH and LH levels prior to day 13, the predicted day of LH surge in the IVF cycle, were reviewed and found to be much higher than normal. Reviewing five other cycles of this patient and finding normal pituitary gonadotrophin file and normal follicular ovarian responses, the authors suggest that *V. agnus-castus* was the causative agent.

In the 1996 study by Merz et al. that primarily examined prolactin secretion in male subjects, initial hormone levels of FSH and LH were measured on days 1 and 13 (beginning and near-end of placebo phase) and from blood samples taken during the prolactin secretion profiling. The authors state that *V. agnus-castus* had no effect on FSH or LH levels, but no other details were provided.

Progesterone/Testosterone Synthesis

In a randomized, placebo-controlled, double-blind study, Milewicz et al. examined the effect of *V. agnus-castus* on prolactin reserve and luteal phase progesterone synthesis in 52 women. The intervention was *V. agnus-astus* 20 mg daily or placebo, for 3 months. Results from the 37 women (20 = placebo, 17 = *agnus-castus*) who completed the study showed that compared to preintervention, the *V. agnus-castus group* had statistically significant increases in luteal phase progesterone synthesis. The study information came from a German publication with an English abstract. Information about inclusion/exclusion criteria, study specifics, study funding, or author disclosures were not available.

In the 1996 study by Merz et al. that primarily examined prolactin secretion in male subjects, initial hormone level of testosterone was measured on days 1 and 13 (beginning and near-end of placebo phase), and from blood samples taken during the prolactin secretion profiling. The authors state that *V. agnus-castus* had no effect on testosterone levels, but no other details were provided.

Infertility

Gerhard et al. studied the influence of a commercially available preparation of *V. agnus-castus* on infertility. Using a randomized, placebo-controlled, double-blind design, 96 women with fertility disorders (31 with luteal insufficiency; 38 with secondary amenorrhea; 27 with idiopathic infertility) received either *V. agnus-castus* or placebo twice a day for 3 months. The dose of *V. agnus-castus* was 30 drops of Mastodynon twice a day (*agnus-castus* or casticin-standardization not mentioned). The outcome measures were: (i) pregnancy or spontaneous menstruation for women with secondary amenorrhea, and (ii) pregnancy or improved luteal hormone levels in women with luteal insufficiency or idiopathic infertility. A total of 66 women were suitable for evaluation. No differences were noted between the placebo and *V. agnus-castus* groups with respect to effect.

PMS and Menopausal Symptoms

In a 1997 multicenter, randomized, double-blind, controlled trial, Lauritzen et al. examined the efficacy and tolerability of a commercially available capsule formulation of *V. agnus-castus* (Agnolyt) compared with pyridoxine in women with PMS. Inclusion criteria were females aged 18 to 45 years, PMS symptoms in luteal phase of menstrual cycle, PMS symptoms with each cycle, PMS symptoms affecting quality of life, and no drug therapy for PMS in 3 months preceding the study. Of 175 participants, 85 were in the *V. agnus-castus* group (took one capsule twice a day, with one capsule containing 3.5 to 4.2 mg of *V. agnus-castus*, the second capsule containing placebo), and 90 were in the pyridoxine group (days 1–15, took one capsule twice a day, each capsule containing placebo; days 16–35, took one capsule twice a day, each capsule containing 100 mg of pyridoxine). Women in both treatment groups had equal reductions in PMS scores (*V. agnus-castus*: 15.2 to 5.1; pyridoxine: 11.9 to 5.1; $p = 0.37$), suggesting no differences in effect.

In 2000, Loch et al. conducted an open label, uncontrolled study examining the efficacy and safety of a new oral *V. agnus-castus* treatment for PMS complaints. Suffering from PMS was the only inclusion criterion and pregnancy was the only exclusion criterion. A questionnaire on mental and somatic PMS symptoms was completed by 857 gynecologists after interviewing 1634 females at the start of Femicur therapy (20 mg daily), and after a period of three menstrual cycles under therapy. Physicians reported that 42% of women reported that they had no more PMS symptoms, 51% showed a decrease in symptoms ($p < 0.001$), and 1% had an increase in number of symptoms. After 3 months of treatment, both psychic and somatic complaints were dramatically lowered. Although 30% of the women still complained about mastodynia after *V. agnus-castus* treatment, most reported complaints of lower intensity. Physicians described the patients' tolerance of this *V. agnus-castus* product as good or very good in 94% of women. Although one of the authors works for the pharmaceutical company that makes Femicur, the article did not contain funding disclosure statements.

In 2000, Berger et al., using a prospective, multicenter trial design, examined the efficacy of an oral, casticin-standardized *V. agnus-castus* therapy on 43 women diagnosed with PMS. Treatment phases consisted of baseline (two cycles, pretreatment), treatment (three cycles), posttreatment (three cycles, no treatment). The dose was 20 mg, but no placebo control was included. At the end of the trial, Moos' menstrual distress questionnaire (MMDQ) scores were reduced by 43% compared with start (statistically significant, $p < 0.001$), but that improvement decreased gradually in the post-treatment phase. At the end of the posttreatment phase, patients had improved compared to the start of therapy ($p < 0.001$) and for up to three cycles thereafter. A group of 20 women had baseline MMDQ scores that were reduced by at least 50% at the end of treatment phase. *Visual analogue scale* (VAS) and global efficacy scales showed similar findings ($p < 0.001$ and global efficacy rated excellent by 38 women). Areas of improvement included symptoms related to pain, behavior, negativity, and fluid retention. The most frequent adverse events were acne, headaches, and menstrual spotting.

In 2001, using a prospective, randomized, double-blind, placebo-controlled, parallel-group comparison design, Schellenberg studied the efficacy and tolerability of *V. agnus-castus* extract on PMS. Participants were female outpatients, 18 years of age or older, of six general medicine clinics and had a PMS diagnosis according to the *Diagnostic and Statistical Manual of Mental Disorders*. Dose of *V. agnus-castus* was 20 mg daily for 3 months. Results showed that the group receiving *V. agnus-castus* had significant improvements ($p < 0.001$) in all symptoms except bloating compared to the placebo group. Sensitivity analyses removing women taking contraceptives did not alter results. Tolerability was good with acne, itching, and mid-cycle bleeding as the adverse events noted.

An uncontrolled study in 2002 by Lucks examined the effects of 3-month dermal application of *V. agnus-castus* essential oil (oil distilled at some point in the shrubs' development of the fruit but while some leaves were still on the plant) on menopausal and perimenopausal symptoms. A 1.5% solution of the essential oil was incorporated in a bland cream or lotion and applied once a day, 5 to 7 days/week, for 3 months. Descriptive outcome measures were self-report via a survey of symptomatic relief (major, moderate, mild, none, worse) and side effects. A total of 33% of women reported major improvement in symptoms, with the most often area of improvement being hot flashes/night sweats. Both improvement and worsening occurred in the areas of emotions and menstruation flow. Subjects who were also on progesterone supplementation reported breakthrough bleeding.

Mastodynia

In a 1987, Kubista et al. reported results from a placebo-controlled study comparing the effects of lynestrenol, *V. agnus-castus* (Mastodynon), and placebo therapy in women with severe mastopathy with cyclic mastalgia. More women in the lynestrenol and *V. agnus-castus* groups than placebo group reported good relief of PMS symptoms (82, 54, 37%, respectively).

In 1998, Halaska and colleagues examined the tolerability and efficacy of *V. agnus-castus* extract on mastodynia/mastalgia (breast pain, breast tenderness). The study was a double-blind, placebo-controlled, parallel-group (50 women each) design. Length of treatment (*V. agnus-castus* [60 drops daily dose] or placebo) was 3 months. Efficacy was determined using a VAS. Results of study showed that the intensity of mastodynia diminished more quickly in the *V. agnus-castus* group with low incidence of side effects.

Luteal Phase Length

In the 1993 randomized, placebo-controlled, double-blind study where Milewicz et al. examined the effect of *V. agnus-castus* on pituitary prolactin reserve, they also examined luteal phase length. Of the 37 women (20 = placebo, 17 = *V. agnus-castus*) who completed the study (1 month prior to, and 3 months treatment), the shortened luteal phases of the *agnus-castus* group became normal. The study information came from a German publication with an English abstract. Information about inclusion/exclusion criteria and study specifics were not available.

Premenstrual Dysphoric Disorder

Premenstrual dysphoric disorder (PMDD) is characterized by markedly depressed mood, anxiety, affective lability, and decreased interest in daily activities during the last week of luteal phase in menstrual cycles of the last year. In 2002, Atmaca et al. conducted an 8-week, randomized, single-blind, rater-blinded, prospective- and parallel-group, flexible-dosing trial to compare the efficacy of fluoxetine with *V. agnus-castus* for the treatment of PMDD in 42 females. Both fluoxetine and *V. agnus-castus* had dose ranges from 20 to 40 mg. Outcome measures included the Penn daily symptom report, Hamilton depression rating scale, clinical global impression (CGI)-severity of illness scale, and CGI-improvement scale. Both drugs were well tolerated. No statistically significant differences between groups were found. The authors concluded that fluoxetine was more effective (a decrease of more than 50% in rating symptoms) for psychological symptoms (depression, irritability, insomnia, nervousness), whereas *V. agnus-castus* helped with physical symptoms (irritability, breast tenderness, swelling, cramps). Lack of placebo-control and short duration of treatment were significant limitations.

Toxicological Effects

No systematic toxicological studies have been conducted, according to the Expanded Commission E Mongraphs.

Adverse Effects and Toxicity

Throughout years of use, *V. agnus-castus* has shown only mild adverse effects. Pruritus, rash (unspecified), urticaria, increased menstrual blood flow, persistent headaches, and gastrointestinal discomfort have been reported. Few adverse events related to chasteberry have been reported to the Food and Drug Administration.

Case Reports of Toxicity Caused by Commercially Available Products

An extensive search of all standard references, as well as reports of studies in humans, shows that there have been no case reports of toxic exposure to *V. agnus-castus* use. However, one case of nocturnal seizures, possibly attributed to *V. agnus-castus,* has been reported. The patient was taking concomitantly black cohosh root (*Cimicifuga racemosa*), *V. agnus-castus*, and evening primrose as well. Thus, attribution of effect to a specific agent was not possible.

In animals, an adverse influence on nursing (lactation) performance has been observed; *V. agnus-castus* could potentially interfere with proper lactation.

Interactions

According to the German Commission E Monographs, drug interactions with *V. agnus-castus* are unknown. However, with animal experiments showing evidence of a "*dopaminergic effect*," it is generally recommended that the effect of *V. agnus-castus* can be diminished in cases when there is concurrent ingestion of dopamine-receptor antagonists (e.g., haloperidol). Similarly, because *V. agnus-castus* inhibits the secretion of prolactin via a dopamine-agonist action, drug interactions may occur with the D_2 family of dopamine-receptor agonists (bromocriptine, pergolide, pramipexole, ropinirole, cabergoline).

Some liquid formulations contain large percentages of alcohol (≥50% vol); health risks from ethanol may exist, and in certain populations, use of the dried extract formulations instead would be advisable.

Reproduction

Although there are no known case reports of toxicity in human reproduction, because of possible endocrine effects, *V. agnus-castus* could disrupt fetal development or proper gestation. A case of ovarian hyperstimulation syndrome and multiple follicular development resulting in no pregnancy occurred in a woman who took *V. agnus-castus* prior to one of her IVF protocol cycles. Tests showed that her serum gonadotropin and hormone evels were out of the desired range.

Regulatory Status

V. agnus-castus is available for use without a prescription in all Member States of the European Union and the United States. In the United States, *V. agnus-castus* is categorized as a dietary supplement. Throughout the world, *V. agnus-castus* is available through pharmacies, health-food shops, mail order companies, supermarkets, and department stores.

19

INHIBITORS OF PHOSPHOLIPASE

Phospholipase A_2 or phosphatide acylhydrolase 2, is an enzyme that catalyzes the hydrolysis of the acyl group attached to the 2-position of intracellular membrane phosphoglycerides. This hydrolysis release arachidonic acid from membrane phosphoglycerides. Arachidonic acid is the precursor of PGs, thromboxanes, and leukotrienes. In regard to the possible mechanisms observed so far, the inhibition of phospholipase A_2 is mediated via lipocortine or by direct interaction with the enzyme itself.

The former mechanism utilizes a protein known as *lipocortine*, the synthesis of which is commanded by steroidal hormones and steroid-like plants known as *triterpenoids*.

Examples of lipocortine-mediated phospholipase A_2 inhibitors that are of therapeutic value and potent anti-inflammatory drugs are cortisone, prednisolone, and betamethasone. The other possible mechanism involves a direct binding with the enzyme itself, a mechanism thus far unused in therapeutics, but with promise. One such compound is also a triterpene: betulinic acid.

When looking for an inhibitor of phospholipase A_2 from medicinal plants, one could look into plant species that are traditionally used as snake-bite antidotes because hemolytic and myolytic phospholipases A_2 are often present in snake venom, which results in damage to cell membranes, endothelium, skeletal muscle, nerves, and erythrocytes.

Other medicinal features to consider when searching for plants with potential as phospholipases A_2 are abortifacient, analgesic, antipyretic, and hypoglycemic uses. Such features are present in the following plant species.

Medicinal Aristolochiaceae

The family Aristolochiaceae is a family of herbaceous plants often used in Asia and the Pacific to counteract snake poisoning, promote urination and menses, mitigate stomachache, and treat dropsy and skin diseases. During the past 20 years, members of this family, especially from the genus Aristolochia have attracted much interest and has been the subject of numerous chemical and pharmacological studies. The anti-inflammatory property of Aristolochia species is probably the result of a direct interaction between aristolochic acid and derivatives of phospholipase A_2. *Aristolochia indica* L., *Aristolochia kaempferi*, and *Aristolochia recurvilabra* Hance are used for the treatment of inflammatory conditions.

A. indica L. Indian *Aristolochia*, also known as Indian birthwort, *ishvara* (Sanskrit), or *adagam* (Tamil), is a bitter climber native to India. The medicinal material consists of the rhizome, which is to resolve inflammation (India), counteract insect poison, and as an antipyretic (Philippines and Vietnam). The rhizome contains aristolochic acid, which inhibits in vitro and dose-dependent phospholipid hydrolysis by the human synovial fluid phospholipase A_2, snake venom phospholipase A_2, porcine pancreatic phospholipase A_2, and human platelet phospholipase A_2.

Aristolochia kaempferi Willd. (*Aristolochia chrysops* [Stapf] E.H. Wilson ex Rehder, *Aristolochia dabieshanensis* C.Y. Cheng and W. Yu, *Aristolochia heterophylla* Hemsl., *Aristolochia kaempferi* f. *heterophylla* S. M. Hwang, *Aristolochia kaempferi* f. *mirabilis* S. M. Hwang, *Aristolochia neolongifolia* J.L. Wu and Z.L. Yang, *Aristolochia mollis* Dunn, *Aristolochia shimadae* Hayata, *Isotrema chrysops* Stapf, *Isotrema heterophyllum* [Hemsl.] Stapf, and *Isotrema iasiops* Stapf), or yellow mouth Dutchman's pipe, *ma tou ling*, *yi ye ma dou ling* (Chinese), is a perennial climber that grows to a height of 1 m in forests, thickets, and the mountain slopes of China, Taiwan, and Japan. The plant is herbaceous and develops small yellow flowers in the summer.

The fruits are cylindrical or ovoid, 3–7 × 1.5–2-cm, dehiscing capsules. The drug consists of the fruit, which is shaped like human lungs, and is therefore recommended in China for all forms of pulmonary infections. Other diseases for which they are prescribed are hemorrhoids, ascite, and heartburn. The plant is known to contain phenanthrene alkaloid derivatives including aristoliukine-C, aristofolin A and E, aristolochic acid-Ia methyl ester, and aristolochic acid, as

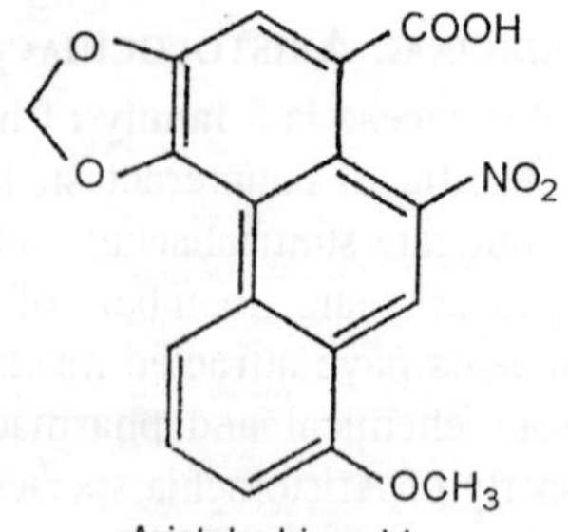

Aristolochic acid

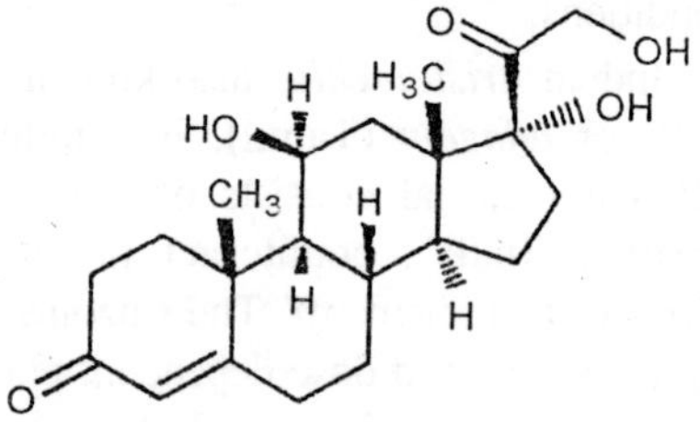

Cortisol

well as kaempferol-3-*O*-rutinoside and quercetin kaempferol-3-*O*-rutinosid.

The plant is known elaborate a series of quite unusual phenanthrene alkaloid derivatives, of which aristoliukine-C, aristofolin A and E, aristolochic acid-Ia methyl ester, and aristolochic acid. Other chemical constituents found in this plant are flavonoid glycosides such as kaempferol-3-*O*-rutinoside and quercetin kaempferol-3-*O*-rutinoside. Exposure to Aristolochiaceae family is associated with the development of cancer in humans. A significant advance is the toxicological effects of aristolochic acid has been provided by the work of Pezzuto et al. They showed that aristolochic acid is a mutagen.

Aristolochia recurvilabra Hance (*Aristolochia debilis* Sieb. et Zucc, *Aristolochia sinarum* Lindl., *Aristolochia longa* L.), or *ch'ing-mu-hsiang, pai-shu, ma dou ling, sam pai liang yin yao* (Chinese), is a climber that grows to a height of 1.5 m in thickets, mountain slopes, and moist valleys to 1500 m altitude in China, Taiwan, and Japan by roadsides, in thickets, and in meadows. The flowers are tubular and dark purple at the throat. The drug consists of the rhizome. It is highly esteemed and was, at one time, worth 300 silver taels. The rhizome can be easily mistaken for ginger. It is used to treat digestive

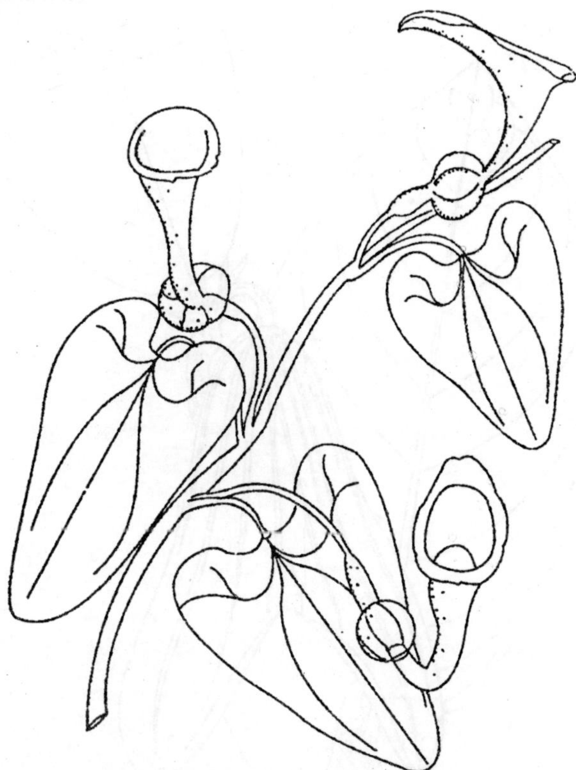

Fig. 19.1. Aristolochiaceae recurvilabra.

disorders, fluxes, diarrhea, dysentry, and snake bites. Levi et al. reported cases of hepatitis following ingestion of teas containing aristolochic acid. Hong et al. showed that a methanol extract of *Aristolochia debilis* is a potent inhibitor of COX-2 activity.

Thottea grandiflora Rottb. is a shrub that grows in the primary rainforests of Malaysia, Thailand, and Singapore. The stems are terete and hairy. The leaves are simple, alternate, thick, glossy, and glaucous underneath and grow up to 25 cm long. The flowers are axillary, 15 cm long, purple, membranaceous, and three-lobed. The fruits are linear follicles. The roots are used to invigorate, break fevers, treat agues, and as a postpartum remedy. The pharmacological potential of this plant is unexplored.

Medicinal Myristicaceae

The Myristicaceae family has attracted a great deal of interest on account of its ability to produce series of unusual phenylacylphenols—

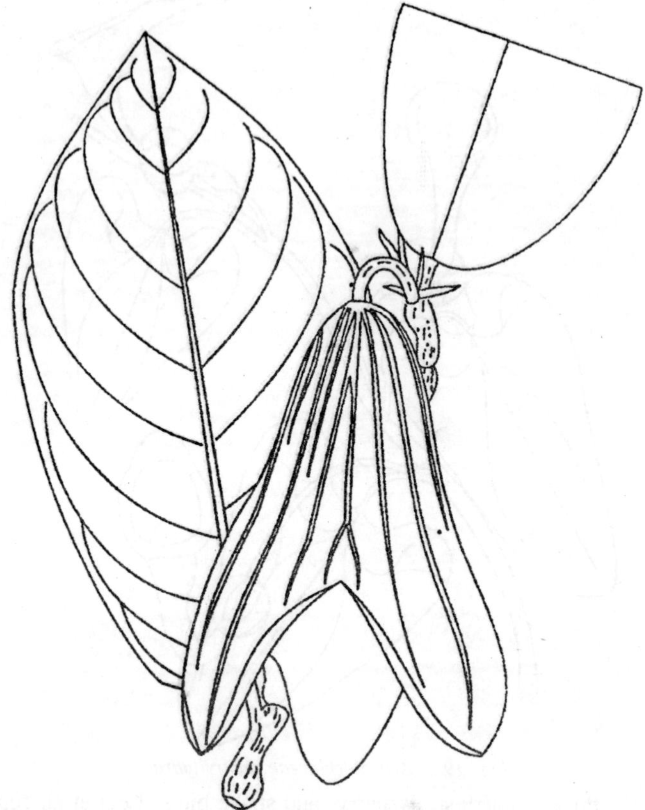

Fig. 19.2. Thottea grandiflora.

of possible symbiotic origin—that might have some potential for the treatment of inflammation. One such compound is YM-26567-1 from *Horsfieldia amygdalinia* (Wall.) Warb. isolated by Mikaye et al.

Horsfieldia amygdalinia (Wall.) Warb (*Myristica amygdalina* Wall, *Horsfieldia tonkinensis* H. Lecomte, *Horsfieldia thorelii* H. Lecomte, *Horsfieldia tonkinensis* var. *multiracemosa* H. Lecomte, *Myristica glabra* auct. non Blume, *Horsfieldia glabra* auct. non (Blume) Warb, *Horsfieldia prunoides* C.Y. Wu), or *feng chui nan* (Chinese), is a timber tree that grows to a height of 25 m in hilly, sparse forests or dense forests of mountain slopes and groves in China, India, Laos, Burma, Pakistan, Thailand, Vietnam, Malaysia, and Indonesia. The bark is grayish-white and exudes sticky blood-like latex. The mature fruits are ovoid to elliptical drupes that are orange and to 2.5 cm long. The seeds are oily and completely enclosed in a crimson tunic. The leaves

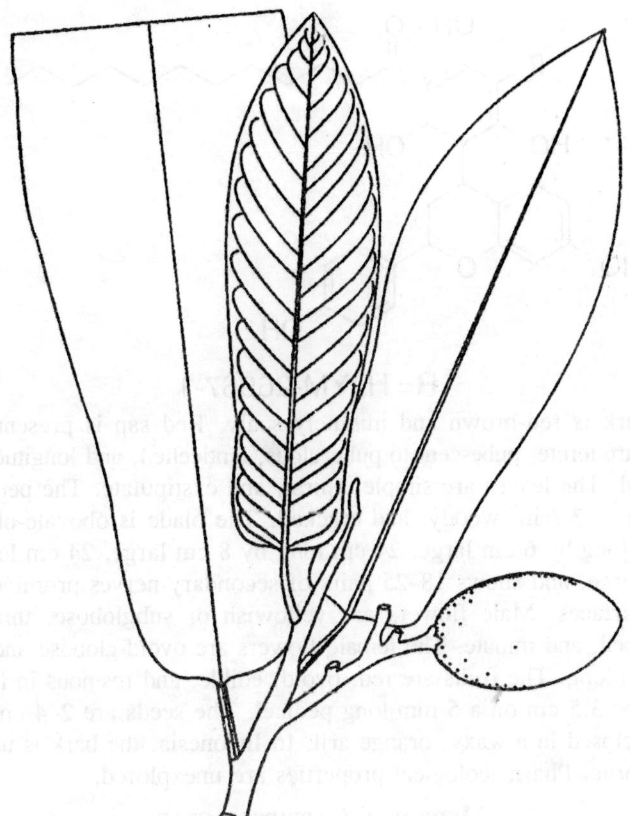

Fig. 19.3. Horsfieldia valida.

and bark are used to make a tea to treat intestinal discomfort, and the bark is used to heal sores and pimples. The anti-inflammatory property of *Horsfieldia amygdalinia* (Wall.) Warb is confirmed in vitro. Mikaye et al. reported that YM-26567-1 from the fruit of this plant competitively inhibits the enzymatic activity of phospholipase A_2. In the course of further screening for YM-26567-1 derivatives, YM-26734 was selected, and inhibited phospholipase A_2 from rabbit platelets with an inhibition concentration 50% (IC_{50}) value of 0.085 m*M*.

Horsfieldia valida (Miq.) Warb. (*Myristica valida* Miq., *Endocomia macrocoma* [Miq.] de Wilde subsp. *prainii* [King] de Wilde; *Horsfieldia merrillii* Warb.; *Horsfieldia oblongata* Merr., *Horsfieldia prainii* [King] Warb., *Myristica prainii* King.), or *yunnan feng chui nan* (Chinese), is a buttressed tree that grows to a height of 25 m and a girth of 50 cm in the primary rainforests of Indonesia, Malaysia, and the Philippines.

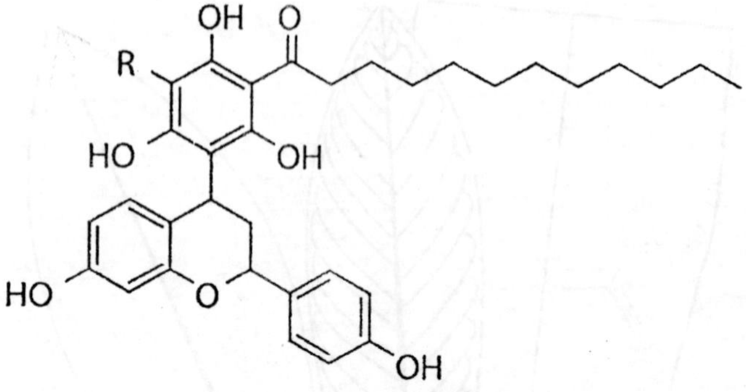

R= H, YM-26567-1

The bark is red-brown and minutely scaly. Red sap is present. The stems are terete, pubescent to puberulous, lenticelled, and longitudinally fissured. The leaves are simple, spiral, and exstipulate. The petiole is 2.3 cm × 3 mm, woody, and cracked. The blade is obovate-oblong, 19 cm long by 6 cm large, 24 cm long by 8 cm large, 24 cm long by 6 cm large, and shows 18–25 pairs of secondary nerves prominent on both surfaces. Male flowers are yellowish or subglobose, three- to five-lobed, and minute. The female flowers are ovoid-globose and 2.5–2.8 mm long. The fruits are red, ovoid, edible, and resinous in flavor, and 6 × 3.5 cm on a 5-mm-long pedicel. The seeds are 2–4 cm long and enclosed in a waxy, orange aril. In Indonesia, the bark is used to treat sprue. Pharmacological properties are unexplored.

Medicinal Caprifoliaceae

The family Caprifoliaceae comprises approx 400 species, of which *Lonicera japonica* Thunb., *Lonicera affinis* Hook and Arn, *Lonicera confusa* DC, *Sambucus javanica* Reinw. ex. Bl, *Sambucus sieboldiana* (Miq.) Graebn, and *Weigela floribunda* (Sieb. and Zucc.) K. Koch. are used to treat inflammatory conditions in Asia and the Pacific. There is an expanding body of evidence to suggest that biflavonoids from this family might hold some potential as phospholipase A_2 inhibitors. One such compound is ochnaflavone from *Lonicera japonica* Thunb.

Lonicera japonica Thunb. (*Lonicera chinensis* Wats, *Lonicera brachypoda* DC. var. *repens* Sieb.), or Chinese honeysuckle, *kim ngam*, *day nhan dong* (Vietnamese), *jen-tung* (Chinese), is a climbing shrub. The flowers are tubular, up to 4 cm long, and white when fresh but yellow when dry. In China, the flowers, stems, and leaves are used in medicine as febrifuge, correctives, and astringents and are used to treat infections and poisoning. The dried flowers are a common sight

Ochnaflavone

in the Chinese pharmacies of Malaysia, where they are prescribed as an antipyretic. In Vietnam, a decoction of stems or flowers is drunk to treat syphilis and rheumatism. The anti-inflammatory and antipyretic properties of *Lonicera japonica* Thunb. are confirmed and involve a biflavonoid, ochnaflavone, strongly inhibited the enzymatic activity of rat platelet phospholipase A_2 (IC_{50} approx 3 μM). This activity was strong and dependent of the pH, noncompetitive, and irreversible. In addition, the inhibitory activity of ochnaflavone is rather specific against group II phospholipase A_2 than group I phospholipase A_2 (IC_{50} approx 20 μM). These results indicate that the inhibition of phospholipase A_2 by ochnaflavone may result from direct interaction with the enzyme.

Sambucus javanica Reinw. ex Bl. (*Sambucus hookeri* Rehd, *Sambucus thunbergiana* Bl.), or *so tiao, chieh ku ts'aois* (Chinese), or

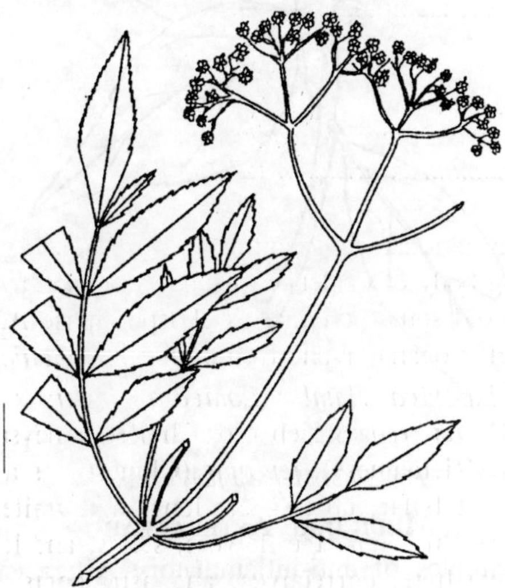

Fig. 19.4. Sambucus javanica.

kambiang beriak (Indonesian), is a deciduous shrub of open spaces of land in town or countryside that are abandoned and where plants can grow freely, village outskirts, and wasteland. The flowers are white, starry, and small, and the fruits are red berries. In Indonesia, the leaves and bark are used to cure itching. The plant is also used to treat rheumatism, assuage pain, reduce fever, and resolve swellings. The pharmacological potentials of this plant are unknown.

Weigela floribunda (Sieb. & Zucc.) K. Koch. (*Diervilla* versicolor), crimson weigela, or Japanese wisteria, is a deciduous shrub that grows up to 2.5 m in Asia and was introduced as an ornamental shrub in the United States. The flower appears from May to June, and is large and purplish. The plant is medicinal in China and Indonesia, where it is used to wash sores. The pharmacological potentials of the plant are unknown.

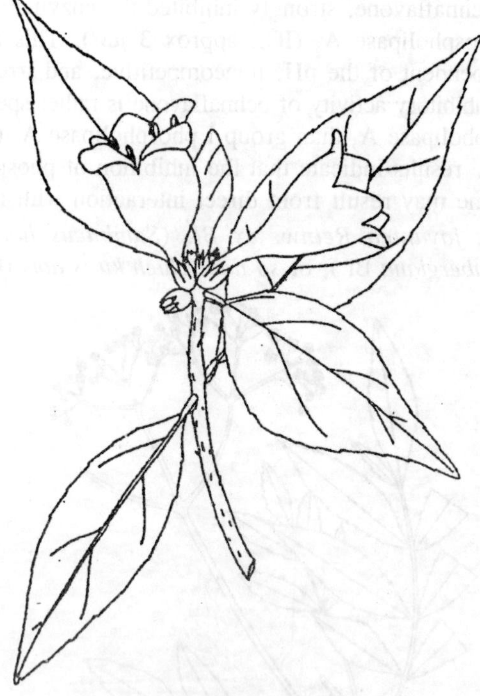

Fig. 19.5. Weigela floribunda.

Medicinal Asteraceae

Classical examples of anti-inflammatory Asteraceae are *Arnica montana* and *Calendula officinalis*, both used in European medicine to treat bruises and contusions. There is an expanding body of evidences to suggest that Asteraceae could be a useful source of anti-inflammatories, such as sesquiterpene lactones and/or triterpene alcohols, the latter being known to inhibit 12-*O*-tetradecanoylphorbol-13-acetate (TPA)-induced inflammation in mice as efficiently as commercial indomethacine by possible inhibition of phospholipase A_2.

One of the most exiting findings in this area is perhaps the isolation of Bt-CD, a neoclerodane diterpenoid from *Baccharis trimera* (Less) DC or *carqueja* (Brazil) used to treat rheumatism and diabetes that shows anti-phospholipase A_2 activity. Note also the anti-phospholipase A_2 and anti-inflammatory activity of *Santolina chamaecyparissus*. *Cirsium japonicum* DC, *Crossotephium chinense* L. Makino, *Inula chinensis* Rupr. ex Maxim., and *Sigesbeckia orientalis* L. are used in Asia for the treatment of inflammatory conditions.

Cirsium japonicum DC (*Cnicus japonicum* Maxim, *Cnicus spicatus*), or Japanese thistle, *azami* (Japanese), *ta chi*, *hu chi*, *ma chi*, *tz'u chi*, *shan nin p'ang*, *chi hsiang ts'ao*, *yeh hung hua*, and *ch'ien*

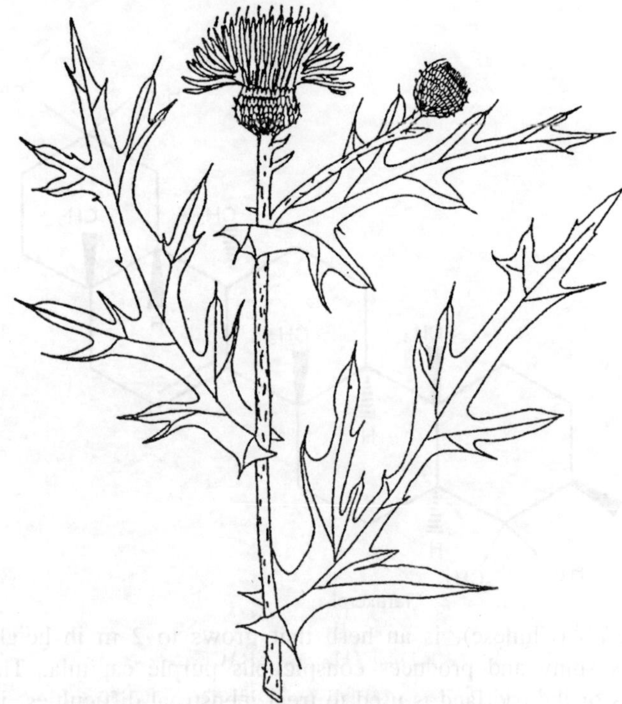

Fig. 19.6. Cirsium japonicum.

Neo-clerodane diterpenoid

Taraxerol

chen ts'ao (Chinese), is an herb that grows to 2 m in height. The plant is spiny and produces conspicuous purple capitula. The drug consists of the root and is used to treat menstrual difficulties, irritable uterus, wounds, and snake bites. A decoction of the aerial part is used

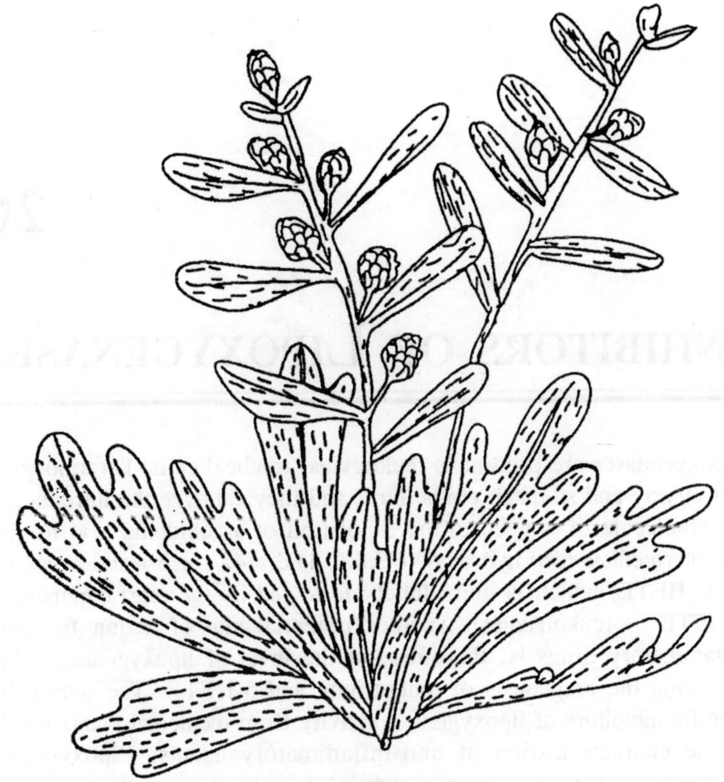

Fig. 19.7. Crossotephium chinense.

to stop bleeding from the nose. In Taiwan, the plant is used to heal burns. In Cambodia and Laos, the root is applied to ulcers and abscesses. The pharmacological properties of this herb are unknown.

Crossotephium chinense L. Makino (*Crossostephium artemisoides* Less, *Artemisia judaica* sensu Lour, *Artemisia loureiro* Kostel.) is a sub-shrub growing in crevices in the rocks in Japan and is cultivated in other Asian countries as pot ornamental. The plant is glaucous with dissected fleshy leaves. In China, the leaves are used to calm itching. In Taiwan, the leaves are applied to contusions and wounds. In Vietnam, Cambodia, and Laos, an infusion of the plant is drunk to treat congestion. The plant is known to elaborate taraxerol, taraxeryl acetate, and taraxerol, which might participate in the medicinal uses. It would be interesting to know whether further studies on this herb discloses inhibitors of phospholipase A_2.

20

INHIBITORS OF LIPOXYGENASES

Lipoxygenases are present in leukocytes, tracheal cells, keratinocytes, and airway and stomach epithelium, and they catalyze the introduction of a molecule of oxygen to the 5-position of arachidonic acid to give the intermediate (5S)-hydroxy- (6E,8Z, 11Z, 14Z)-eicosatetraenoic acid or 5- HETE, which is immediately followed by the rearrangement of 5-HETE to leukotrienes. Another potential site of action for anti-inflammatory drugs is, therefore, at the level of lipoxygenases, thus inhibiting the biogenesis of leukotriene and 5-HETE. The search for specific inhibitors of lipoxygenase activity from medicinal plants results in the characterization of anti-inflammatory agents. Lipoxygenase inhibitors might hold some potential for the treatment of asthma, psoriasis, arthritis, allergic rhinitis, cancer, osteoporosis, and atherosclerosis. The evidence currently available suggests the families Myrsinaceae, Clusiaceae, and Asteraceae have potential as sources of lipoxygenase inhibitors.

MEDICINAL MYRSINACEAE

The family Myrsinaceae consists of 30 genera and about a 1000 species of tropical plants that have attracted a great deal of interest for their quinones and saponins, which have exhibited a large spectrum of pharmacological activities. About 40 species of plants classified within the family Myrsinaceae are medicinal in the Asia–Pacific region, particularly for the treatment of inflammatory conditions. One of these medicinal herbs is *Ardisia villosa* Roxb.

Ardisia villosa Roxb., or *xue xia hong* (Chinese), is a shrub that grows up to 3 m tall in the wild in China, Taiwan, Thailand, and Malaysia. The stems are stoloniferous, blackish, rusty villous, or hirsute

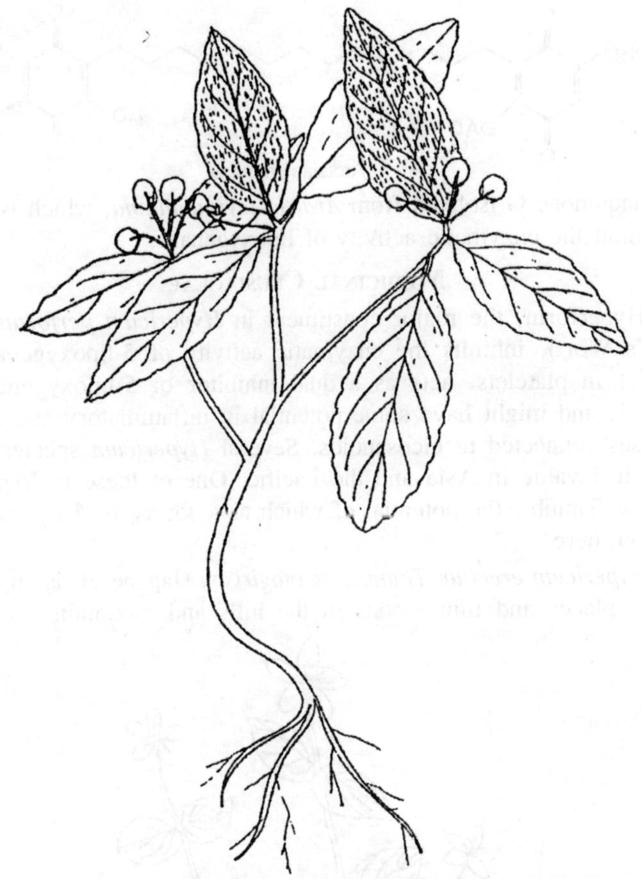

Fig. 20.1. Ardisia villosa.

almost throughout. The leaves are simple, spiral, and exstipulate. The blade is selliptic-lanceolate, somehow fleshy, light green, and marked with numerous blackih dots. The flowers are lavender or pink. The fruits are dark red or blackish with globose berries. The plant is used in China to treat contusions and rheumatic and neuralgic pains. In Malaysia, a decoction of leaves is used as bath to treat dropsy; the roots are used to reduce fever and treat cough. An interesting feature of *Ardisia* species, and the Myrsinaceae family in general, is the production of a very unusual series of dimeric benzoquinones known as ardisiaquinones, which are known to inhibit the enzymatic activity of 5-lipoxygenases, a feature that could explain the frequent use of *Ardisia* species to treat inflammatory conditions. One such compound is

Ardisiaquinone G

ardisiaquinone G isolated from *Ardisia teysmanniana*, which is known to inhibit the enzymatic activity of lipoxygenase.

Medicinal Clusiaceae

Hyperforin, the major constituent in *Hypericum perforatum* (St. John's Wort), inhibits the enzymatic activity of 5-lipoxygenase and COX-1 in platelets, acts as a dual inhibitor of 5-lipoxygenase and COX-1, and might have some potential in inflammatory and allergic diseases connected to eicosanoids. Several *Hypericum* species are of medicinal value in Asia and the Pacific. One of these is *Hypericum erectum* Thunb., the potential of which as a source of 5-lipoxygenase is given here.

Hypericum erectum Thunb., or *otogirisou* (Japanese), is an herb of grassy places and thin woods in the hills and mountains of Japan,

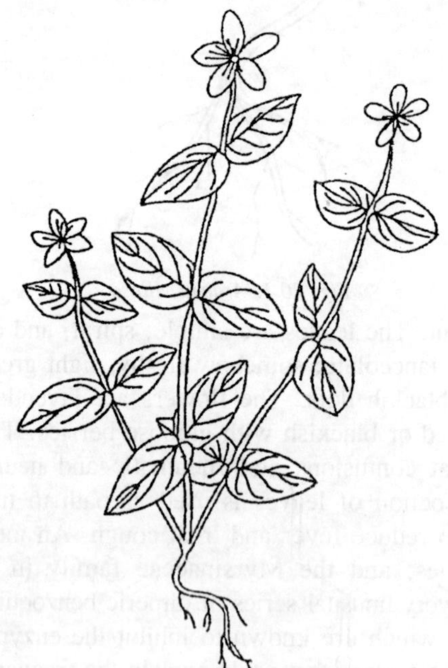

Fig. 20.2. Hypericum erectum.

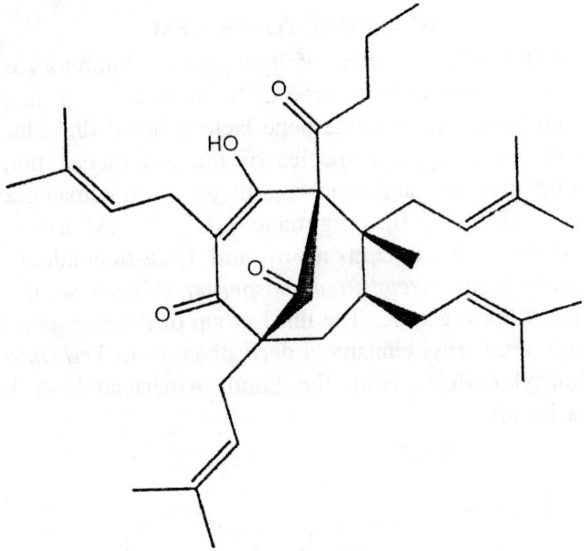

Hyperforin

Korea, and China. The plant is a lithe herb with decussate leaves and yellow flowers. In Japan, the juice expressed from the leaves is used to heal cuts and sooth bruises. A decoction of the fruits is used to stop bleeding. In Vietnam and Cambodia, a paste of the aerial parts is applied to dog bites and bee stings, and is used internally for the treatment of malarial fever. *Hypericum erectum* Thunb. is an important herb in Chinese medicine as an anti-hemorrhagic agent, astringent, and antibiotic that is known to contain antiviral phloroglucinol derivatives, as well as the anti-hemorrhagic compounds otogirin and otogirone. Also, because the plant is known to elaborate a series of polyprenylated phloroglucinol derivatives including erectquione A, B, C, its potential as a lipoxygenase inhibitor would be worth assessing.

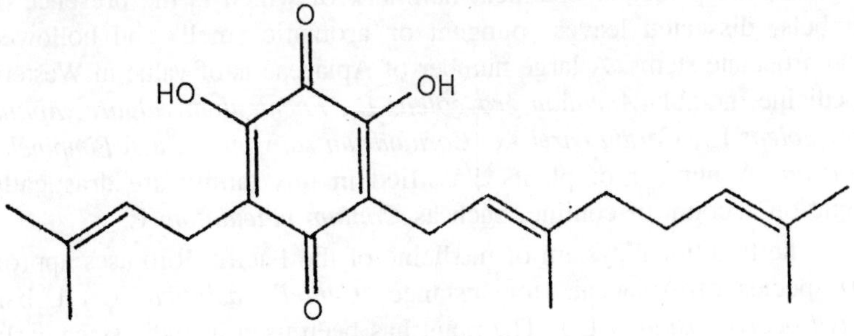

Erectquione A

Medicinal Asteraceae

One of the richest sources of lipoxygenase inhibitors is perhaps the family Asteraceae, where three different types of principles have been characterized. The sesquiterpene lactone helenalin, which can be isolated from several plant species of the Asteraceae family, is a potent anti-inflammatory and antineoplastic agent. In human granulocyte, helenalin inhibited 5-lipoxygenase (IC_{50} 9 m*M* after 60 min preincubation) in a concentration- and time-dependent fashion. Polyacetylenes from *Artemisia monosperma* showed some levels of activity against lipoxygenase. The third group of lipoxygenase inhibitors in this family are bornyl cinnamoyl derivatives from *Verbenisa* species, such as bornyl caffeate from the South American herb *Verbenisa turbacensis* Kunth.

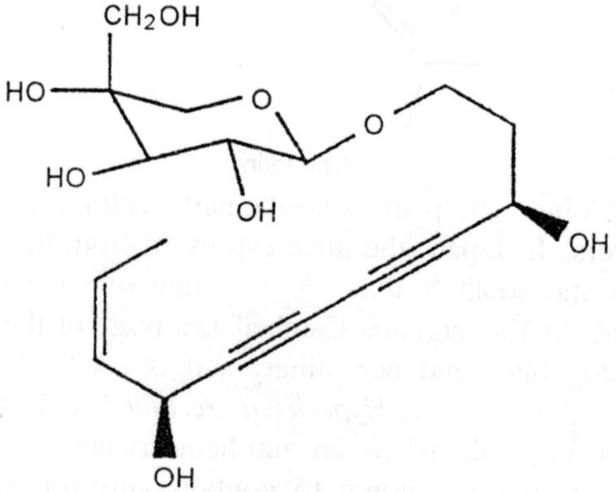

Polyacetylene

Medicinal Apiaceae

The family Apiaceae is a large group of flowering plants which comprises some 250 genera of herbs, mostly growing in temperate regions, the principal botanical hallmark of which is the presence of umbels, dissected leaves, pungent or aromatic smell, and hollowed and articulate stems. A large number of Apiaceae is of value in Western medicine, notably *Anethum graveolens L.*, *Foeniculum vulgare*, *Apium graveolens* L., *Carum carvi* L., *Coriandrum sativum* L., and *Pimpinella anisum*. A number of plants classified in this family are drastically toxic on account of coniine, such as *Conium maculatum* L.

The traditional system of medicine of the Pacific Rim uses approx 80 species of Apiaceae, for instance, *Centella asiatica* (L.) Urban (*Hydrocotyle asiatica* L.). The plant has been used in India since early times for skin diseases and as a diuretic. It has long been a popular

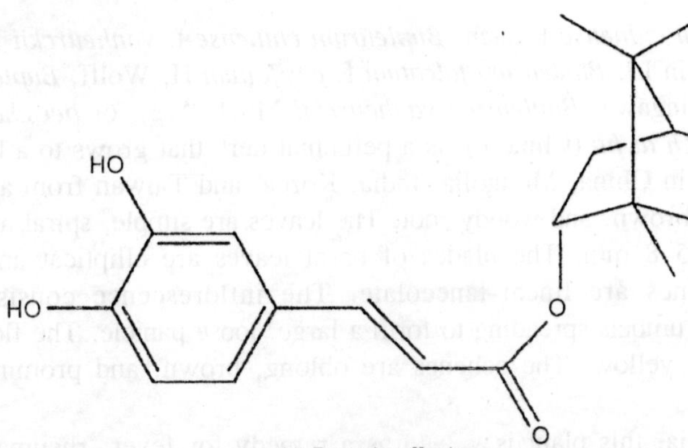

(-)-Bornyl caffeate

remedy in India for leprosy and syphilis. However, large doses are said to have narcotic action. The plant was used also by the surgeons of Napoleon's army.

Bupleurum chinense DC (*Bupleurum falcatum* L. var *scorzoneraefolium* (Willd.) Ledeb, *Bupleurum octoradiatum* Bge.

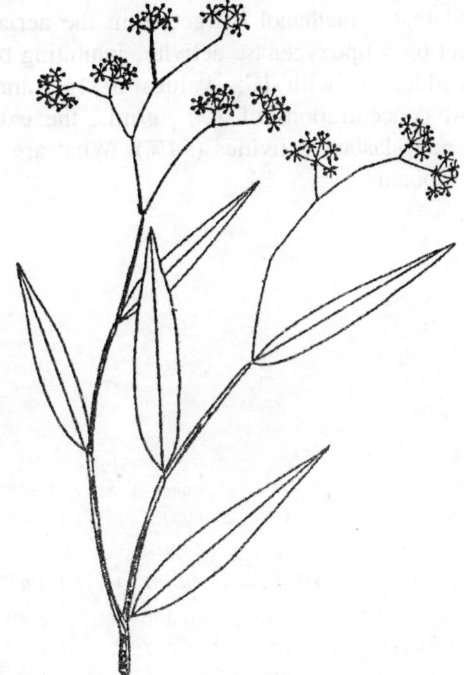

Fig. 20.3. Bupleurum chinense.

Bupleurum chinense Franch, *Bupleurum chinense* f. *vanheurckii* R. H. Shan & Yin Li, *Bupleurum falcatum* f. *ensifolium* H. Wolff, *Bupleurum togasii* Kitagawa, *Bupleurum vanheurckii* Muel- Arg), or *bei chai hu, tz' u hu, ch'ai hu* (Chinese), is a perennial herb that grows to a height of 90 cm in China, Mongolia, India, Korea, and Taiwan from a stout elongate, brown, and woody root. The leaves are simple, spiral and 4–7 cm × 5–8 mm. The blades of basal leaves are elliptical and the cauline ones are linear-lanceolate. The inflorescence consists of numerous umbels spreading to form a large, loose panicle. The flowers are bright yellow. The achenes are oblong, brown, and prominently ribbed.

In Asia, this plant is valued as a remedy for fever, rheumatism, gout, and inflammatory illnesses. In China, the roots are used as febrifuges, deobstruents, and carminatives, and are used to assuage muscle pains, thoracic and abdominal inflammations, puerperal fever, and diarrhea.

A significant advance in the understanding of the anti-inflammatory properties of *Bupleurum fruticescens* has been provided by Prieto et al. The showed that a methanol extract from the aerial parts had a significant effect on 5-lipoxygenase activity, inhibiting both LTB_4 and 5(*S*)-HETE production, with IC_{50} values of 112 and 95 μg/mL, respectively. At concentrations of 200 μg/mL, the extract inhibited COX-1 (90%) and elastase activities (54%). What are the principles involved here, saponin?

21

Inhibitors of Elastase

The seeds and vegetative part of plants contain several sorts of inhibitors of insect, fungal, mammalian, and endogenous proteinases. These inhibitors may be involved in plant defense mechanisms against predators and participate in the development of the plant itself. Peptidic proteinase inhibitors are well studied in the families Fabaceae, Poaceae, Asteraceae, and Solanaceae. Non-proteinaceous inhibitors of serine protease are, in comparison, less known. Among serine proteinases are human neutrophils and macrophages, which digest degrade elastin, cartilage proteoglycans, fibronectin, and foreign materials ingested during phagocytosis.

In normal physiological conditions, it is inhibited by α-1-protease inhibitor of plasma. Damage to connective caused by leakage of elastases leads to damage associated with inflammatory diseases, such as pulmonary emphysema, adult respiratory distress syndrome, septic shock, cystic fibrosis, carcinogenesis, chronic bronchitis, and rheumatoid arthritis.

Compounds that directly inhibit elastase or its release from human neutrophils are of enormous pharmaceutical and cosmetological interest in the development of new anti-inflammatory drugs. A possible source for elastase inhibitors are the medicinal Asteraceae and Droseraceae, particularly those used as traditional medicine in Asia.

Medicinal Asteraceae

The family Asteraceae is a prolific source of sesquiterpene lactones, among which, melampolides have been shown to inhibit the enzymatic activity of elastases. Melampolides are a common member of the *Melampodiinae* subtribe. Examples of medicinal Asteraceae known to elaborate melampolides are *Sigesbeckia orientalis* L. and *Mikania cordata* (Burm.f.).

Sigesbeckia orientalis L., or sigesbeckia, commonly known as St. Paul's wort, *sa phaan kon* (Thai), *hi lien*, *chu kao mu*, *hu kao*, *kou kao*, and *nien hu ts'ai* (Chinese), is an annual, branched herb that grows up to 1.2 m tall in Asia and the Pacific Islands. The capitula are bright yellow. The plant has the reputation of "smelling like a pig" in China, where it is used to treat fever, snake bites, skin diseases, loss of appetite, chronic malaria, numbness of the extremities, and cancerous sores. In Taiwan, the plant is used to reduce swellings. In the Philippines, a decoction of the plant is used to heal wounds. A

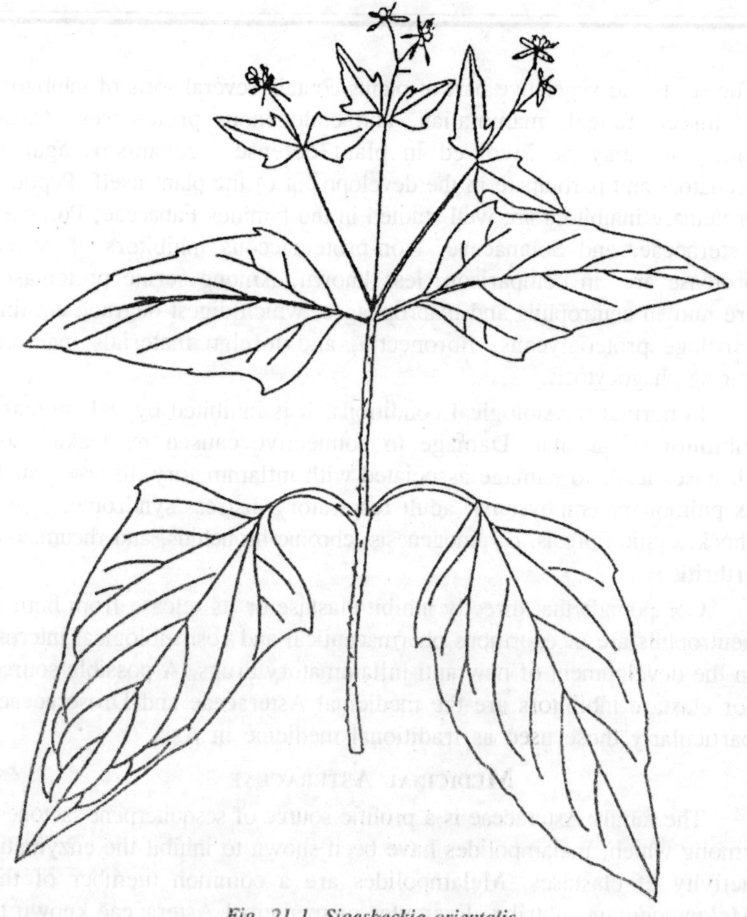

Fig. 21.1. Sigesbeckia orientalis.

patent showed the ability of the plant to stimulate wound healing, to promote healing, and to restore elasticity to damaged skin. The dermis is thick, supple, and sturdy layer of connective tissue that encompasses a dense meshwork of collagen and elastin fibers, which are responsible for elasticity, tone, and texture. When the coils of collagen and elastin suffer cuts and crosslinking damage and the skin losses much of its strength and elasticity, wrinkles appear. This initial research led to an investigation of *Sigesbeckia orientalis* L.'s ability to restore normal quantities of collagen and elastin fibers in abnormal stretching of the dermis (pregnancy, change in weight) from a linear scar or from some endocrine disorders. Are melanpolides involved here?

Sigesbeckia glabrescens Mak., or *hi chum*, is used in Korea to treat liver and kidney diseases, asthma, allergic disorders, costiveness, deafness, and blindness. In China, the plant is prescribed for rheumatic

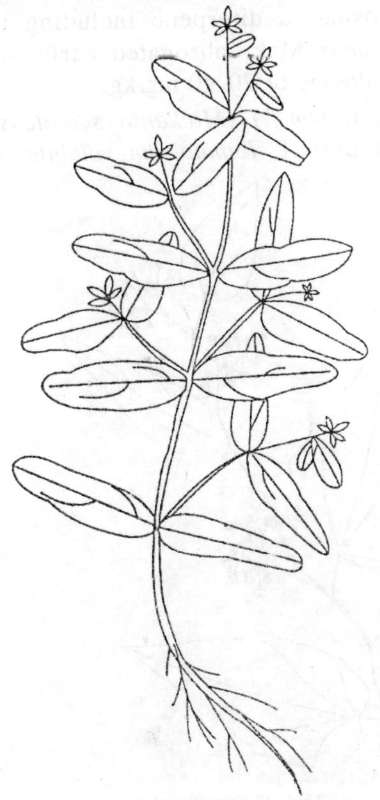

Fig. 21.2. Sigesbeckia globrescens.

pain, numbness, weak bones, and to wash boils. The anti-inflammatory property of *Sigesbeckia glabrescens* Mak. is confirmed experimentally, as an intraperitoneal injection of an aqueous extract of the plant inhibited compound 48/80 induced systemic anaphylaxis in mice. The extract dose-dependently inhibited the release of histamine from peritoneal mast cells by compound 48/80. The plant has a strong antianaphylactic activity by inhibition of histamine release from mast cells. The extract dose-dependently inhibited the active systemic anaphylaxis and serum IgE production induced by immunization with ovalbumin and interleukin (IL)-4-dependent IgE production by lipopolysaccharide (LPS)-stimulated murine whole spleen cells. Note that serine protease enzymes induces the release of significant amounts of histamine from mast cells, and that the antihistaminic effect described earlier could result from a possible inhibition of elastase by melampolides, but this remains to be confirmed.

Note that darutoside, a diterpene including isolated from *Siegesbeckia glabrescens* Mak. abrogated early pregnancies in experimental rats at a dosage of 20–40 mg/kg.

Mikania cordata (Burm.f.) (*Mickania scandens* [L.] Willd, *Eupatorium caudatum* Burm.f, *Eupatoirum volubile* Vahl, *Mikania*

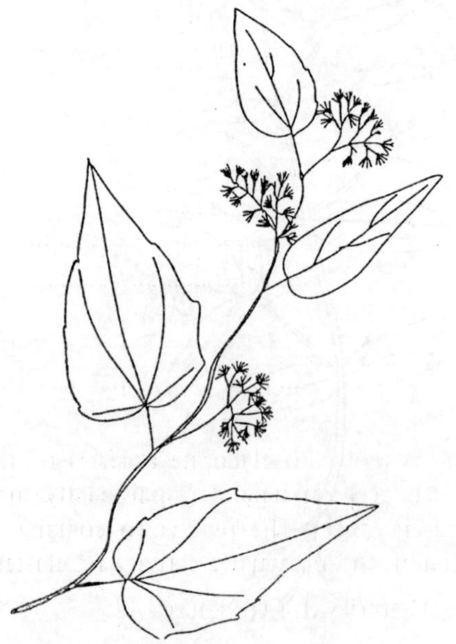

Fig. 21.3. Mikania cordata.

Mikanolide

Deoxymikanolide

volubilis [Vahl] Willd, *Mikania chenopodifolia* Willd), or river vine, heartleaf hem vine, or climbing hemp vine, is a climber native to tropical America. The plant grows throughout Southeast Asia to the Bismarck Archipelago. The leaves are cordate, and the capitula are grouped in panicles. In Taiwan, the plant is used to resolve swellings. In Malaysia, it is used to calm itches, and in Indonesia it is used to heal wounds.

Mikania cordata is known to elaborate a series of sesquiterpene lactones, among which deoxymikanolide significantly inhibits acetic acid-induced writhing in mice. The plant also contains a series of melampolides that inhibit the enzymatic activity of elastase.

Medicinal Droseraceae

The family Droseraceae consists of four genera and about 100 species of perennial herbs, of which *Drosera burmannii* Vahl, *Drosera rotundifolia* L, *Drosera indica* L., and *Drosera peltata* Sm. are used in Asia for the treatment of cough. Naphthoquinones and flavonoids, which occur in this family, have not been fully studied for pharmacology, and it appears that flavonoids inhibit human neutrophil elastase, hence the potential for the treatment of inflammation.

Drosera rotundifolia L., or round leaf sundew, is a little perennial herb that can reach 35 cm in height. The plant is found in temperate bogs and swampy areas. The leaves are simple, fleshy, broadly ovate and arranged into rosettes. The leaves are covered with sticky, shiney, red tentacles. The flowers are pink.

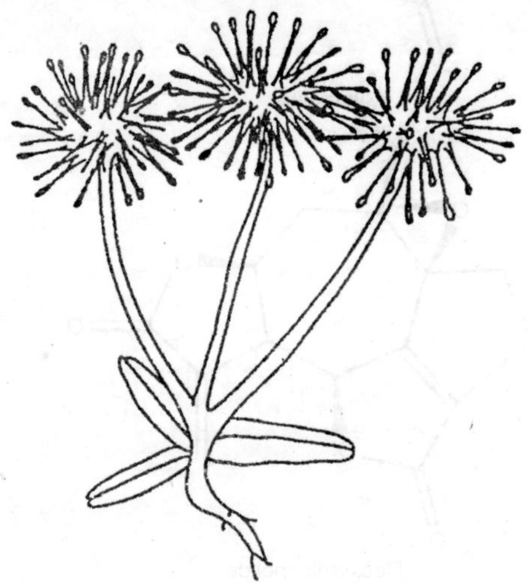

Fig. 21.4. Drosera rotundifolia.

The plant has been traditionally used in Europe to treat chronic bronchitis, asthma, and whooping cough, and the entire air-dried plant, or *Drosera*, was listed in the *French Pharmacopoeia* in 1965 (tincture, 1 in 5; dose 0.5–2 mL), and in 1880, Murray described its uses in the Royal Hospital for whooping cough. In Japan, a decoction of the plant is used to treat cough. This effect is probably mediated by flavonoids such as hyperoside, quercetin, and isoquercitrin, which are known to abound in the plant. Quercetin from *Drosera madagascariensis* inhibits human neutrophil elastase with an IC_{50} value of 0.8 μg/mL, as well as hyperoside (IC_{50} 0.15 μg/mL) and isoquercitrin (IC_{50} 0.7 μg/mL).

22

Inhibitors of Nitric Oxide Synthetase

NOS is an important enzyme involved in the regulation of inflammation, vascular tone, neurotransmission, and cancer. NO is generated via oxidation of the terminal guanidine nitrogen atom from L-arginine by NOS. NO is a very toxic free radical that can cause substantial tissue damage in high concentrations, especially in the brain. In stroke, for example, large amounts of NO are released from nerve cells to cause damage to surrounding tissues including neurones and myocytes. NO is also released during inflammation and is involved in the growth of tumors; it is understood that endogenously formed NO induces the malignant transformation of mouse fibroblasts. Among NOSs, inducible NOS is involved in the overproduction of NO and is expressed in response to IL-1β, tumor necrosis factor-α, and LPS, the genetic expression of which is notably commanded by the NF-κB macrophages. Molecules capable of inhibiting inducible NOS and/or induction of NF-κB activation may be of therapeutic benefit in various types of inflammation. Such molecules could be of sesquiterpenic nature as discussed under the following subeadings.

Medicinal Asteraceae

There is an expanding body of evidence to suggest that sesquiterpene lactones inhibit the synthesis NO synthetase. One such compound is an ambrosanolides-type sesquiterpene known as cumanin characterized from *Ambrosia psilostachya*. This sesquiterpene inhibit the enzymatic activity of NO synthetase with an IC_{50} value of 9.38 μM. Another example is the well-known artemisinin, a sesquiterpene used as an alternative

Cumanin

drug in the treatment of severe and multidrug-resistant malaria, which inhibits NO synthesis in cytokine-stimulated human astrocytoma T67 cells.

Other sorts of NO inhibitors are triterpenes, such as ursolic acid and 2-α-hydroxy ursolic acid and 2-α-hydroxy ursolic acid from *Prunella vulgaris* L., inhibit the production of NO by murine leukaemic monocyte macrophage cells, RAW 264.7, cultured in vitro. The IC_{50} values were 17 μM for ursolic acid and 27 μM for 2-α-hydroxy ursolic.

Inula chinensis Rupr. ex Maxim. (*Inula japonica* Thunb., *Inula britannica* L.), or *hsuan fu hua*, is indigenous of northern China, Mongolia, Korea, and Japan. It is a perennial herb that grows to a

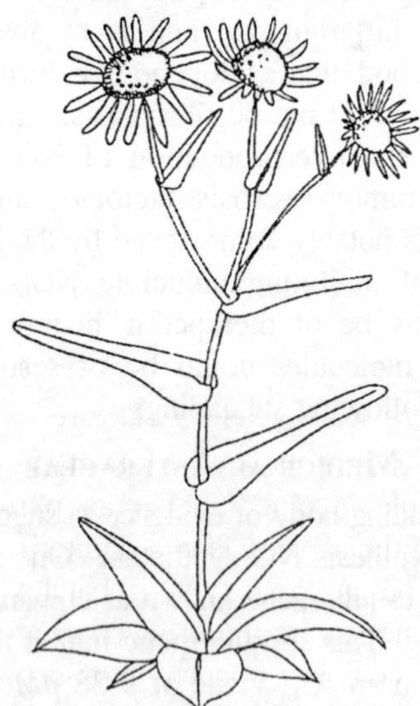

Fig. 22.1. Inula chinensis.

height of 60 cm. The drug consists of the flowers dried in the sun, are used in China as analgesic, to treat swellings, sore throat, cough, vomiting, fullness of chest and as a deobstruent and laxative, diuretic, depurative, tonic, and carminative. Hernandez et al. characterized from *Inula viscosa* a sesquiterpene lactone, inuviscolide, which reduces the phospholipase A_2-induced edema with an inhibitory dose at which half of the phospholipase A_2-induced edema was reduced, ID_{50}, value of 98 mmol/kg. Han et al., studied the mechanism of action of 1-*O*-acetyl-4R,6S-britannilactone, a sesquiterpene isolated from the flowers of *Inula britannica* and showed that this substance suppressed NO and PGE2 synthesis in RAW 264.7 macrophages through the inhibition of iNOS and COX-2 gene expressionvia a blocking the binding of NF-κB to the promoter in the target genes. Other sesquiterpenes able to inhibit the enzymatic activity of inducible nitric oxide synthase from the genus *Inula* are bigelovin, 2,3-dihydroaromaticin and ergolide, which potently inhibits the activity on LPS-induced NOS in murine macrophage RAW 264.7 cells with an IC_{50} value of 0.46 m*M*, 1.05 and 0.69 μM, respectively.

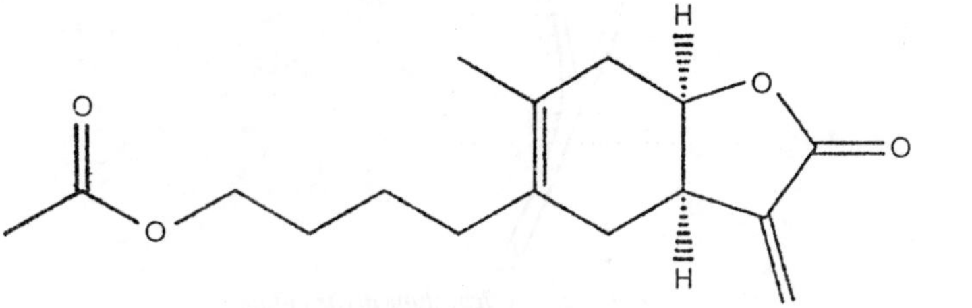

1-O-acetylbritannilatone

Carpesium divaricatum Sieb. et Zucc., or *gankubisou* (Japanese), is an herb that grows to a height of 1 m in shady and damp waste places, roadsides, and hillsides in China, Japan, and Korea. The leaves are lanceolate, and the inflorescences consist of yellow, cylindrical capitula.

The plant has been used in traditional Korean herbal medicine for its antipyretic, analgesic, and anti-inflammatory properties vermifuge.

The active principle involved in the antipyretic, analgesic, and anti-inflammatory traditional uses is a sesquiterpene known as 2β,5-epoxy-5, 10-dihydroxy-6α-angeloyloxy-9β-isobutyloxy-germacran-8α, 12-olide. This sesquiterpene lowers the production of NO by LPS/IFN-γ-stimulated RAW 264.7 cells in a concentration-dependent manner, with an IC_{50} value of approx 2.16 m*M*. This carence in NO is not owed to inhibition of the enzymatic activity. In addition, Kim et al., showed

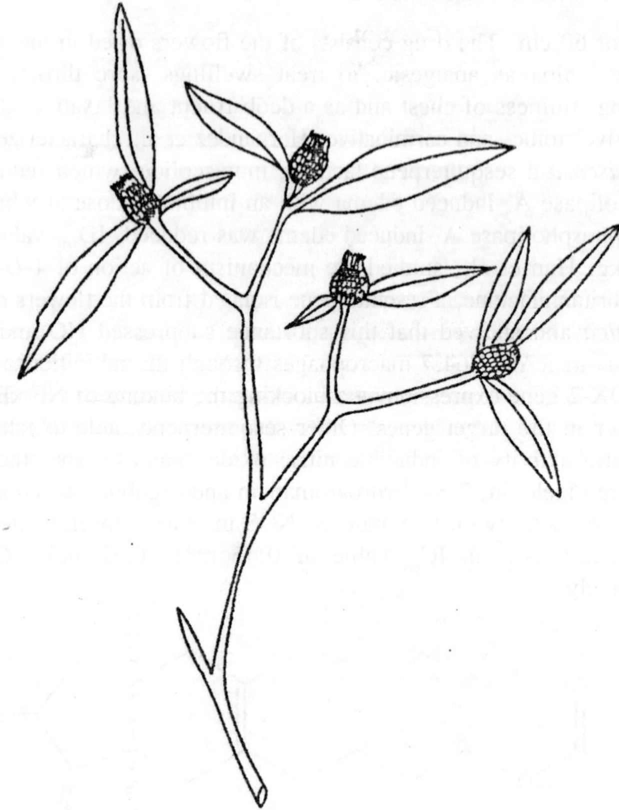

Fig. 22.2. Carpesium divaricatum.

that the cells exposed to the sesquiterpene had lower level in iNOS protein and mRNA suggesting inhibition of nuclear factor-κB (NF-κB) activation through a mechanism involving the inhibition of iNOS gene expression via inhibition of NF-κB DNA binding.

Medicinal Lauraceae

The family Lauraceae consists of 50 genera and 2000 species of trees, shrubs, and herbs, of which 70 are of medicinal value in the Asia–Pacific region. Lauraceae are well-known for elaborating isoquinoline alkaloids and sesquiterpenes, the latter most likely representing a vast source of material for the search for NOS. Examples of such compounds are costunolide and dehydrocostunolide found in the leaves of *Laurus nobilis* (bay leaf, laurel), the leaves of which are widely used as a spice, antiseptic, stomachic, and to treat rheumatism in traditional European medicine. The potential of *Neolitsea zeylanica* Nees (Merr.) as a potential source of NOS inhibitor is discussed here.

Neolitsea zeylanica Nees (Merr.) (*Tetradenia zeylanica* Nees, *Litsea zeylanica* Nees) or shore laurel, *tejur* (Malay), Or *nan ya xin mu jiang zi* (Chinese), is a tree that grows up to 20 m tall in forests and thickets from sea level up to 1000 m in Burma, Malaysia, Sri Lanka, Borneo, the Philippines, India, China, and Australia. The young stems are glabrous. The leaves are simple, alternate, or crowded at apex of stems. The blades are ovate-oblong or oblong and glaucous beneath. The flowers are small and arranged in axillary, subsessile, four- to five-flowered umbels. The fruits are subglobose, 8 mm–1.5 cm in diameter, and seated on a disc-shaped, wavy, marginated perianth.

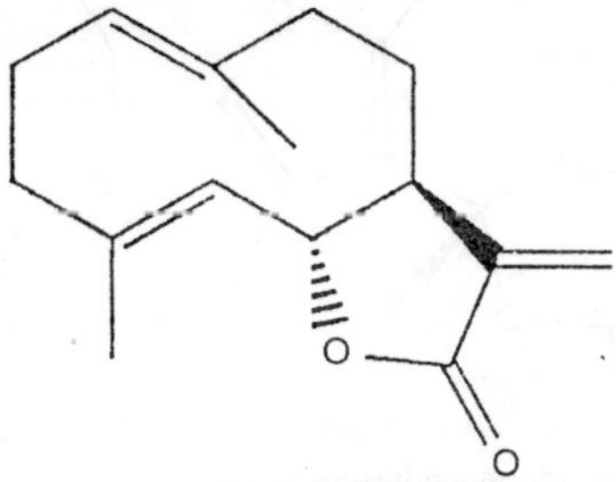

Costunolide

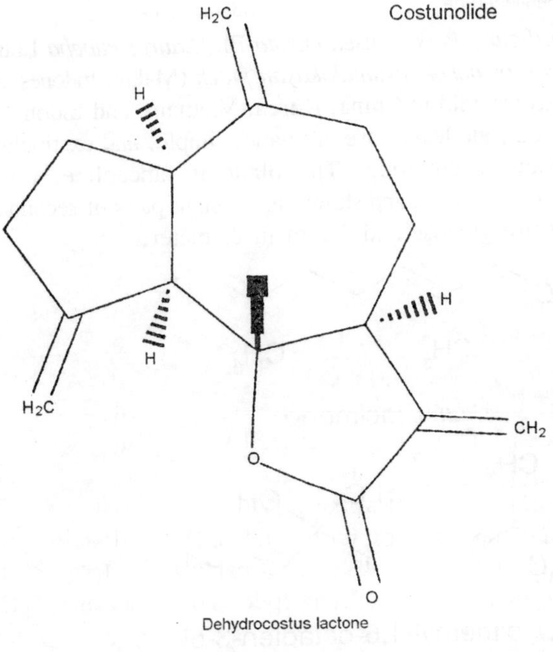

Dehydrocostus lactone

In Malaysia, a paste of the roots is applied to fingers to treat eruptions. The plant is known contain some sesquiterpene lactones including neolinderane, zeylanine, zeylanicine and zeylanidine, the potential of which as an inhibitor of NOS would be worth investigation because pseudoneolinderane and linderalactone inhibited the production of superoxide anion generation by human neutrophils in response to fMLP/CB. The IC_{50} values for pseudoneolinderane and linderalactonewere 3.21 and 8.48 μg/mL, respectively.

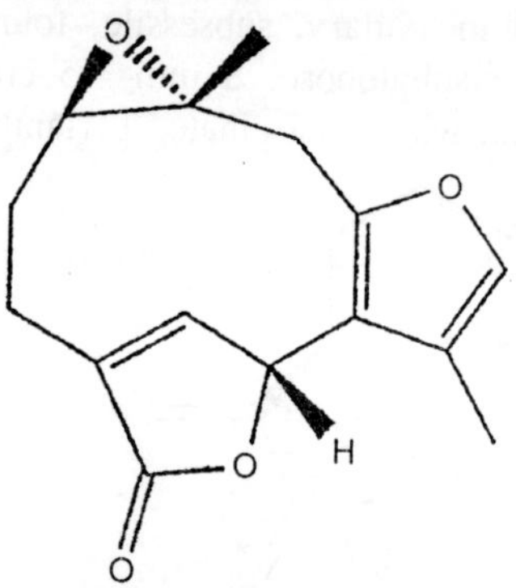

pseudoneolinderane

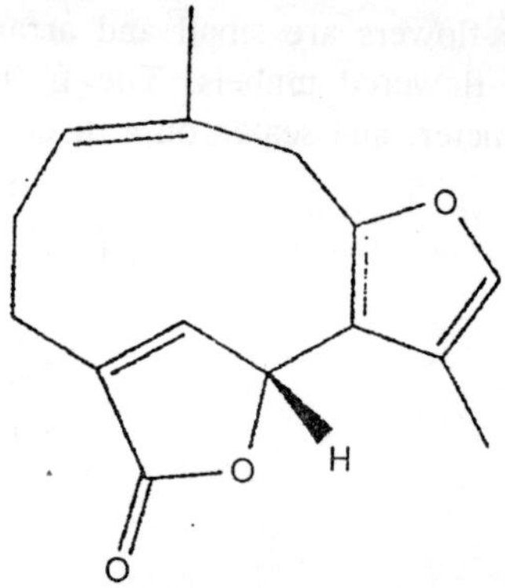

linderalactone

Litsea cubeba (Lour.) Pers. (*Litsea citrata* Bl., *Laurus cubeba* Lour., *Daphnidium cubeba*), or *pokok myuniak kayah puteh* (Malay, Indonesian), is a shrub which grows wild in China, Korea, Vietnam, and Indonesia. The stems are smooth; the leaves are aromatic, simple, and exstipulate. The petiole is about 1 cm long. The blade is lanceolate, thinly coriaceous, 12–4 cm × 3–1 cm and shows six to eight pairs of secondary nerves. The fruits are globose and 3 mm in diameter.

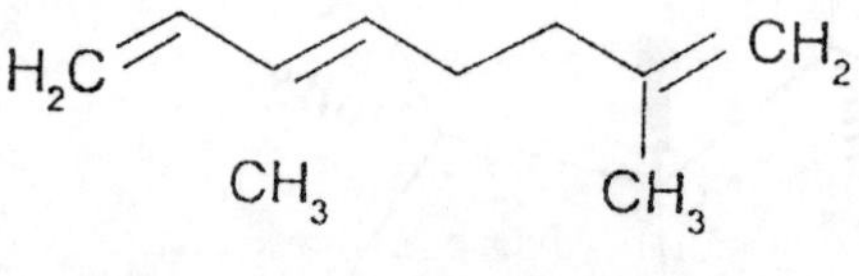

*cis*α–ocimene

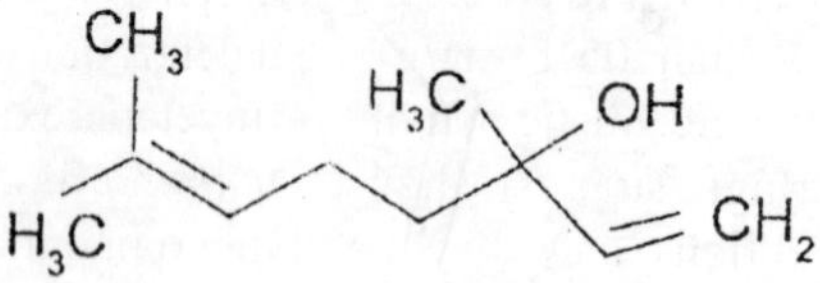

3,7-dimethyl-1,6-octadien-3-ol

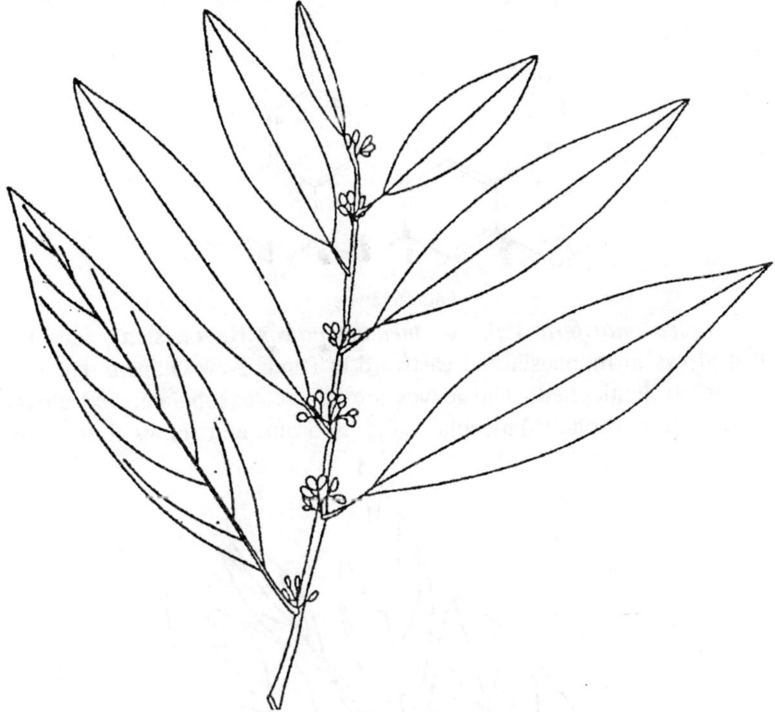

Fig. 22.3. Litsea cubeba.

In China, the seeds are eaten to promote digestion and treat cough and bronchitis. In Vietnam, Cambodia, and Laos, a decoction of the plant is used to treat mental disorders such as hysteria and forgetfulness. In Taiwan, the plant is used to treat athlete's foot and other skin diseases.

The plant is strongly aromatic on account of an essential oil which comprises *cis*-α-ocimene (25.11%), 3,7-dimethyl-1,6-octadien-3-ol (16.85%), and *trans*-nerolidol (13.89%), hence the use of the plant in aromatherapy. A methanolic extract of bark of *Litsea cubeba* (Lour.) Pers. and its fractions (0.01 mg/mL) from bark inhibit NO and PGE_2 production in LPS-activated RAW 264.7 macrophages without significant cytotoxicity at less than 0.01 mg/mL concentration. The methanol extract decreased the enzymatic activity of myeloperoxidase (0.05 mg/mL). These findings suggest that *L. cubeba* is beneficial for inflammatory conditions and may contain compound(s) with anti-inflammatory properties. Can we expect the vasorelaxant laurotetanine isolated from the plant to exert such activity?

Laurotetanine

Litsea odorifera Val., or *medang pawas* (Indonesian), is a tree that grows in Indonesia and eastward to Papua New Guinea. The stem is slightly lenticelled. The leaves are simple, exstipulate, and glossy. The blade is broadly lanceolate, 7.5 × 5 cm, and shows four to five

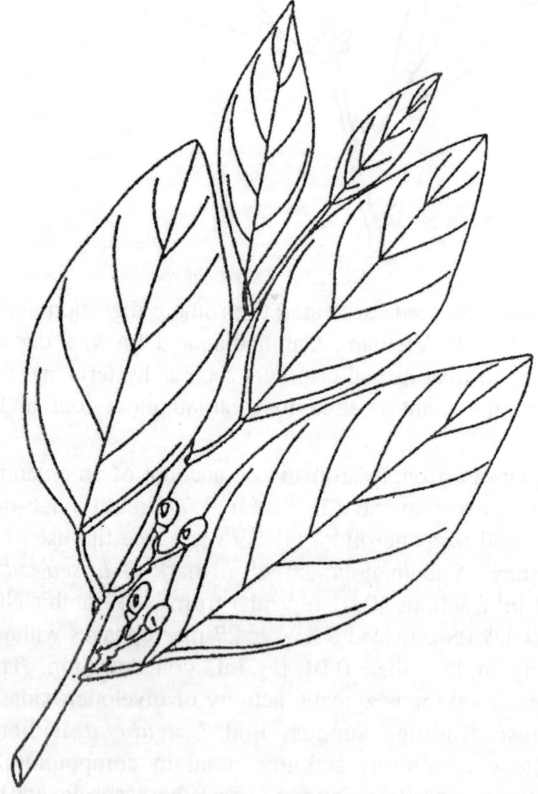

Fig. 22.4. Litsea odorifera.

pairs of secondary nerves. The fruits are to 1 cm long, dark green with white spots, glossy, and ovoid. The plant is used to treat biliousness, to promote lactation, and to heal boils and furuncles. The pharmacological potential of this plant is unexplored, and it would be interesting to know whether further study reveals evidence of nitric oxidase inhibition.

MEDICINAL SOLANACEAE

The family Solanaceae consists of about 85 genera and 2800 species of plants, of which, 80 are of medicinal value in the Asia–Pacific region. Solanaceaeare well known for their parasympatholytic tropane alkaloids, such as hyoscyamine. Classic examples are *Atropa belladonna* L. (belladona herb), *Datura stramonium* L. (stramonium), and the dried leaves and flowering tops of *Hyoscyamus niger* L. (hyoscyamus), which have been used as antispasmodic drugs. In the family, the genus *Physalis* is known to produce 16,24-cyclo-13,14-secosteroidal terpenes called physalins, which might be of interest as inhibitors of NOS. An example of medicinal *Physalis* is *Physalis alkekengi,* a medicinal plant of the Asia–Pacific region.

Physalis alkekengi, or Chinese lantern, alkekengi, bladder cherry, ground cherry, strawberry tomato, winter cherry, *suan chiang*, or *teng leng ts'ao*, is an ornamental perennial herb that grows to a height of 80 cm in Eurasia. The leaf blade is narrowly to broadly ovate. The flowers are mostly white, with a greenish or yellowish eye, and are rotate or campanulate. The fruits are shiny, orange-red, globose, 1–1.5 cm in diameter. The berries are enclosed in an inflated calyx that resembles a little lantern. The plant is used in China to break fever, promote urination, and treat cough. The seeds are used to promote labor. *Physalis alkekengi* is known to elaborate a series of 16,24-cyclo-13,14-secosteroidals known as physalins, such as physalins N and O. Physalins B, F, and G from *Physalis angulata* L. lower NO, tumor necrosis factor-α, IL-6, and IL-12 release by macrophages stimulated with LPS and IFN-γ. It would be interesting to learn whether further studies on Solanaceae, and *Physalis* species in general, disclose any molecule of therapeutic value in treating inflammation.

23

BIOCHEMICALS PROTECTING HERBAL PLANTS

Pesticides occupy a rather unique position among the many chemicals that man encounters daily, in that they are deliberately added to the environment for the purpose of killing or injuring some form of life. Ideally their injurious action would be highly specific for undesirable target organisms and noninjurious to desirable, nontarget organisms. In fact, however, most of he chemicals that are used as pesticides are not highly selective but are generally toxic to many nontarget species, including man, and other desirable forms of life that coinhabit the environment. Therefore, lacking highly selective pesticidal action, the application of pesticides must often be predicated on selecting quantities and manners of usage that will minimize the possibility of exposure of nontarget organisms to injurious quantities of these useful chemicals.

Toxicologic evaluations of the hazard of handling and use of pesticides have for many years focused primarily on preventing injury to man, and common laboratory animals have served as the experimental models for man's biochemical, physiologic, and pathologic responses to these chemicals. Problems of species differences in susceptibility have always left some doubt concerning assignment of safe dosages for man on the basis of studies on common laboratory animals, but this approach appears to have been reasonably successful in protecting the *general population* in that there has not emerged any clear association between increasing use of pesticides and incidence of chronic diseases. However, as discussed subsequently, occupational exposures have resulted in chronic or persistent neurologic disease states in the case of a few compounds.

Acute poisoning by pesticides do occur. They are usually the result of occupational exposures or of careless use, misuse, or mishandling the pesticides. The mortality rate attributed to poisoning by pesticides has been estimated at 0.65 per one million population in the United States, but it has also been estimated that there are 100 nonfatal poisonings for each fatal one. In spite of the fact that a clear association between chronic diseases and pesticide exposures is not apparent, new and sensitive toxicologic and analytic methods have raised many questions concerning the possibility to subtle effects that would be difficult to recognize unless one directed investigations specifically to reveal them. A review of the status of epidemiologic studies on pesticide toxicology pointed out design and interpretive pitfalls that give cause to question whether our knowledge is adequate to assess the degree of injury or lack of injury to man's health resulting from past or current uses of pesticides.

Furthermore, increased awareness and concern for ecologic implications of the use of pesticides have begun to direct the attention and research of toxicologists toward studies on wild species as well as on man and domestic animals and laboratory animals that are selected as test models to represent man. The toxicology of pesticides, therefore, must take into account problems relating to both their injurious effects directly upon man and their effects on other species of animals in the environment from which man derives pleasure as well as food or which are essential to maintain a proper ecologic balance.

It is not uncommon for people to equate *pesticides* with *insecticides*. This is erroneous since the term "pesticide" is a general classification and includes a variety of chemicals with different uses. Pesticides chemicals have in common the capability of destroying life of some forms and are classified as pesticides because the organisms against which they are directed are deemed to be undesirable by the person or society that applies them. Indeed, insecticides represent one group of pesticides that are used in large quantities and have a history of causing toxic effects in man, but among the other types of pesticides one can find several potent, injurious agents. In terms of quantities used, the *herbicides*, chemicals used to destroy unwanted plants, rival the insecticides. Another common misconception is that pesticides imply a unity of action, that they all act similarly. This of course is not true. There is as great a diversity in their types of action and primary target tissues as there is diversity in their chemistry and physicochemical properties. There are a large number of pesticides whose acute toxicity is manifested through functional or biochemical action in the central and peripheral nervous systems, but there are others in which nervous system involvement does not occur or is merely secondary to primary effects in other organ systems. The literature on pesticides reveals great disparities in the extent of knowledge concerning specific mechanisms of action. For some groups of compounds the mechanism of toxic action is well understood at the molecular level. For others there is essentially no information concerning mechanisms of toxicity. Similarly the full gamut of toxic dose-response ranges is represented by pesticide chemicals. Even within a similar chemical class, individual compounds ranging from extremely toxic to practically nontoxic may be found. Obviously, therefore, one cannot generalize either qualitatively or quantitatively concerning the toxicity of pesticides.

Economic and Public Health

As with the use of any potentially injurious chemical substance, the use of pesticides must take into consideration the balance of the benefits that maybe expected versus the possible risk of injury to human health or to degradation of environmental quality. It is indeed extremely difficult to quantify the risk-benefit equation relating to the use of pesticides. In some cases the prospect of mass starvation due to destruction of food crops by inserts and noxious weeds versus the question of possible injury to a few members of the population as a result of use of insecticides may clearly indicate an advantage of pesticide use in terms of numbers of people whose health and welfare are protected. Similarly where vector-borne diseases represent a major threat to the health of large populations of humans and where the use of chemical pesticides to destroy the vectors of these diseases is a successful procedure, the application of these chemicals seems to be clearly indicated On the other hand, widespread distribution of chemicals in the environment to control what may be primarily a nuisance situation raises questions as to whether the benefits to be achieved really justify any risk, however minimal, that human health may be jeopardized.

If one extends these considerations beyond purely a concern for human health and considers the question of ecologic balance, the risk-benefit equation takes on different proportions. In the first case, with the exception of possible exposures of the persons who handle the concentrated pesticides, the human population may not be exposed to any significant quantity of the chemical. However, when these chemicals are distributed over widespread areas of land and aquatic surfaces, there is a distinct possibility that desirable species in the environment, other than man, will receive potentially toxic doses of the chemicals. This may not appear to have any direct effect on man's health and welfare; however, if such effects lead to a serious ecologic imbalance, indirect effects on man are possible. Perhaps the best known of all pesticides, DDT, exemplifies a situation of a product that when introduced as an insecticide in 1942 appeared to hold immense promise of benefit to agricultural economics and protection of public health against vector-borne disease. It was hailed as the miracle insecticide and for two decades was used with little concern for injury, and indeed little evidence that injury was produced. However, during the third decade of its use, effects on the environment, effects in nontarget species other than man, began to arise serious doubts concerning its continued usefulness. Now three decades after its patent many countries of the world have critically restricted the use of DDT because of evidence of environmental damage.

Control of Vector-Borne Disease

Pesticides of various types are used in the control of insects, rodents, and other pests that are involved in the life-cycle of vector-borne disease such as malaria, filariasis, yellow fever, viral encephalitis, typhus, bubonic plague, Rocky Mountain spotted fever, rickettsialpox, etc. The success of DDT in reducing the incidence of malaria in many parts of the world has been dramatic. To cite one example, in the Latina province of Italy in 1944 there were 175 new cases of malaria; in 1945 a DDT spray control program was initiated and by 1947 there were only five new cases of malaria, and by 1949 no new cases of malaria appeared.

This is only one example of a success story for DDT. The story has been repeated and continues to be repeated in some areas. Worldwide estimates of the lives saved by using DDT to destroy insects that transmit malaria and other diseases are numbered in the millions and the illnesses prevented are numbered in the hundreds of millions.

Agricultural Productivity

In many parts of the world excessive loss of food crops to insects and other destructive pests contribute to an obvious health problem—starvation. In these countries use of chemicals for controlling these pests clearly seems to have a favourable cost-benefit relationship. In lands of plenty such a clear health benefit may be less obvious. Then, attempts to evaluate the cost-benefit ratios are often reduced to economic considerations. It has been estimated that in 1963 the use of pesticides in the United States resulted in an increase in the value of farm production of about 1.8 billion dollars. This was achieved with an expenditure of about 0.44 billion dollars for control chemicals and procedures. Thus, one can estimate that the net economic benefit was an approximate 1.4-billion-dollar contributed to the gross national product.

Urban Pest Control

Although the total usage of pesticides, in term of pounds applied, is largest in those applications related to agriculture or forestry, these toxic chemicals are also used in urban areas. In addition to the use of pesticides by government service agencies, as in mosquito and rodent control programs and weed control on highways and utility rights of way, there is a rather large use of pesticides by individual home owners and gardens. For example, during a one-year period in Salt Lake Country, Utah, of the total of 200,865 lb of pesticides used, 102,49C lb were used for domestic or household applications. The balance was used by farmers, commercial applicators, fruit growers, and government agencies, and for mosquito abatement, and on livestock. There are, however, great contrasts in these proportions, as illustrated by the statistics of Arizona. The domestic usage for the state accounted for only about 0.6 per cent of the total compared to over 50 per cent of the total in Salt Lake Country, Utah.

It is clear that the opportunities for exposure to pesticides are great. Because the use of pesticides is associated primarily with agricultural operations, major concern is usually for the food we eat. However, it is quite possible that less controlled and less regulated uses of pesticides may offer the greatest opportunity for exposure to toxicologically significant quantities.

Environmental Contamination

It is apparent that there are many sources of exposure of humans and other nontarget species to pesticides by direct contact with materials at the site of application. In recent years, however, it has become increasingly apparent that exposures to pesticides far remote from the source of application are also possible. This results from the translocation of the chemicals from their sites of application through the various media of the environment. The extent to which translocation within the environment occurs will depend to a large degree on the physicochemical properties of the pesticides. Perhaps one of the most important factors is the extent of and time required for degradation of chemicals to simpler nontoxic forms. Since several of the organochlorine insecticides and some of the heavy metals are the most persistent types of pesticides, these compounds have been the object of most concern for problems of translocation and biomagnification. For example DDT is only slowly metabolized by biologic systems. Some of the metabolites are extremely resistant to further degradation, but retain some of the biologic activities of the parent compound. In addition, the partition coefficient for DDT in fat-soluble substances, relative to aqueous media, is very high. Therefore, this chemical will be concentrated through a food chain since it tends to partition into lipoidal biologic materials in increasing concentrations until, at the top of the food chain pyramid, a potentially hazardous concentration may exist.

Other nonbiologic modes of translocation include vaporization and drift by airborne routes so that the materials are carried by prevailing wind patterns far remote from their site of application. Subsequently, they may be precipitated out by rainfall onto land and surface waters in areas in which the pesticides have not been applied directly. Application to the soil may result, ultimately, in suspension of the pesticides, adsorbed on soil particles, and airborne translocation as dust. The extent to which pesticides will remain in soil after application depends upon a number of factors; such as soil type, moisture, temperature, pH, microorganism content, degradability of the pesticide itself, and the extent of cultivation and cover crops. In general, the organochlorine insecticides are most persistent in soils (with the exception of heavy metals, which of course are not further degraded), followed by certain of the herbicides and with the phosphate insecticides and carbamate insecticides and herbicides being the least persistent. An understanding of the potential for persistence and translocation, therefore, must take into consideration not only the biologic aspects of pesticides but also an analysis of their behaviour under various physical and chemical characteristics of the environment. As will be pointed out subsequently, chemical changes of the parent insecticides that result from either physicochemical reactions in the environment or biologically catalyzed reactions may lead to products with either greater or lesser toxicity and with either greater or lesser potential for biotranslocation.

Production and Use Statistics

Before the mid-1940s the primary pesticides in use were botanical in origin and compounds of heavy metals. Subsequently, there has been a marked increase in total pesticide usage and a rapid proliferation of synthetic organic compounds. There are now approximately 900 chemicals that are registered for sale as pesticides against about 2,000 pest species. The U.S. production of pesticides in 1971 was approximately 1.2 billion lb.

Shifts in uses of major classes reflect not only developments in agricultural practice but also the effect of regulatory restrictions and the development of resistance by the pests to certain classes of chemicals.

Human Poisonings

As stated initially, pesticides have a relatively good record in the United States in terms of fatalities resulting from exposure. The United States escaped major incidents of mass acute fatal poisonings, but this is not the case when one considers the worldwide record. There have been several reports of various disease conditions or altered clinical test values resulting from chronic exposure to pesticides, but these conditions are generally reversible and thus cannot be classified as true chronic injury. The relatively small numbers of cases in which progressive chronic disease has been associated with pesticide exposure preclude establishment of cause-and-effect relationships and prevent the conclusion that the widespread use of pesticides has contributed to an increasing incidence of chronic disease. This is not to say there is room for complacency in this regard. As new methods of toxicologic evaluation reveal subtle effects previously unknown and as this information is applied to well-designed epidemiologic studies, it may be found that pesticides have produced currently undetected effects on health. In our present state of knowledge, however, we must deal with the evidence at hand and hope that increased awareness on the part of the medical profession and of the public will stimulate further exploration of any possible injurious effects.

Most of the epidemiologic studies that have been conducted to search for possible associations between disease and pesticide exposure have been done on sample populations that would be expected to be high-risk groups, such as persons occupationally exposed in the manufacturing, formulating, or application of the materials. This appears an obvious choice of study groups; however, failure to find effects in these groups need not preclude that effects occur. For example, persons who experience discomfort or mild illnesses may voluntarily remove themselves from occupations involving the use of pesticides. In addition, as will be discussed later, laboratory animal research has shown that certain types of adaptation occur with continuous and frequent exposures to pesticides. Whether or not this is a factor that can influence the detection of effects in workers with different durations of exposure remains to be demonstrated. As discussed below, however, there is ample evidence that exposure to pesticides has resulted in acute fatal poisonings and reversible illnesses.

Injuries from occupational exposures reported under the requirements of the State Workmen's Compensation Law in California have provided statistical compilations of the extent of injuries due to pesticides and other agricultural chemicals. The rate for all occupational disease reports in agricultural workers reports in agricultural workers in 1969 was 8.5 per 1,000 workers, more than three times the rate for all industry (2.6 per 1,000). There were 727 occupational disease reports attributed to agricultural chemicals in California in 1969. Thirty-two per cent of these involved organic phosphate insecticides, 10 per cent herbicides, 8 per cent halogenated hydrocarbon insecticides, 6 per cent fertilizers, and 44 per cent miscellaneous or unidentified chemicals. Of the 175 cases diagnosed as systemic poisonings, organophosphate insecticides were responsible for 80 per cent, and they were involved in 47 per cent of another 160 reports of digestive and other non-localized symptoms of illness. This high contribution of systemic poisonings due to organic phosphates continued the record of several years. Parathion was the agent most frequently involved. Clearly, workers involved in direct agricultural operations were a high-risk group, and clearly, organophosphorus insecticides were high-risk compounds. Although, as a class herbicides ranked second as a cause of occupational disease, less than 5 per cent of these reports involved systemic poisoning.

Routes of Exposure

Analysis of residues on masks or on pads placed on exposed skin surfaces of workers involved in pesticide applications indicated that the dermal route offers the greatest potential for occupational exposure. The type of pesticide formulation applied was also a factor in the relative contribution of the respiratory route of exposure. When aerosols were used, an average of 2.87 per cent of the total (dermal and respiratory) exposure was by the respiratory route, compared with 0.23 per cent for dilute sprays and 0.94 per cent for dusts. Different degrees of hazard were associated with different jobs. Thus, indoor house spraying was much more hazardous than outdoor spraying of several types. In an airplane spraying operation the relative hazard differed depending on the particular job. For example in the airplane spraying of a fruit orchard the loader received about three times as much as the pilot and $4^2/_3$ times as much as the flagman. Of course, the hazard to applicators is dependent not only on the extent and route of exposure, but on several other factors such as the relative rates of absorption from the skin and lungs, particle sizes of dust and aerosols, and the inherent toxicity of the materials. Wolfe and coworkers (1967) found, in their studies of a wide variety of spraying operations involving 11 different pesticides, that the highest means value for the percentage of toxic dose received per hour of work was 44.2 per cent for workers who loaded airplanes with 1 per cent TEPP (tetraethyl pyrophosphate) dust. Although there were several illnesses associated with this operation, these authors considered the incidence quite low in view of the relative hazard. They suggested that three factors might account for this: the number of hours per day (or week) that the worker is actually engaged in loading airplanes is low; knowledge of the high toxicity of TEPP may prompt more diligent use of protective clothing and respiratory protective devices; and only a small percentage of the dry dust impinging on exposed skin is likely to be absorbed.

Oral ingestion is the most frequent route of exposure in cases of nonoccupational poisonings. Dermal exposures have resulted in deaths of small children who come in contact with presumably empty containers for highly toxic pesticides. Respiratory exposure as well as dermal of the general population is possible as a result of drift from agricultural operations. Household use of pesticide aerosol "bombs," vaporizers, pest strips, and other aerosol or vapor-generating devices is a potential source of respiratory exposure in nonoccupational settings. Hayes (1969) reported that 19 different organophosphorus insecticides that have resulted in human poisonings there were 20 compounds in the organochlorine class, five different carbamates, four botanicals, three inorganic elements, and six miscellaneous compounds for a total of 57 different insecticides. Eight herbicides were responsible for human poisonings, seven fungicides, six rodenticides, one molluscicide, and one nematocide for a total 80 different compounds.

Insecticides

Only select examples of the various classes of insecticides will be discussed here. For additional discussion of their chemistry and metabolism the reader should consult the extensive report by Menzie (1969). Comprehensive complication of chemical and common names, structures, and LD 50 values in rats may be found in Gaines (1969) and Frear (1969). Acute toxicity data for fish and wildlife are available in several reports. Summaries of results of subacute and chronic feeding studies for many compounds have been made available in the monograph by Lehman (1965). Several books and monographs that are devoted exclusively to pesticides provide much more extensive coverage than is possible here. Handbooks prepared by Hayes (1963) and by Morgan (1976) provide information on clinical toxicology and emergency treatment for many pesticides.

Organophosphorus Insecticides

As discussed earlier, insecticides (of the several classes of pesticides) have most frequently been involved in human poisonings and organophosphorus compounds have most frequently been the offending agents.

Historic considerations

The first organophosphate insecticide was tetraethyl pyrophosphate (TEPP). It was developed in Germany as substitute for nicotine, which was in short supply in that country during World War II. Related extremely toxic compounds such as ethyl N-dimethyl phosphoroamido-cyanidate (tabun) and isoprophyl methylphosphonofluoridate (sarin) were kept secrete by the German government as potential chemical warfare agents. These, and other extremely toxic compounds, are the so-called nerve gas chemical warfare agents.

TEPP, although an effective insecticide, was highly toxic to mammals and are rapidly hydrolyzed in the presence of moisture. Further efforts to find more stable compounds for use in agriculture led to the synthesis by Schrader in 1944 of parathion (E605; O,O-diethyl O-*p*-nitrophenyl phosphate). Because it exhibited a wide range of insecticidal activity and suitable physical and chemical properties such as low volatility and sufficient stability in water and mild alkali, parathion became one of the most widely used organophosphorus insecticides. It continues to be used extensively in agriculture, but because of its high mammalian toxicity, by all routes of exposure, other less hazardous compounds have begun to take its place. Parathion has the dubious distinction of being the pesticide most frequently involved in fatal poisonings. During the last two decades the agricultural chemistry industry has developed many other organic triesters of phosphoric acid and phosphorothioic acid that have been registered for use as insecticides.

Shortly after parathion became available for study, acute toxicity studies on experimental animals revealed signs of poisoning that resembled excessive of cholinergic nerves. These could be alleviated by atropine, a cholinergic blocking agent. This suggested inhibition of acetylcholinesterase of nerve tissues as the mechanism of toxic action, as had been demonstrated for related organophosphate triesters, and was confirmed by the finding that tissues of rats poisoned by parathion had markedly reduced cholinesterase activity and increased free acetylcholine in their brains. Thus, the biochemical basis for nerve tissue, became known soon after its introduction as an insecticide. Subsequent development and research on other organophosphate insecticides have revealed that they all, in sufficient doses, inhibit acetylcholine-esterase *in vivo* and thus share a common mechanism of acute toxic action. The chemical mechanism of cholinesterase inhibition is discussed in more detail later in this chapter and in several extensive reviews and monographs.

Signs and symptoms of acute poisoning

Signs and symptoms of acute systemic poisoning by organophosphate insecticides are predictable from their biochemical mechanism of action. Thus inhibition of acetylcholinesterase results in accumulation of endogenous acetylcholine in nerve tissue and effector organs with consequent signs and symptoms that mimic the muscarinic, nicotinic, and central nervous system actions of acetylcholine. Acetylcholine is the chemical transmitter of nerve impulses at endings of postganglionic parasympathetic nerve fibers, somatic motor nerves to skeletal muscle, preganglionic fibers of both parasympathetic and sympathetic nerves, and certain synapses in the central nervous system.

Muscarinic receptors for acetylcholine are found primarily in smooth muscles, the heart, and exocrine glands. Signs and symptoms of organophosphorus insecticide poisoning that results from stimulation of these receptors include tightness in the chest and wheezing expiration due to bronchoconstriction and increased bronchial secretions, increased salivation and lacrimation, increased sweating, increased gastrointestinal tone and peristalsis with consequent development of nausea, vomiting, abdominal cramps, diarrhea, tenesmus and involuntary defecation, bradycardia that can progress to heart block, frequent and involuntary urination due to contraction of smooth muscle of the bladder, and constriction of the pupils (miosis).

Nicotinic signs and symptoms result from accumulation of acetylcholine at the endings of motor nerves to skeletal muscle and autonomic ganglia. Muscular effects include easy fatigue and mild weakness followed by involuntary twitching, scattered fasciculations and cramps with progression to generalized fasciculations, and muscular weakness that affects the muscles of respiration and contributes to dyspnea and cyanosis. Nicotinic actions at autonomic ganglia may, in severe intoxication, mask some of the muscarinic effects. Thus tachycardia may result from stimulation of sympathetic ganglia to overcome the usual bradycardia to muscarinic action on the heart. Pallor, elevation of blood pressure, and hyperglycemia also reflect nicotinic action at sympathetic ganglia.

Accumulation of acetylcholine in the central nervous system is believed to be responsible for the tension, anxiety, restlessness, insomnia, headache, emotional instability and neurosis, excessive dreaming and nightmares, apathy, and confusion that have been described after organophosphate poisoning. Slurred speech, tremor, generalized weakness, ataxia, convulsions, depression of respiratory and circulatory centers, and coma are other central nervous system effects.

The immediate cause of death in fatal organophosphate poisoning is asphyxia resulting from respiratory failure. Contributing factors are the muscarinic actions of bronchoconstriction and increased bronchial secretions, nicotinic action leading to paralysis of the respiratory muscles and the central nervous system action of depression and paralysis of the respiratory center.

Localized effects

Localized effects at the site of exposure may be seen in the absence of obvious signs and symptoms of systemic absorption as described above. Exposure to vapours, dusts, or aerosols can exert local effects on the smooth muscles of the eyes and respiratory tact resulting in early miosis and blurred vision due to spasm of accommodation in the first case and bronchoconstriction in the case of respiratory exposure. Secretory glands of the respiratory tract, as well as smooth muscles, may be affected by minimal inhalation exposure to the organophosphates leading to watery nasal discharge, nasal hyperemia, sensation of tightness in the chest, and prolonged wheezing respiration. Local effects of dermal exposure include localized sweating and fasciculations at the site of contact. Gastrointestinal manifestations are usually the first to appear after oral ingestion and some of them may be due to local anticholinesterase action in the gastrointestinal tract.

Systemic effects

Systemic effect are, in general, similar irrespective of route of absorption, but the sequence and time may differ. Respiratory and ocular symptoms would be expected first after exposure to airborne organophosphates, while gastrointestinal symptoms and localized sweating would likely be first to appear after oral and dermal exposure, respectively. However, these generalizations may not hold for compounds that must be metabolically activated. The onset of symptoms after exposure to organophosphate compounds is usually rapid, within a few minutes to two or three hours. The duration of symptoms is generally from one to five days. In fatal untreated poisonings, deaths, usually occur within 24 hours. It should be recognized that, in addition to the usual factors of route or exposure, concentrations of active material, etc., the quality of sings and symptoms, their rate of onset, and their durations may differ markedly for different compounds by virtue of differences in rat of biotransformation, distribution, and affinities for acetylcholinesterase. For example, in five cases of attempted suicide by ingestion of dichlofenthion, severe cholinergic crises did not appear until 40 to 48 hours but they persisted for 5 to 48 days in the three survivors. This extremely prolonged course was associated with persistent residues of this insecticide in the blood and fat of the patients. Dichlofenthion has a higher octanol/water partition coefficient that most organophosphorus insecticides, and the prolonged course of the poisonings was due to a slow release of the insecticides from adipose tissue reservoirs.

Organophosphate insecticides in common use are rapidly metabolized and excreted, and subacute or chronic poisoning by virtue of accumulation of the compounds in the body does not occur. However, because several of the organophosphates produce slowly reversible inhibition of cholinesterase *accumulation of this effect* can occur. Signs and symptoms of poisoning that resemble those produced by a single high dose will occur when the accumulated inhibition of cholinesterase produced by smaller, repeated doses reaches a critical level. Cessation of exposure normally results in complete recovery. Chronic complaints associated with poisoning by organophosphates have been reported as due to sequelae of severe acute poisoning. A few compounds have produced delayed and persistent peripheral neuropathy, apparently unrelated to anticholinesterase action.

Delayed neurotoxic effects

These are produced by several phosphate triesters. Although this can result from a single toxic dose, the neuropathology is generally delayed in onset. Most notorious of the compounds that produce this effect is triorthocresyl phosphate (TOCP). This compound is not a potent anticholinesterase, and it is not used as an insecticide. However, a number of compounds that are used as insecticides can produce this effect and it is common practice to screen for this action in safety evaluation tests. The function disturbances associated with phosphate triester neuropathy begin in the distal parts of the lower limbs in both man and other sensitive animals. Mild sensory disturbances and motor weakness with ataxia occur, progressing in severity and extent to increased weakness and flaccidity of the legs and varying amounts of sensory disturbance. Upper limbs may also become involved. After several days to a few weeks the peak of the process is reached and thereafter improvement in the functional disturbance begins. Recovery is slow and not always complete.

Although hens and man seem to be the most sensitive species to the organic phosphate triester neuropathy, studies on various compounds have shown that dogs, cats, calves, monkeys, sheep, pigs, horses, pheasants, ducks, and rats will also sustain this effect. For screening for possible production of this effect by pesticides, hens are usually used as the experimental animal. Because of potent anticholinesterase actions of many pesticides, it is often impossible to administer sufficient doses to the animal to produce the neuropathic effect. To overcome this and to screen for the neuropathy, a common procedure is to administer atropine to protect against the acute cholinergic action. Using this procedure Gaines (1969) found that 22 to 30 organophosphorus pesticides tested and three out of nine carbamate insecticides produced leg weakness in atropinized hens under sufficient time and dosage conditions. With all but three of the compounds, however, the onset of leg weakness occurred within 24 hours, and for most compounds the hens recovered within a months. Aldridge and Johnson (1971) consider this rapid onset and relatively rapid recovery to result from a different mechanism than for TOCP and other long-acting neurotoxins.

Metabolism

Toxicity Relationship. Several biotransformation reactions that organophosphorus insecticides undergo have been discussed in several reviews and monographs. In this section selected biotransformation reactions are discussed as illustrations of the development of knowledge that has led to an understanding of factors that affect the susceptibility of animals to poisoning by these compounds.

Activation

The early organophosphorus anticholinesterases such as TEPP and DEP were phosphate triesters and were potent inhibitors of cholinesterase both *in vivo* and *in vitro*. The development of parathion introduced the phosphorothionates. The majority of compounds now in use as insecticides contain the (=S) thiono moiety, and are either phosphorothionates (e.g., parathion, methyl parathion) or phosphorodithioates (e.g., azinphosmethyl, malathion). Early in research on parathion and its oxygen analog, paraoxon, it became apparent that in addition to conferring greater stability against nonenzymatic hydrolysis, substitution of =S for =O on the phosphorus compound altered its toxic properties. Parathion was less toxic to animals than paraoxon, and several factors that altered the toxicity of parathion in rats did not affect paraoxon's toxicity; although both compounds inhibited acetylcholinesterase and produced similar cholinergic signs of poisoning. Further studies showed that highly purified parathion did not inhibit cholinesterase *in vitro*, and that the inhibitory activity of less purified samples could be attributed to contamination with the S-ethyl and S-phenyl isomers of parathion or with its oxygen analog, paraoxon. Subsequently it was demonstrated that paraoxon was the active anticholinesterase formed from parathion in intact rats.

There are other activation reactions, involving a few compounds, in which parents insecticides are converted to more potent anticholinesterase agents. They include oxidation of phosphoroamidates and thioether oxidation by mixed function oxidases.

Inactivation

In addition to the requirement for an oxo (=O) group to be present for anticholinesterase activity, metabolic modification of the alkyl and

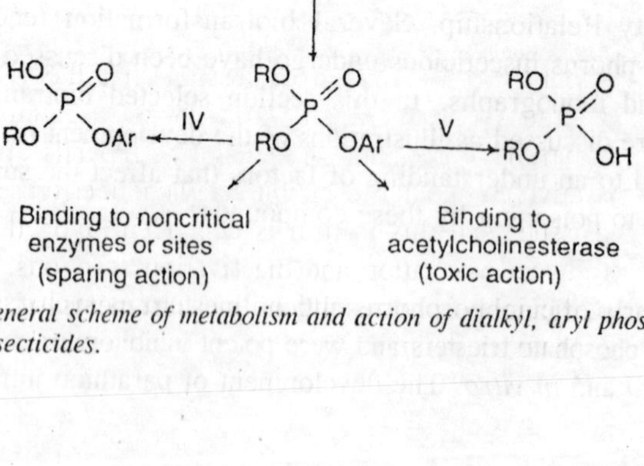

Fig. 23.1. General scheme of metabolism and action of dialkyl, aryl phosphorothioate insecticides.

aryl substituents can also influence activity. Reactions II, III, IV, and V are enzymatic detoxification reactions that yield products that do not inhibit acetylcholinesterase. Largely as a result of *in vitro* studies, it was proposed that reaction V, catalyzed by paraoxonase (A-esterase), was the major pathway of detoxication of parathion. This enzyme is widely distributed among several tissues in rats and other mammals. It does not require addition of cofactors for measurements of activity *in vitro* and probably hydrolyzes several other organophosphates (P=O compounds), but apparently does not hydrolyze the P=S compounds directly. Thus, the proposed enzymatic mechanism of detoxification of parathion and other phosphorothionate insecticides was for many years, based on the concept that hydrolytic detoxication (reaction V) followed the formation of the oxygen analogs (reaction I). However, studies using ^{32}P-labeled parathion have shown that the arylphosphorus bond can be cleaved (reaction III) without prior oxidation to paraoxon.

Another detoxification pathway involves the hydrolysis of carboxyester or carboxyamide linkages in some insecticides by tissue or plasma carboxylesterases Malathion and dimethoate examples. Products or the hydrolysis of the carboxyester of the carboxyester or amide groups do not inhibit cholinesterase, and enzymatic formation of these products has been demonstrated *in vivo* and *in vitro* studies. In several species of mammals, this appears to be the major pathway of detoxification for these insecticides, and their selective insecticidal action is due to a relative lack of these hydrolytic enzymes in insects. The importance of this reaction in mammals as a detoxification pathway has been demonstrated in studies in which animals pretreated with other organophosphate compounds that strongly inhibit carboxylesterases become more susceptible to the acute toxicity and anticholinesterase action of malathion. Pretreatment with triorthocresyl phosphate (TOCP), a strong inhibitor of carboxylesterase but weak anticholinesterase, reduced the LD 50 of malathion in rats from 1100 to 10 mg/kg, a 110-fold potentiation.

It is apparent from the above discussion that the relationships between enzymatic metabolism and toxicity of organophosphorus insecticides is extremely complex. The toxicity depends upon the net availability of active compound to inhibit acetylcholinesterase at critical sites in nerve tissue, and this in turn is dependent upon the dynamic relationships between activation and inactivation reactions. There are not always predictable from results of measurements of relative of enzyme reactions under optimum conditions *in vitro*, particularly when both activation and inactivation reactions are catalyzed by enzyme systems with common cofactor requirements, tissue distributed, and intracellular location.

Acetylcholinesterase inhibition and reversal

There is abundant evidence that both the organophosphorus and carbamate insecticides (discussed subsequently) produce their acute toxic actions by inhibiting acetylcholinesterase. In addition to the fact that it has been demonstrated that many of these compounds are potent inhibitors *in vitro*, several lines of *in vivo* evidence support this mechanism. The consequence of acetylcholinesterase inhibition is accumulation of acetylcholine at effector sites, and the protection against acute poisoning offered by atropine and other cholinergic blocking agents supports the mechanism. Additionally, induced reversal of cholinesterase inhibition by chemical compounds, such as the oxime derivatives, results in alleviation of symptoms of poisoning. A combination of pharmacologic antidotes (atropine) and biochemical antidotes (oximes) is potentiative in its antidotal activity.

The rate of recovery of free and active acetylcholinesterase following poisoning by organophosphorus and carbamate insecticides varies with different compounds. In general, the carbamates are usually considered reversible inhibitors of cholinesterase, and their duration of action is relatively short. In addition, because of the reversal of inhibition by dilution of the enzyme (as would occur if one sampled a tissue and diluted it with buffer during preparation for assay), determination of acetylcholinesterase inhibition by carbamates *in vivo* poses some technical difficulties. Unless care is taken, it is quite possible to observe the typical signs of anticholinesterase poisoning following carbamates; but by the time tissues are removed and prepared for assay, decarbamylation or reversal of enzyme-carbamate complex may have occurred and inhibition is undetectable. Therefore, in suspected cases of poisoning, where the history and signs and symptoms suggest a carbamate exposure, but clinical tests show a normal or nearly normal blood cholinesterase value, one must be guided by the history before concluding that the poisoning was not the result of a carbamate insecticide.

The case for organophosphate poisoning is somewhat different in that the compounds are in general much more slowly reversible inhibitors. However, even within this class there are marked differences in the persistence of inhibition following toxic doses of the compound. Spontaneous reversal of enzyme inhibition by organophosphates as well

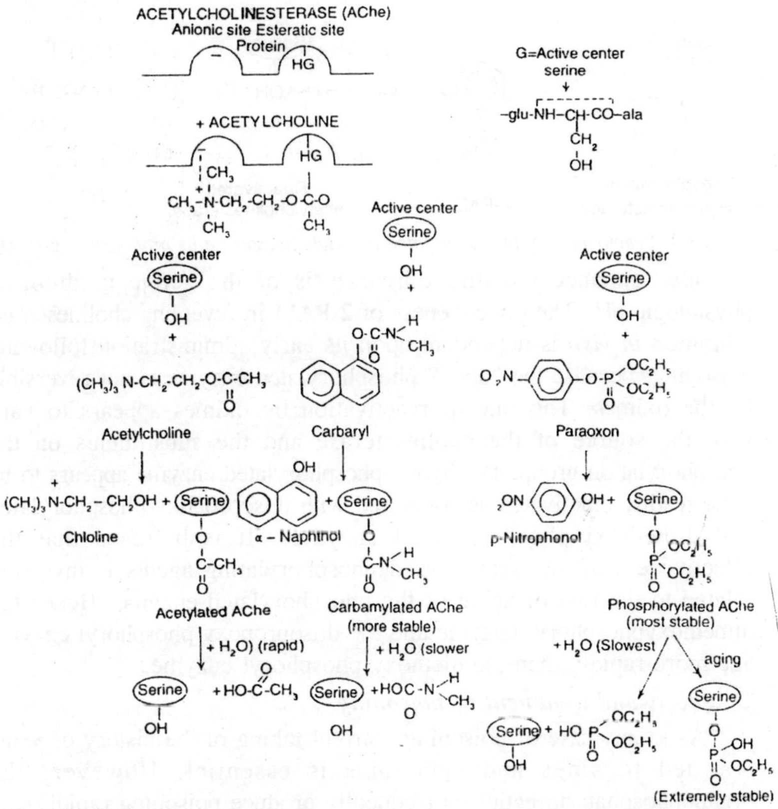

Fig. 23.2. Scheme of hydrolysis of acetylcholine by acetylcholinesterase and reactions of the anticholinesterase insecticides carbaryl and paraoxon.

as carbamates can occur at varying rates, depending upon the insecticide, by hydrolysis of the phosphorylated cholinesterase. The rate of reactivation *in vitro* of mouse brain and diaphragm acetylcholinesterase inhibited *in vivo* was five to ten times greater for azinphosmethyl and parathion-methyl than for azinphosmethyl and parathion-ethyl.

Fortunately, there are available chemicals that will accelerate the hydrolysis of the phosphorylated enzyme, and hence accelerate regeneration of active acetylcholinesterase. The most successful compounds are oxime derivatives, and the best known of these is 2-pyridine aldoxime methiodide which is now a standard part of the therapy of organophosphorus poisoning. In addition to the capacity of 2-PAM to accelerate the dephosphorylation of acetylcholinesterase it

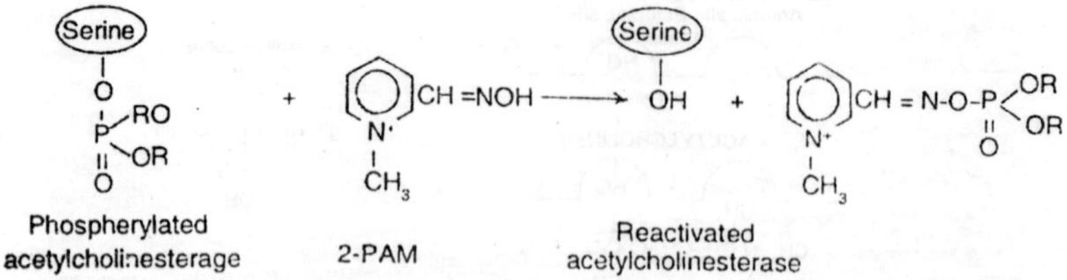

Serine — O — P(=O)(RO)(OR) + 2-PAM (pyridinium CH=NOH, N·CH$_3$) ——→ Serine — OH + pyridinium CH = N-O-P(=O)(OR)(OR), N·CH$_3$

Phospherylated acetylcholinesterage   2-PAM   Reactivated acetylcholinesterase

Fig. 23.3. Reactivation of phosphorylated acetylcholinesterase by pralidoxine (2-PAM).

can also enhance the direct hydrolysis of the active inhibitor at physiologic pH. The effectiveness of 2-PAM in reversing cholinesterase inhibition *in vivo* is dependent upon its early administration following poisoning, because the "aged" phosphorylated enzyme is not reversible by the oximes. The rate of reactivation by oximes appears to vary with the source of the cholinesterase and the substituents on the phosphorylation group. Diethyoxy-phosphorylated enzyme appears to be most readily reactivated as compared with diisopropoxy-phosphorylated and dimethoxy-phosphorylated enzymes. It is believed that the effectiveness of the oximes as dephosphorylating agents is inversely related to the rate of aging of the phosphorylated enzyme. Hence the dimethoxyphosphoryl enzyme and the diisopropoxy phosphoryl enzyme age more rapidly than the diethoxy phosphoryl enzyme.

Diagnosis and treatment of poisoning

As in any case of poisoning, careful taking of the history of vents that led to sings and symptoms is essential. However, the organophosphate insecticides frequently produce poisoning rapidly and if in sufficient doses, may have a rapid fatal outcome. It is important, therefore, to be guided by the characteristic signs and symptoms and take emergency action even though a complete history may not have been obtained.

In very severe case the treatment should include (1) artificial respiration, preferably by mechanical means, and (2) atropine sulfate, 2 to 4 mg intravenously as soon as cyanosis is overcome. This may be repeated at five to ten-minute intervals until signs of atropinization appear. Note that this dosage of atropine is greater than that usually used for other purposes, but because people poisoned by anticholinesterase compounds have increased tolerance for atropine, it is a safe dose, used carefully by an astute physician. (3) Following atropinization, treatment before time is spent in decontaminating the skin, stomach, or eyes as may be indicated; however, decontamination must be followed promptly. The skin should be washed with an alkaline soap, which will not only remove, but also help hydrolyze, the phosphate ester. Appropriate clinical procedures for evacuating the stomach and cleansing the eyes may be indicated. A case history of successful treatment of poisoning by dicrotophos, in which a total of 3911.5 mg of atropine and 92 g of pralidoxime chloride was given over a 23-day period, illustrates the importance of vigorous treatment in severe cases of poisoning.

In more usual and less severe cases the procedure should be as follow: Administer atropine SO_4, 1 to 2 mg, if symptoms appear. If excessive secretions occur, keep the patient fully atropinized by giving atropine sulfate every hour up to 25 to 50 mg in a day. Proceed with decontamination of the skin and removal of the poison from the stomach or eyes as the second step in this case. In these less severe poisonings 2-PAM administration should be instituted if the patient fails to respond satisfactorily to atropine, followed, of course, by symptomatic treatment. The doses indicated above are those suggested for adults. Anyone expecting to face the possibility of dealing with severe poisoning by organophosphate insecticides should consult more detailed descriptions of diagnosis and therapy.

Knowledge of the biochemical action of the organophosphate insecticides has provided a means for a relative specific clinical test for diagnosis of excessive exposure to these compounds Routine measurements of blood cholinesterase activity are frequently made in workers engaged in occupations where exposure to phosphate insecticides is a possibility. As discussed in several reports the inhibition of the activity of plasma or red cell cholinesterase is reasonably well correlated with the severity of exposure and poisoning. Measurement of the cholinesterase activity of the blood only indirectly reflects the extent of biochemical lesion at critical sites in nerve tissues or effector organs, however. Depending upon the compound, the relative inhibition of plasma pseudocholinesterase and erythrocyte acetylcholinesterase may differ. Since the red cell enzyme is apparently identical to that in nerve tissue, assays on red cells are usually considered more reflective of nerve tissue activity. Rather marked inhibition of red cell and plasma cholinesterase may be present in the absence of symptoms. Total inhibition of plasma and 60 to 70 per cent inhibition in red cell activity has been noted in the absence of overt signs of poisonings. However, the relationship between inhibition of blood cholinesterase activity and symptoms differs with different compounds and may reflect differences in distribution of the inhibitions. Relationships between blood and nerve tissue cholinesterase inhibition and signs of poisoning for various compounds in experimental animals have been reviewed by DuBois (1963) and Wills (1972).

Tolerance to acute, sublethal effects of some organophosphates

This has been demonstrated in experimental animals. In these experiments the phosphates were administered repeatedly or fed in the diet at sublethal doses for several days. Initially, acute cholinergic signs and symptoms were observed. In time, however, the animals no longer responded with obvious signs after each dose, and their general appearance, growth, and behaviour appeared normal. However at sacrifice, these apparently normal animals had markedly inhibited blood and nervous tissue cholinesterase activity and elevated levels of acetylcholine in their brains. Adaptation or compensation to central nervous system and behavioural effects of anticholinesterase insecticides also occur in rats in spite of continued brain acetylcholinesterase inhibition and elevated acetylcholine levels.

Experiments by Brodeur and DuBois (1964) suggest that the apparent tolerance involves development of a refractoriness of cholinergic receptor sites. Tolerant animals were resistant to the acute toxicity of carbachol, which has direct effect on cholinergic receptors. Adaptation to high concentrations of acetylcholine has been observed to occur at the neuromuscular junction and at ganglia within a few minutes to a few hours, in contrast to the several days required for adaptation in the subacute experiments cited above. There are also reports that tolerance to reduced cholinesterase activity also occurs in man. Stavinoha and associates (1969) found that two different strains of rats that had adapted to low acetylcholinesterase activity in the brain different with respect to the levels of acetylcholine in the brain; one strain had normal levels of acetylcholine during adaptation while the other had elevated concentrations. They concluded there was no apparent correlation between the concentration of brain acetylcholine and adaptation. Although the mechanism suggested by Brodeur and DuBois (1964) of a refractoriness of cholinergic receptor sites is attractive, other possibilities related to the rate of production, release and destruction of acetylcholine could be considered.

Carbamate Insecticides

The acute toxicities of the carbamate insecticides also vary through a wide range. Unlike the organophosphates, most of the aromatic carbamate-ester insecticides have low dermal toxicities. However, one cannot generalize that carbamates are without dermal toxicity as illustrated by the extreme toxicity of aldicarb by both the oral and dermal routes. This compound, because of its extreme toxicity, is recommended only for limited use in greenhouse operations. The carbamates are not broad-spectrum insecticides, and some of the common household insect pests such as the housefly and German cock, each are relatively immune; however, bees are extremely sensitive to these insecticides. For several of the compounds, the LD 50 values for houseflies and German cockroaches are, on a body weight basis, greater than the LD 50s for rats.

Action and mechanism

The mode of action of the carbamates, like the organophosphates, is inhibition of acetylcholinesterase and the signs and symptoms of poisoning are typically cholinergic with lacrimation, salivation, miosis convulsions, and death. As indicated previously, however, the carbamates are relatively rapidly reversible inhibitors of cholinesterase. Atropine sulfate is the recommended antidote for poisoning by carbamate insecticides. Administration of 2-PAM is not recommended and at least for some compounds, seems to be specifically contraindicated since there have been reports that it aggravates the toxicity of carbaryl. In addition to the typical cholinergic signs of poisoning, experiments in rats showed that some of the less toxic carbamate insecticides when administrated intravenously produced a pronounced anesthetic effect with respiratory failure as the most critical determinant of the intravenous toxicity. This anesthetic action was rapid in onset. However, if artificial respiration was applied for two to five minutes animals resumed spontaneous respiration. Cholinergic signs then gradually developed. No pronounced anesthetic effects were observed with the carbamate insecticides when they were administered by the intraperitoneal or oral routes. This anesthetic effect has also been noted with several organophosphate insecticides and also appears to be unrelated to their anticholinesterase action.

Metabolism-toxicity relationships

Studies of the correlation between toxicity and *in vitro* anticholinesterase activity of a series of monomethylcarbamates showed that there was good correlation between *in vitro* inhibition and intravenous LD50s in rats, but the *in vitro* anticholinesterase action was poorly correlated with oral LD50s. The carbamate insecticides are direct inhibitors of acetylcholinesterase (i.e. they do not require metabolic activation), and the lack of correlation between the oral toxicity and *in vitro* anticholinesterase activity appeared to reflect differing rates of detoxication of the compounds. Hydrolysis of the

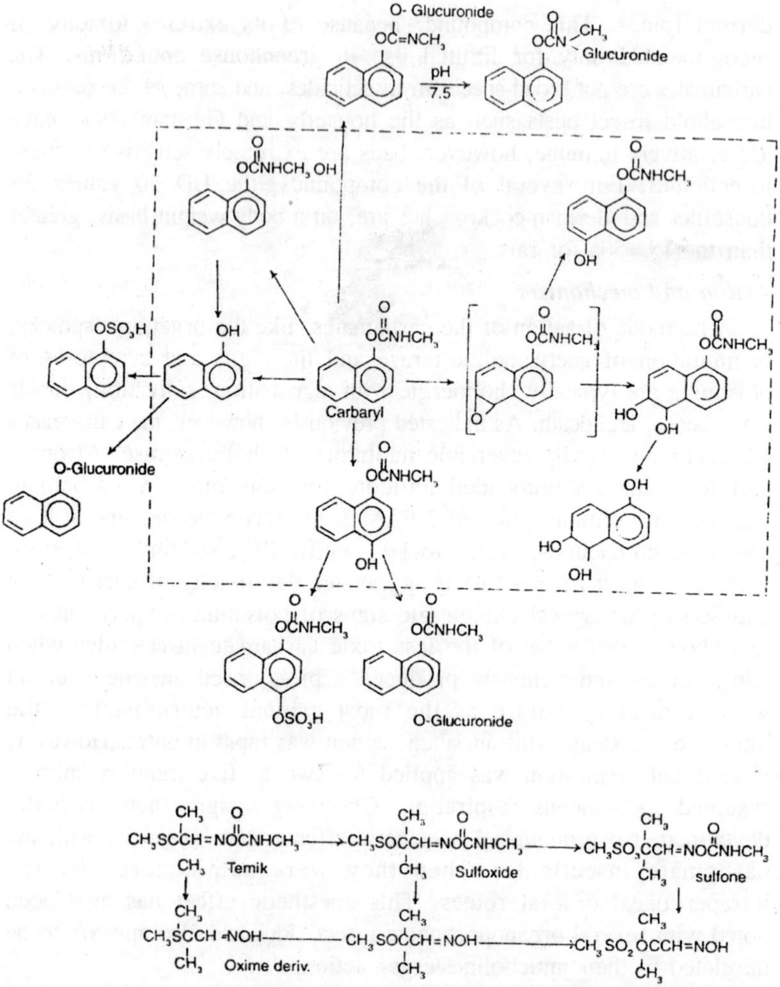

Fig. 23.4. Examples of metabolism of carbamate insecticides. A–Metabolism of carbaryl pathways within dashed rectangle demonstrated with liver microsomes in vitro. B–Metabolism of Temik.

carbamic acid ester linkage results in metabolites that lack anticholinesterase activity. The biotransformation pathways for typical carbamate insecticides are shown. Although hydrolysis occurs to some extent with all compounds, various oxidation steps that are catalyzed by mixed function oxidases also occur. The products formed by these reactions are not always less toxic than the parent compounds, but the parent compounds themselves, do have anticholinesterase action.

Cholinesterase inhibition and symptoms

Studies of the relationship between cholinesterase inhibition and signs and symptoms of poisoning in rats showed that with dosages that did not produce any noticeable symptoms (0.25 to 1.0 mg/kg, intramuscularly, of propoxur) the activity of both brain and plasma cholinesterase was reduced the brain and plasma cholinesterase activities to 50 per cent of normal level. At higher dosages (10 to 50 mg/kg) the degree of inhibition of both brain and plasma cholinesterase closely followed the severity of symptoms that were produced, with brain cholinesterase being slightly more inhibited than plasma. Studies on human volunteer were also conducted to determine the relationship between the inhibition of erythrocyte cholinesterase and onset of sings of poisoning. The lowest erythrocyte cholinesterase activity (27 per cent of normal) was observed at 15 minutes after ingestion of 1.5 mg/kg of propoxur in a 90 kg adult man. At this time no sings were observed, but moderate discomfort, that was described as pressure in the head was present. Blurred vision and nausea developed three minutes later, and 20 minutes after ingestion the man was pale and his face was sweating, pulse rate was 140 minutes compared to 76 before ingestion, and both systolic and diastolic blood pressures were increased. Following these symptoms, nausea, repeated vomiting, and profuse sweating developed. The symptoms lasted from about the thirtieth until the fortyfifth minute after ingestion, and during this period erythrocyte cholinesterase activity recovered from a level of 50 to 55 per cent of its normal value. Sixty minutes after ingestion the patient showed signs of improvement but felt nauseated and tired; pulse and blood pressure were normal. Two hours after ingestion the patient felt completely recovered. This rapid disappearance of symptoms was accompanied by further rapid recovery of erythrocyte cholinesterase activity. Studies on both rats and men indicated that the lethal dose of a carbamate insecticide is a considerably greater multiple of the dose causing the first signs of poisoning than for the organophosphorus insecticides. As a result, overexposure to carbamates might be expected to give early warning of poisoning in the form of appearance of slight symptoms, when, if heeded and exposure terminated, could prevent exposure to acutely dangerous quantities.

Other actions of carbamates

One of the least acutely toxic carbamate insecticides, carbaryl, has reportedly produced teratogenic effects in experimental animals. Although in most species the doses for effects on fetuses were near the maternal toxic doses, in beagle dogs the teratogenic dose was found to be only about a tenth of the toxic to the mother, hen given as single daily doses in gelatin capsules. Weil and coworkers (1972) reviewed the considerable literature on studies of reproductive and teratogenic action of carbaryl and concluded that the sensitivity of dogs to teratogenic action was related to the fact that dogs did not metabolize carbaryl to l-naphthol, a major metabolic pathway in most other species including man.

Cloudy swelling of cells in the proximal convoluted tubules of the kidneys was noted in rats and dogs fed 400 ppm of carbaryl in their diets for several months. Of related interest, it has been reported that the urinary amino acid-nitrogen: creatinine ratios were increased in a group of human volunteers who ingested daily of carbaryl of 0.12 mg/kg/day of several weeks. Although the exact relationships between the histologic changes in experimental animals and the biochemical changes in man is not established, they would seem to be related effects and the dosage relationships suggest that man may be much more sensitive to injurious effects of carbaryl on the kidney.

Organochlorine Insecticides

The organochlorine insecticides include the chlorinated ethane derivatives, of which DDT is the best known examples; the cyclodienes, which include chlordane, aldrin, dieldrin, hepatchlor, endrin, and toxaphene; and the hexachlorocyclohexanes, such as lindane. From the mid-1940s to the mid-1960s the organochlorine insecticides enjoyed wide use in agriculture, soil, and structure insect control, and in malaria control programs. However, they have, as a class, come into disfavour because they are very persistent in the environment and tend to accumulate in biologic as well as nonbiologic media. As a class the organochlorine insecticides are often considered to be less acutely toxic, but of greater potential for chronic toxicity, than the organophosphate and carbamate insecticides. However, there is a wide range of acute toxicities of individual compounds, from extremely toxic to slightly toxic. The organochlorine insecticides can also be classed as neuropoisons. However, their mechanism of action is not the same as that of the phosphates and carbamates. Indeed the precise mechanism is unknown for most of them.

DDT

DDT has been the best known, the cheapest, and probably one of the most effective of the synthetic insecticides. It was synthesized as early as 1874 but its insecticidal effectiveness was not discovered until 1939, and it was patented for this use in 1942. DDT was used extensively during World War II in control of lice and other insects by application directly to humans. There is no evidence that harm to these people resulted from this direct application. Indeed there seems to be no documented, unequivocal report of fatal human poisoning from DDT in spite of its widespread use and availability. Acute, nonfatal poisonings have occurred as a result of accidents or suicide attempts. Statistical associations between levels of storage of DDT and its metabolites and certain types of chronic disease in man have been reported however, causal relationships have not been established and other reports indicate no association between tissue DDT levels and chronic disease. There is no question, however, that the general population has sustained exposure to DDT and derivatives, and as a result practically everyone born since the mid-1940s, when DDT was introduced into commerce, has had a lifeline of exposure and storage of some quantity of this insecticide in fatty tissues. Thus chronic exposure to DDT has resulted in an accumulation of residues in man and other animals, but the health significance of these residues is not currently apparent and remain to be further evaluated.

On the other hand, there is convincing evidence that DDT and metabolites accumulate in natural food chains by a process of biologic concentration in ecosystems. As a result, organisms at the top of these natural food chains may sustain injury from DDT or its metabolites that are present as a result of gradual accumulations of residues in organisms that make up their food sources. Both field and laboratory studies have provided evidence that reproductive success in certain species of wild birds is adversely affected by exposure to DDT or its metabolites. Additionally, fish and some lower aquatic organisms are extremely sensitive to the acute toxicity of DDT.

The prospect of possible ecologic imbalance from continued use of DDT, the uncertainty as to the effect, if any, of continued prolonged exposure and storage of low levels of DDT in humans, and the development of resistant strains of insects have promoted the Environmental Protection Agency to markedly restrict the use of DDT in the U.S.A. Several other countries have taken similar actions. However, because of its relatively low cost, unavailability of substitutes that are both safe and effective, and its continuing presence as an environmental contaminant in spite of curtailed use, there continues to be interest in its toxicity.

Signs and symptoms of acute and subacute poisoning

Signs and symptoms of poisoning in man and animals resulting from high doses of DDT include paresthesia of the tongue, lips, and face; apprehension hypersusceptibility to stimuli; irritability; dizziness; disturbed equilibrium; tremor; and tonic and colonic convulsions. Motor unrest and fine tremors associated with voluntary movements progress to coarse tremors without interruption in moderate to severe poisoning. Symptoms appear several hours after large doses, and in animals poisoned with fatal doses death occurs in 24 to 72 hours. It has been estimated that a dose of 10 mg/kg will cause signs of poisoning in man. Although there are rather marked species differences in susceptibility to acute poisoning by oral ingestion, when the compound is given by intravenous administration, the dose and time required for poisoning are quite similar for a wide variety of species including insects. Unlike most of the organophosphate insecticides, DDT is poorly absorbed after dermal exposure, especially when applied in the powder form. This poor absorption from the skin probably accounts for the rather good safety record of DDT in spite of its wide and sometimes careless use by applications and formulators.

Although the functional injury produced by high doses of DDT is referable to effects in the central nervous system, there is little pathologic changes in the cells and tissues of the central nervous system in acute poisonings. Inhalation of the dust results in irritation in the lungs, but primary pathologic changes that result from exposure to high, but nonfatal, doses, or from subacute or chronic feeding, are observed in the liver. With large doses centrolobular narcosis of the liver has been reported. Smaller doses result in liver enlargement, which in rodents is somewhat characteristic in that the cells and mitochondria themselves are enlarged. Histologic changes in the livers of male rats fed diets containing 5 to 15 ppm or more for six months include hypertrophy, inclusion bodies, and cytoplasmic granulation of a characteristic type in which the granules orient themselves around the periphery of the cell. These changes were not seen in female rats fed less than 200 ppm in the diet, however, and liver necrosis was observed only at dietary levels of 1,000 ppm or more Severe, unremitting tremors were observed at levels of 1,000 ppm, and nervousness, hyperactivity, and occasional tremors were observed at 200 and 400 ppm. The histologic changes in the liver appeared to be characteristically restricted to rodents and were not seen in experiments on primates. These changes were reversible with cessation of exposure. Cockerels given subcutaneous injections of DDT daily for 90 days had reduced testicular size, and direct estrogenic effects have been observed in female rats given single doses of 50 mg/kg of DDT.

Site and mechanism of toxic action

The locus of primary toxic action of DDT is believed to be sensory and motor nerve fibers and the motor cortex. The mechanism of action is still incompletely known; however, recent evidence indicates that DDT is capable of altering the transport of sodium and potassium ions across the membranes of nerve axons. Studies on isolated neurons and nerve fibers have shown that DDT blocks potassium efflux across the membrane. This action results in an increased negative after potential. Narahashi (1969) studied the effect of DDT on giant nerve fibers of the squid and lobster by means of the voltage clamp technique. He concluded that DDT slows the turning-off process of sodium conductance across the nerve membrane and inhibits the turning-on process of the potassium conductance. The molecular mechanisms for these effects are uncertain, but two possibilities have been suggested. Matsumura and O'Brien (1966) suggested that a charged-transfer complex between DDT and constituents of nerve fibers might account for the altered nerve axon membrane permeabilities. This hypothesis was based upon the findings of specific DDT-binding components in cockroach nerves. It has also been shown that DDT inhibits Na^+, K^+, and Mg^{2+} adenosine triphosphatase activity in the nerve-ending fraction of rat brain *in vitro*. The degree of inhibition of this enzyme by various toxic and nontoxic analogs of DDT corresponded, in general, to their *in vivo* toxicities. This suggests a possible interference in energy metabolism required for ion transport across nerve membranes.

Distribution and storage

DDT and one of its major metabolic products, DDE, have high fat: water partition coefficients and, therefore, tend to accumulate in adipose tissue. Studies in both man and laboratory animals indicate there is a log-log relationship between the daily intake and the residues of DDT and DDT-derived material in adipose tissue. At a constant rate of intake, however, the concentration of the insecticide in adipose tissue reaches an equilibrium and remains relatively constant. Following cessation of exposure, DDT is slowly eliminated from the body. Elimination has been estimated at a rate of approximately 1 percent of stored DDT excreted per day. During the years of its most extensive use in the late 1950s and early 1960s, the average of DDT in fat was about 5 ppm. Total storage of DDT derived from material was about

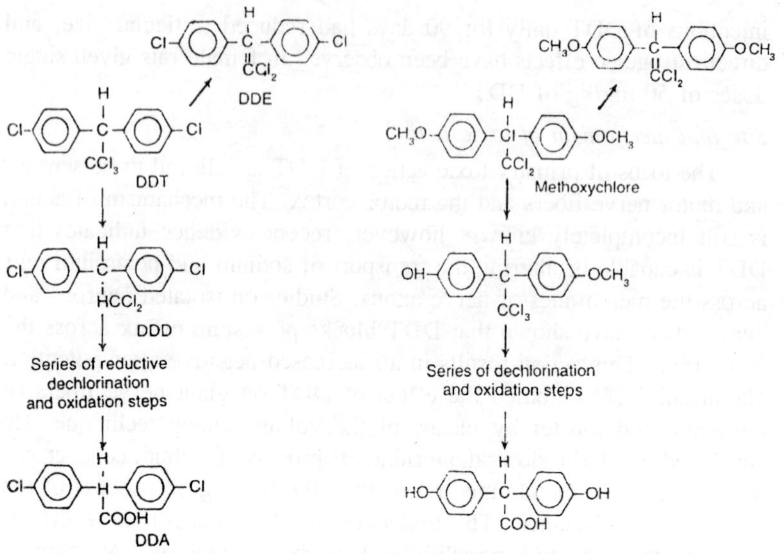

Fig. 23.5. Summary comparison of major metabolic pathways for DDT and methoxychlo..

15 ppm; this consisted primarily of DDT and its lipophilic metabolite; DDE. With declining use of DDT, there appears to have been a reduction in these levels so that the average adipose tissue level for man in the late 1960s was 1 to 2 ppm of DDT and a total of about 9 ppm of total DDT derived materials. Corresponding in time with these observations, analyses of whole meals indicated that the average amount of DDT that an adult in the United States obtained from food decreased from approximately 0.2 mg in 1958 to only about 0.04 mg per day in 1970.

Because lipid storage of DDT is, in a sense, a detoxication mechanism (it removes the compound from reactive sites of action) the insecticide can accumulate to relatively high concentration in adipose tissue when ingested by various species at low dosage rate over prolonged periods of time. This contributed to the so-called biomagnification of DDT in which a series of organisms in a food chain accumulate greater and greater quantities in their fat at each higher trophic level. Ultimately a species at the top of a food chain, e.g., carnivorous birds, may be a adversely affected. Because of the nature of reproduction in birds, they may be considered a more susceptible species. Eggshell thinning has been demonstrated both in the field and in laboratory studies to result from ingestion of DDT and related chlorinated hydrocarbon insecticides. Increased breakage of thin-shelled eggs probably has contributed to population declines of these fish-eating birds.

Another action of DDT that may contribute to effects on wild bird populations is the capacity of DDT and related materials to enhance the metabolism of estrogens. This could create an endocrine imbalance that affects the egg-laying and nesting cycle in such a way that total reproductive success and survival of young during the nesting season may be reduced.

An example of biomagnification related to human exposures was reported for nursing infants by Quimby and coworkers (1965). From an analysis of DDT content of typical meals, it was estimated 0.08 ppm of DDT. This would result in an infant dosage of 0.0112 mg/kg per day or approximately 20 times as much as the infants' mothers. Although this indicates the possibility of biomagnification involving humans there remains no evidence that infants have been harmed by these quantities.

Methoxychlor

Methoxychlor is a chlorinated ethane derivative that has enjoyed increasing use as an insecticide as the use of DDT has declined. The attractiveness of methoxychlor is that it is practically nontoxic to mammals and compared to DDT has relatively low persistence. Of course, it also has some less desirable insecticidal properties than DDT. Compared to oral LD50 values for rats in the range of 100 to 250 mg/kg for DDT, the LD50 for methoxychlor is 6,000 mg/kg. While DDT has been estimated to be stored in fat at an average of 10 to 20 times its chronic intake, and the half-life of stored methoxychlor in rats is one to two weeks compared with an estimated six months to a year for DDT. Although methoxychlor is slowly metabolized to a small extent by pathways similar to those for DDT the major and much more rapid pathway of metabolism is by O-demethylation and subsequent conjugation and excretion. These pathways are catalyzed by microsomal enzymes in mammals and by enzymes in soil organisms and other biota. Consequently, methoxychlor presents much reduced problems of persistence in the environment and biomagnification. Research by on other analogs of DDT suggests the possibility of development of rapidly degradable compounds that have as effective insecticidal properties as DDT but with reduced persistence in the environment.

Chlorinated cyclodiene insecticides

These compounds are also neuropoisons, and many of the signs and symptoms of poisoning resemble those produced by DDT. Unlike

DDT, however, these compounds tend to produce convulsions before other less serious signs of illness have appeared; Persons who have been poisoned by cyclodiene insecticides report headache and nausea, vomiting, dizziness, and mild chronic jerking. On the other hand, patients occasionally have convulsions with no warning symptoms. Unlike the situation with DDT there have been a number of fatalities resulting from acute poisoning by the cyclodiene insecticides.

Davies and Lewis (1956) reported 14 case histories of acute endrin poisoning resulting from an ancient in which at least 49 persons were made ill from eating bakery foods that had been prepared with endrin-contaminated flour. The source of the contamination was a railroad transport cart that had been used to transport bags of flour and that had, some two months previously, been used to transport a leaking container of a concentrated solution of endrin in xylene. The syndrome associated with these poisoning was referred to as fits and consisted of several, and in some cases sudden and unforewarned convulsions.

Several human fatalities have resulted from drinking emulsions or solutions of dieldrin. Garrestton and Curley (1969) described an incident in which a four-years-old boy and his two-year-old sister ingested a 5 per cent solution of dieldrin. Generalized convulsions began within 15 minutes after ingestion and the younger child died before medical assistance could be obtained. At autopsy there were no gross abnormalities apparent. The older child sustained convulsive seizures for 7.5 hours, but these were ultimately controlled with a high dose of anticonvulsants and he survived. Dieldrin distribution studies in this child showed that dieldrin strongly binds to serum proteins in a ratio of 440:1 (bound:unbound) plasma dieldrin. Dieldrin partitioned into fat as fat biopsies showed ratios of fat to serum concentrations of 174:1 at three days after poisoning and 2,200:1 at 179 days after poisoning. Liver function tests indicated some liver injury present for several months after the acute poisoning. Similar studies of a nonfatal case of acute chlordane poisoning in a child revealed signs of poisoning that were similar but the half-life of chlordane in the body appeared to be less than for dieldrin. Studies on persons exposed to dieldrin indicated that 20 mg/100 ml of blood is the approximate threshold at which symptoms of intoxication occur. Delayed and sudden appearance of symptoms of acute dieldrin poisoning several weeks or months after last exposure have been demonstrated in experimental animals and occupationally exposed men. Abnormal EEG recordings have been observed for months after exposure to dieldrin.

Increased incidence of liver tumors in mice fed dieldrin has been observed in chronic feeding studies. On the other hand, Deichmann and MacDonald (1971) found that overall tumor incidence in rats fed aldrin (20 to 50 ppm) or dieldrin (20 to 50 ppm) was lower than in controls and no different from controls in endrin-fed (2 to 12 ppm) rats. A panel review of several studies related to tumorigenicity of aldrin and dieldrin led to a conclusion that the available data did not meet criteria required to detect carcinogenic activity. Another panel, however, concluded that aldrin, dieldrin, and heptachlor (as well as DDT) could be judged "positive" for tumor induction on the basis of adequate tests in one more species of laboratory animal. A working group of the International Agency for Research on Cancer concluded that dieldrin was hepatocarcinogenic in mice, but that conflicting reports prevented conclusion of carcinogenicity of aldrin and heptachlor. To a large extent, because of suspicion of carcinogenicity, the manufacture and use of these compounds have been severely curtailed. No convincing evidence that these compounds or any other insecticide in use has contributed to increased incidence of tumor in man has emerged, and the subject of carcinogenic potential of the organochlorine insecticides remains an area of controversy and continued research.

Aldrin and dieldrin have been reported to produce various effects on reproduction in a variety of species, e.g., decreased fertility and decreased viability of the young, but the dietary concentrations required for these effects were as high as or higher than those that produced other effects such as histologic changes in livers of adult animals and were thought to be related to hormonal imbalance.

Action, metabolism, and storage

Acute poisoning by the chlorinated cyclodienes can also be classified as neurotoxicity. Generally they are considered central nervous system stimulants; however, their precise site and mechanism of action are incompletely known. Biochemical studies have shown that in animals poisoned with dieldrin and other cyclodienes there was an alteration of brain amino acid ratios and an increased level of ammonia in the brain. These actions might explain the central nervous system effects; however, other convulsive agents produce similar effects, and it is not clear whether the biochemical changes in the brain were the cause or the result of convulsions produced by the insecticides. It has been reported that in brains of rats poisoned with dieldrin, gamma butyrobetaine and related compounds were released from brain mitochondria. It was suggested that they might be responsible for the effects of dieldrin, because intracranial injections of the betaine esters caused violent and fetal convulsions. Other treatments that produce convulsions also led to a release of betainecoenzyme A esters These treatments include electroshock, ammonium chloride, and comphor. Although the release of betaine esters as a common underlying mechanism for the convulsive effects of a variety of agents may be attractive, it also may the result of postconvulsive action initiated by different mechanisms for different agents.

An important difference between DDT and the chlorinated cyclodienes that should be noted is that cyclodienes are absorbed from the intact skin. The difference between the oral dermal LD5 values for the cyclodienes is much less than the difference for DDT. Whereas the cyclodienes may not be pose any appreciably greater risk than DDT to the general population that might be exposed to small quantities of these materials in their food, from the standpoint of the occupational exposure, working the concentrated solutions of the cyclodienes would be more hazardous than working with concentrates of DDT.

Aldrin and heptachlor are metabolized by microsomal enzymes to their corresponding epoxides. Because the epoxides are equally or more toxic by acute dosage than the corresponding parent compounds, it has been suggested that epoxide formation represents an activation reaction. However, it is also felt that the parent compounds are toxic in their own. The epoxides of aldrin and heptachlor are lipid-soluble and it is the epoxides i.e., dieldrin and heptachlor epoxide, that are stored in the adipose tissue of man and other animals. Evidence that epoxidation occur readily in a variety of species is derived from the fact analysis of residues in animals that have been exposed to the parent compounds aldrin and heptachlor reveals only storage of the epoxide forms. The epoxides of these compounds may be further metabolized to more hydrophylic substances as the dihydrols, which can be conjugated and excreted in the urine. Biliary and fecal excretion of the cyclodiene insecticides also occur.

Toxaphene

In recent years this insecticides has ranked first in quantity used in the United States with estimated annual production of the order of 75 to 95 million lb. Toxaphene is described as the mixed isomers of chlorinated camphene containing 67 to 69 per cent chlorine. Thus, in spite of its commercial use as an insecticide for over 25 years, its exact chemical structure has been largely unknown, and it has been listed by the empiric formula $C_{10}H_{10}Cl_8$. Recently, the active ingredients of toxaphene have been the object of extensive investigation that has revealed that it includes more than 170 C_{10} compounds with six to ten chlorine atoms. Identified compounds include several endo-exo isomers of hexa-, hepta-, and nona- chlorobornanes and chlorobornenes of widely varying biologic activity. In view of the extremely high toxicity of the 8-octachlorobornane, it is obvious that the proportion of this (and other highly toxic isomers) present in technical toxaphene could greatly influence the toxicity to both target and nontarget species. Piperonyl butoxide, an insecticide synergist and mixed-function oxidase inhibitor, potentiated the toxicity of heptachlorobornane in both mice and houseflies. The other compounds were potentiated to a moderate degree in houseflies but not in mice. Heptachlorobornane undergoes reductive dechlorination by reduced microsomal cytochrome P-450 and *in vivo* in flies and rats. Enzymatic dehydrochlorination and oxidation of carbon substituents no doubt also help account for the extensive dechlorination that occur in rats. Such extensive metabolism probably also accounts for the relatively low persistence of toxaphene in comparison to other chlorinated hydrocarbon insecticides.

Chronic exposure of laboratory animals to toxaphene in their diet resulted in degenerative or other changes in liver and kidneys, generally at concentrations in excess of 25 ppm. Terpene polychlorinates closely related to toxaphene, increased the incidence of hepatomas in one strain of mice. Thus toxaphene, like most of the other related chlorinated insecticides, comes under suspicion of having potential for tumorigenic action.

Lindane

The gama isomer of hexachlorocyclohexane (HCH) sometimes called benzene hexachloride (HHC) products signs of poisonings that resemble those produced by DDT, i.e., tremors, ataxia, convulsions, and prostration, with stimulated respiration. Violent tonic and clinic convulsions occur in severe cases of acute poisoning. Fatty changes in the liver kidney tubule degeneration have been noted in fatal cases. Technical grades of HCH used in insecticidal preparations actually contain a mixture of isomers. The γ and α isomers are convulsant poisons, while the β and δ isomers are central nervous system depressants and the ε and η isomers appear to be inactive. The mechanism of neurotoxic action has been demonstrated. One interesting but unproven hypothesis reviewed by O'Brien (1967) suggested that the differing actions of the isomers could be related to their binding and goodness-of-fit into pores of a "hypothetic lattice in axonic membranes.

Technical HCH and several of the isomers contained therein have been found to produce liver cell tumors in mice when fed in the diet at high concentrations for most of the animal's lifetime.

Residues of HCH have been found in human fat and milk. Although the α, β, and γ isomers were all found as residues, the α and γ isomers are more rapidly metabolized and the β isomer accounted for 90 per cent of total HCH is isomer residue. Intraperitoneally administered HCH was eliminated in rats at a rate of 5 to 10 per cent of the dose per day. Gamma HCH was metabolized in rats by progressive dehydrochlorination, glutathione conjugation, and aromatic hydroxylation to yield 2,4-dichlorophenyl-mercapturic acid and conjugates of 2,3,5- and 2,4,5-trhchlorophenols that are excreted in the urine.

Mirex and kepone

Mirex has been used extensively in the southeastern United States for control of the fire ant. The acute toxicity of mirex to rats indicated that it was less toxic than DDT. However, the chronicity factor (defined as the single dose LD50 in mg/kg divided by 90-dose LD50 in mg/kg per day was much greater for mirex than for DDT. The respective chronicity factors for mirex, DDT, and dieldrin in rats were 60.8, 5.6, and 12.8. Rats fed mirex in the diet for 166 days had minimal pathologic changes in the liver with 5 ppm and definite enlargement of liver cells, cytoplasmic inclusions, and biliary stasis with 25 ppm. Female rats given 25 ppm of mirex in the diet gave birth to fewer and less viable offspring than control rats and one-third or more of the offspring of mirex-led rats developed cataracts (Gaines and Kimbrough, 1970). A total of 5 ppm in the diet had no effect on rats' reproduction. Mice given 1,000 mg/kg mirex subcutaneously in a single dose developed tumors of various types, and oral administration of 10 mg/kg/day for three weeks followed by feeding 26 ppm in the diet for 18 months resulted in a 40 per cent incidence of hepatomas. Rats fed 50 to 100 ppm of mirex in their diet had a dose-dependent, increased incidence of hepatic megalocytosis, cellular alterations, and neoplastic nodules, with a significantly increased incidence of hepatocellular carcinoma only in males at the high dietary level.

Mirex stimulates hepatic microsomal oxidative metabolism and causes proliferation of the smooth endoplasmic reticulum of the liver. No evidence of metabolism of mirex *in vivo* and *in vitro* has yet been found and it is stored in adipose tissue. Hence, the possibility that environmental contamination with mirex may lead to exposure to Kepone has increased concern about the adverse health and environmental effects of both these compounds. Both mirex and Kepone are highly persistent and have high lipid: water partition coefficients and have been shown to bioconcentrate several thousand fold in food chains.

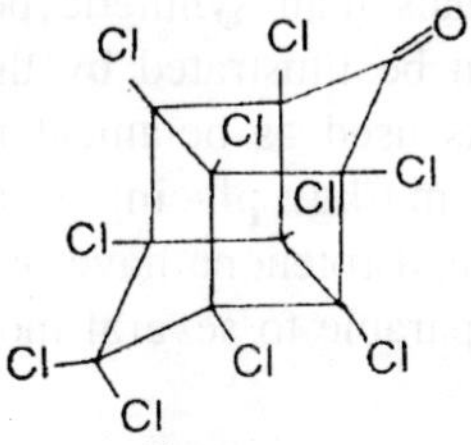

Cl Cl O Cl Cl Cl Cl Cl Cl Cl Cl

Kepone

The toxic effects of Kepone, as seen in humans, were described earlier in this chapter. It is encouraging that a means for hastening the excretion of stored Kepone has been developed. This involves the use of an anion-exchange resin, cholestyramine, which when given orally to patients, enhanced fecal excretion of Kepone by three- to eighteenfold, reduced the half-life of stored Kepone dramatically, and enhanced the rate of recovery from the toxic manifestations, as judged by recovery toward normal sperm counts. The rationale for the use of cholestyramine relates to the biliary-enterohepatic circulation, which cycles Kepone, hence cholestyramine, by binding the insecticide, interrupts the reabsorption phase and shifts the equilibrium from reabsorption and storage to fecal excretion.

The toxic effects of Kepone noted in excessively exposed workers, namely tremor, liver, injury, and altered reproductive potential, had been previously in laboratory animals. Studies at the National Cancer Institute revealed an increased incidence of hepatocellular carcinomas in mice and rats fed Kepone in the diet.

Treatment of organochlorine insecticide poisoning

Treatment of acute poisoning by all of the organochlorine insecticides is largely symptomatic. Phenobarbital has been recommended as an antidote to control convulsions produced by DDT and other compounds. However, intravenous diazepam, because of its lesser respiratory depression, is recommended to sedate and control convulsions associated with most of the organochlorine insecticides. Calcium gluconate has also been useful in controlling convulsions produced by DDT. As with, all exposure, attention should be given to removal of unabsorbed poison from the gastrointestinal tract and the skin. Oil-based cathartics should be avoided, however, as they may increase adsorption.

Botanical Insecticides

It is commonly felt that insecticides derived from natural products are less toxic to mammals than synthetic pesticides. The fallacy of this view, however, can be illustrated by the oral LD50s to rats of the three major products used as botanical insecticides: nicotine has an LD50 of 10 to 60 mg/kg, placing it amongst the most toxic insecticides; pyrethrum and rotenone have oral LD50s in the range of 100 to 300 mg/kg, comparable to several moderately toxic synthesis.

Nicotine

Nicotine acts to stimulate nicotinic receptors in automic ganglia, at the neuromuscular junction, and in some pathways of the central nervous system. Its action at these sites mimics the normal transmitter acetylcholine. Poisoning in vertebrates is followed by symptoms of salivation and vomiting (from ganglionic stimulation), muscular weakness and fibrillation by stimulation at the neuromuscular junction, and ultimately, clonic convulsions and cessation of respiration (effects in the central nervous system). Treatment for nicotine Poisoning is by use of anticonvulsants. Nicotine is oxidized and hydroxylated by microsomal oxidases, which yield less toxic metabolic products. Because it is the principal alkaloid in tobacco, nicotine has been studied extensively for its pharmacologic actions and detailed discussions of its pharmacology are available in textbooks of that science and in a comprehensive review on the effects of tobacco.

Rotenoids

A preparation extracted from tuber root, *Derris elliptica*, was used by primitive people to paralyze fish. It was from this use that its possibility for application as an insecticide developed. The active principle of the Derris species is the compound rotenone plus as many as 13 related derivatives. Poisoning by rotenone in man is rare, and it has been used by direct application for head lice, scabies, and other ectoparasites. Local effects include conjunctivitis, dermatitis, pharyngitis, and rhinitis. Orally, rotenone preparations produce gastrointestinal irritation, nausea, and vomiting. The estimated fatal oral dose for 70-kg man is from 10 to 100 g. Inhalation of the dust is more hazardous, and it can cause respiratory stimulation followed by depression with fits and convulsions. A biochemical mode of action for rotenone in insect tissues, which also occurs in mammalian tissues, is the inhibition of the oxidation of reduced NAD ($NADH_2$ to NAD). The consequence of this blockage is that oxidation of substrates via the NAD system, such as glutamate, alphaketoglutarate, and pyruvate, are blocked by rotenone.

Pyrethrum

Pyrethrum is one of the oldest insecticides known to man, and the active principle of pyrethrum flowers are pyrethrin I and II and cinerin I and II. Pyrethrum extract is used in many household insecticides because of its rapid knock-down action. The estimated fatal oral dose for man of pyrethrum is 50 g/70 kg; fatal poisoning of a child occurred as the result of eating 15 g of pyrethrum concentrate. Signs and symptoms of poisoning by pyrethrum may take several forms. Contact dermatitis is the most common. Cases of asthmatic-like reactions have been reported in some individuals who had a previous history of asthma with a broad allergic background. Severe anaphylactic reactions with peripheral vascular collapse and respiratory difficulty are considered a rare accompaniment of the dermatologic reactions. With massive doses ingested orally, nervous system symptoms may occur, which include excitation and convulsions leading to paralysis and accompanied by muscular fibrillation and diarrhea. Death is due to respiratory failure.

Preparations containing synthetic pyrethroids are less likely to result in allergic reactions. Allethrin one of the synthetic pyrethroids, inhibited both sodium potassium conductances in squid and cockroach giant axons. It exerts four actions on nerve membrane: slightly depolarizes the membrane, increases the negative afterpotential, induces repetitive after discharges, and eventually blocks the action potential.

HERBICIDES

The production and use of chemicals for destruction of noxious weeds have increased markedly during the last decade. Herbicides rival or exceed insecticides in quantity and value of sales. Because plants differ markedly from animals in their morphology and physiology, it might be expected that herbicides would present little hazard of chemical toxicity to vertebrates. Indeed some compounds have very low toxicity in mammals, but even among the herbicides there are highly toxic chemicals, and a number of these have caused fatal poisoning in man.

Chlorophenoxy Compounds

The compounds 2,4-dichlorophenoxyacetic acid (2,4-D) and (2,4,5-T) as their salts and esters are probably the most familiar chemicals used as herbicides. They are used in agriculture for control of broad-leaf weeds and in the control of woody plants along highways and utilities' rights of way. They exert their herbicidal action by acting as growth hormones in plants. They have no hormonal action in animals but their mechanism of toxic action is poorly understood. Animals killed by massive doses of 2,4-D are believed to die of ventricular fibrillation.

At lower doses, when death is delayed, various signs of muscular involvement are seen including stiffness of the extremities, ataxia, paralysis, and eventually coma. Sublethal doses, singly or repeated, lead to a general unkempt appearance without specific signs except a tenseness and muscular weakness. Feeding studies in animals indicate that repeated exposures to doses just slightly smaller than the single toxic dose are tolerated, indicating little cumulative effect. In a case of suicide, an oral dose of not less than 6500 mg led to death. It has been estimated that the oral dose required to produce symptoms in man is probably about 3 to 4 g. Profound muscular weakness was noted in a patient recovering from an episode of acute poisoning by 2,4-D. Peripheral neuritis was reported for three men who had recent heavy occupational exposure to 2,4-D. Pathologic changes in experimental animals killed by the chlorophenoxy compounds are generally nonspecific with irritation of the stomach and some liver and kidney injury.

The chlorophenoxy herbicides have produced contact dermatitis in man, and as mentioned earlier, a rather severe type of dermatitis, chloracne, has been observed in workmen involved in the manufacture 2,4,5-T. This effect appears to be due primarily to the action of a contaminant, 2,3,7,8-tetracholorodibenzo-ρ-dioxin.

Concern about the toxicology of 2,4,5-T and related compounds centers primarily on teratogenic action in experimental animals. The first studies to reveal this action were, it is now known, conducted with a sample of 2,4,5-T that contained a high level (about 30 ppm) of a contaminant 2,3,7,8-tetrachlorodibenzo-ρ-dioxin. This contaminant is formed during the synthesis of the trichlorophenol precursor as shown below.

1,2,3,4,5-Tetra-Chlorobenzene $\xrightarrow[\text{CH}_3\text{OH, NaOH}]{170^\circ\text{C}}$ 2,4,5-Trichloro-phenate sodium + … +

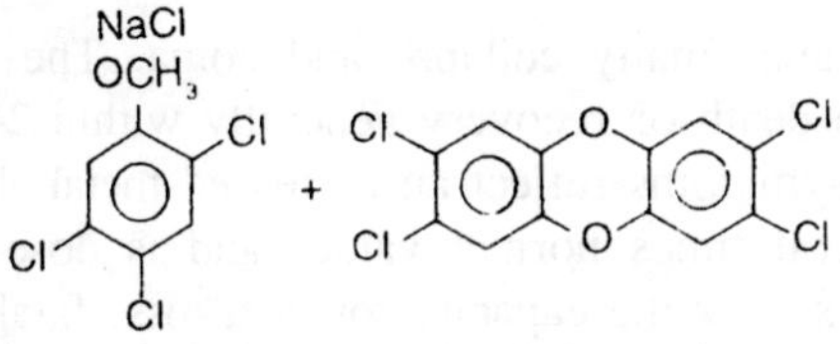

NaCl

OCH_3

2,4,5 - Trichloro-anisole + 2, 3, 7, 8-Tetrachloro-dibenzodioxin

Tetrachlorodioxin (TCDD) is an extremely toxic chemical with LD50s of 0.022 and 0.045 mg/kg for male and female rats and only 0.006% mg/kg for female guinea pig. For female guinea pig, the ratio of the LD50 of 2,4,5-T to the LD50 of the dioxin is 630,000. For female rats the acute oral LD50 for tetrachlorodioxin is about 10,000 times less than the oral LD50 for 2,4,5-T. The daily dose of the dioxin given to pregnant rats during the gestational period that resulted in fetal toxicity was only about 1/400 of the material LD50 of dioxin, or about 1/4,000,000 of the single oral LD50 of 2,4,5-T to female rats. It would appear, then, that the concentration of dioxin as a contaminant in 2,4,5-T is a major factor in determining its teratogenicity. In addition to its extreme acute toxicity and its teratogenic action. TCDD has recently been reported to induce tumor in laboratory rodents fed very low concentrations (5 ppt to 5 ppb) in the diet.

The 2,4,5-T teratogenesis experiments illustrate an important principle for evaluation of the safety of commercial products; that is, one must be concerned not only with major active component, but with minor contaminants that may be prevent as a result of their formation during the manufacture or as the recent of degradative reactions occurring in the development. Presently, the TCDD content is regulated in 2,4,5-T at 0.1 ppm or less.

The acute toxicities of chlorophenoxy herbicides and various enters and salts have been summarized by Rowe and Hymas (1954). The LD50s ranged from 300 to > 1,000 mg/kg in several experimental species tested, with the exception that dogs were relatively more sensitive (LD50 of 100 mg/kg for 2,4,5-T isopropylester).

Dinitrophenols

Several substituted dinitrophenols alone or as salts of aliphatic amines or alkalies are used in weed control. Human poisonings by dinitro orthocresol (DNOC) have been reported. Signs and symptoms of acute poisoning in man include nausea, gastric upset, restlessness, sensation of heat, flushed skin, sweating, rapid respiration, tachycardia, fever, cyanosis, and finally collapse and coma. The illness runs a rapid course with death or recovery generally within 24 to 48 hours. These signs and symptoms reflect an increased metabolic rate, which may exceed several times normal values and is dose-dependent. If heat production exceeds the capacity for heat loss, fatal hyperthermia may result. Chronic exposure to dinitro-orthocresol may also produce fatigue, restlessness, anxiety, excessive sweating, unusual thirst, and loss of weight. A yellow staining of the conjunctiva has been noted, and cataract formation is another possible sequela of chronic dinitro-orthocresol exposure. Blood levels of DNOC below 10 ppm are considered of trivial importance; levels of 11 to 20 ppm indicate appreciable absorption; and above these blood levels toxic manifestations are likely. Levels greater than 50 ppm are critically dangerous. After removal of the poison from the skin or gastrointestinal tract, treatment consists of ice baths to reduce fever and administration of oxygen to assure maximal oxygenation of the blood. Fluid and electrolyte therapy may be necessary to replace loss by sweating. Atropine sulfate is absolutely contraindicated in cases of poisoning by dinitrophenolic compounds, and therefore care should be taken to avoid a misdiagnosis of organophosphate poisoning. Symptoms of poisoning and their severity are enhanced when the environmental temperature is high. In very cool weather blood levels as high as 50 ppm have been tolerated without symptoms. The oral LD50 of DNOC in rats is approximately 30 mg/kg.

It will be noted that the nitrocresol compounds produce symptoms of toxicity similar to those produced by dinitrophenol and therefore probably act by uncoupling of oxidative phosphorylation as has been proposed for dinitrophenol. Compounds that produce uncoupling of oxidative phosphorylation also have the peculiar property of rapidly producing rigor mortis after death. Studies on the toxicology of substituted nitrophenols used in agriculture may be found in report by Spencer and coworkers (1948).

Bipyridyl Compounds

Paraquat is the best-known compound of this class of herbicides, which are increasing in use. Over 200 cases of accidental or suicidal fatalities resulted from paraquat poisoning have been reported during the past decade. Pathologic changes observed at autopsy in all of these

$$\left[CH_3-\overset{+}{N}\langle\bigcirc\rangle-\langle\bigcirc\rangle\overset{+}{N}-CH_3\right]2Cl^-$$

fatal human poisoning showed evidence of lung, liver, and kidney damage. Some cases had myocarditis, and one case showed transient neurologic signs. The most striking pathologic change was a widespread cellular proliferation in the lungs. This pathology was also evident in a suicide case in which the paraquat was injected subcutaneously. In this case the victim died in respiratory distress, and the main pathologic findings at autopsy were in the lungs. Hence, paraquat produces lung damage even when administered by routes in which exposure of the lung is secondary. Although ingestion of paraquat results in gastrointestinal upset within a few hours after exposure, the onset of respiratory symptoms and eventual death by respiratory distress may be delayed for several days. In a case involving a six-year-old child the concentration of paraquat present in the liver and kidney at necropsy was 208 mg per 100 g of kidney. One accidental case involved an individual who mistakenly took a mouthful of the herbicide from a "snout" bottle, and although he spat it out almost immediately, 14 days later cyanosis and severe dyspnea developed. The patient who administered paraquat by subcutaneous injection had chest radiograph changes three days after administration, but did not develop respiratory symptoms for an additional 11 days. Davies et al. (1977) suggest, on the basis of pharmacokinetic studies in dogs and humans, that because paraquat in the systemic circulation is rather rapidly cleared via the kidneys, accumulation of toxic amounts in the lung is secondary to kidney injury. They indicate that the presence of more than 0.2 μg/ml of paraquat in plasma, accompanied by impaired renal function in the first 24 hours after dosing, will usually result in fatal lung injury. On this basis, treatment of paraquat poisoning must be instituted early and involves (1) removal of paraquat from the alimentary tract by gastric lavage and use of cathartics; (2) prevention of further absorption by oral administration of Fuller's earth (30 per cent w/v); and (3) removal of absorbed paraquat by hemodialysis or hemoperfusion. A very similar course of treatment was recommended by Cavalli and Fletcher (1977) who evaluated 96 published cases of paraquat poisoning, 70 of them fatal. They indicate that treatment, in order to be effective, should be initiated within ten hours of ingestion. Ten to fifteen milliliter of commercially prepared concentrate of paraquat is estimated as a lethal oral dose for adults, and massive overdoses of the order of 50 ml are very difficult to treat.

A great deal of concern and public interest is the toxicology of paraquat was stimulated by revelation of its use in a herbicide spray program to control illicit production of marijuana and heroin. High residues of paraquat were found in marijuana cigarettes. It was estimated that 0.26 μg of paraquat could be inhaled by smoking a marijuana cigarette contaminated with 1,000 ppm. It was suggested that a slow buildup of lung "scarring" might occur in persons inhaling even these low quantities. There presently is little or no documentation to support these allegations, although direct inhalation of such a progressive lung toxin as paraquat is obviously to be avoided.

The toxicology of bipyridyl herbicides was initially reviewed by Conning and associates (1969) and recently by Smith and Heath (1976). In animal studies all species examined showed the same response after a single large dose of paraquat given by mouth or by subcutaneous or intraperitoneal injection. There was an early onset of hyperexcitability, which in some cases led to convulsions or incoordination. The animals died over a period of ten days after administration. Early deaths were not associated with any specific systemic pathology. Later death that occurred at two to five days after administration usually were accompanied by severe pulmonary congestion and edema with hyaline membrane formation and inflammatory infiltrates. Animals that survive the pulmonary edema associated with a single dose occasionally show progression of lung lesions of fibrosis and eventual death from respiratory failure. As in man, a single dose may produce pulmonary fibrosis in the dog. The feeding of 0.03 per cent or more of paraquat in the diet of experimental animals led to the production of pulmonary fibrosis in most of the animals. Studies of organ cultures of lungs treated with paraquat revealed extensive necrosis of alveolar cells. Inhalation of paraquat aerosols for several hours produces severe congestion, alveolar edema, and bronchial irritation two to three days after the exposure. However, it the animal survives during this period there is, surprisingly, no further chronic fibrosis produced.

The LD50 for paraquat in guinea pigs, cats, and cows is in the range of 30 to 50 mg/kg. Rats appear to be somewhat more resistant with an LD50 of about 125 mg/kg. The LD50 for man is estimated at about 40 mg/kg. Studies of several species indicate that absorption of paraquat from the gastrointestinal tract is relatively low, in no cases exceeding 20 per cent of the administered dose. There is a rapid disappearance from the blood with 90 to 100 per cent of the dose excreted in the urine within 48 hours. Since there is a long delay until onset of respiratory signs, this compound has been classified among the "hit-and-run" type of toxic agents. Exposure of the skin to solutions of dipyridyls results in erythemia and a mild reactive hyperkeratosis, which may be associated with pustule formation.

Diquat produces acute and chronic effects that differ from those produced by paraquat in that marked effects on the lung are not observed. This has been attributed to an energy-dependent system in the lung that selectively concentrates paraquat. Oral doses near the LD50 produce hyperexcitability leading to convulsions and distention of the gastrointestinal tract with discolouration of intestinal fluids. The only pathology associated with long-term feeding of diquat at levels of 0.05 per cent was the production of cataracts in about ten months. A related compound, chlormequat, has as its target organ the kidney. In both rats and dogs, kidney lesions were the only striking pathology noted in both acute and chronic studies.

It has been suggested that the mechanism of the herbicidal action of the dipyridyls is mediated by free radical reactions, and a similar mechanism has been proposed for the action in mammals. Gage (1968) showed that free radicals could be produced from paraquat and diquat incubated in the presence of reduced NADP and liver microsomes. Proposed biochemical mechanisms of paraquat toxicity are discussed in detail in a recent proceedings of a conference on this subject. The formation of free radicals via a cyclic single reduction-oxidation of paraquat predominates. Since initial reduction of oxidized paraquat uses NADPH, the possibility that paraquat competes for and deprives other systems (essential for cell integrity) of this biologic reducing agent is one aspect of the toxic mechanism. A more comprehensive mechanism that has been proposed involves the reoxidation of reduced paraquat by molecular oxygen with the concomitant production of superoxide radicals that dismulate nonenzymatically to single oxygen. These attack unsaturated lipids of cell membranes and produce lipid hydroperoxides, which may form lipid-free-radicals with consequent membrane damage or which may be reduced by GSH-dependent systems that depend on NADPH for GSH regeneration. The early event of paraquat-induced increased superoxide production is the underlying rationale for the proposal that administration of purified superoxide dismutase may be valuable in therapy of paraquat poisoning.

Carbamate Herbicides

This class of herbicides contains a large number of aromatic and aliphatic esters, which for the most part have relatively low acute toxicities. The compound propham is a typical example of this class of herbicides. Its LD50 by oral administration in rats and rabbits was of the order of 5,000 mg/kg. Feeding rats dietary concentrations of 1,000 ppm for three months produced no signs of effects on general condition and growth, fertility, or pathologic changes. Barban is somewhat more toxic than propham with an oral LD50 to 600 mg/kg for rats and rabbits and 24 mg/kg for guinea pigs. Daily oral administration of 75 mg/kg for 22 days produced some loss of weight, while half of this quantity produced on toxic action. Feeding experiments with rats showed no toxic action, of 150 ppm in the diet for 18 months. Barban, however, is a potent skin-sensitizing agent in man, and allergic reactions and rash may develop on subsequent contact.

Substituted Urea

Like the carbamate herbicides the substituted urea are, as a class, rather nontoxic by acute oral administration. Monuron and diuron are typical examples, with LD50 values in rats of over 3,000 mg/kg. Chronic toxicity studies suggest that monuron has carcinogenic potential. An increased incidence of lung tumors was observed in male mice of one of two strains tested by oral administration in one study. In another study an increased incidence of hepatomas was observed when mice were given 6 mg per animal weekly by gavage, but this study was subject to question as the survival of controls was not fully reported. In two separate studies, rats were fed monuron in their diets for 18 to 24 months. In one study no increased tumor rate over controls was observed, while in the second study 7 per cent of monuron-fed rats developed tumors at various sites while control rats were reported to be tumor free.

Triazines

Most member of this class of herbicides also have low oral scute toxicities ranging above 1,000 mg/kg. Simazine was nontoxic to a variety of animal species including mice, rats, rabbits, chickens, and pigeons. Rats survived daily doses of 2,500 mg/kg for four weeks. Simazine is, however, more toxic to sheep and cattle. Sheep were killed by three daily dose doses of 250 mg/kg, 14 daily doses of 100 mg/kg, or 31 daily doses of 50 mg/kg. Cattle were killed by three daily doses of 250 mg/kg. The acute toxicity of atrazine to rats is greater than for simazine; however, cattle and sheep appear to be more resistant to atrazine than to simazine.

The herbicide amitrole (3-amino-1H-1,2,4-triazole), although not classified as a triazine, is structurally somewhat similar. This compound also has a very low acute oral toxicity to rats and mice (ranging from 15,000 to 25,000 mg/kg). However, amitrole is a rather potential antithyroid agent, and feeding levels of 2 ppm in the diet resulted in significant effects on thyroid function. These functional changes occurred after only one week of feeding of amitrole and goiters can be induced by amitrole with long continuous administration. Amitrole given to rats in the diet at 100 ppm for two years resulted in the development of thyroid adenomas and adenocarcinomas. This has resulted in prohibition of this compound for use as a herbicide where residues might occur on food crops. Amitrole inhibits peroxidase activity in livers and thyroids, and the mode of action in producing thyroid tumors appears to be related to the goitrogenic effect of amitrole with resultant increased TSH (thyroid-stimulating hormone) since other antithyroid agents that result in TSH stimulation also can produce thyroid tumors experimentally. The amitrole case illustrates an important principle in toxicology, that is, the fallacy of assuming safety purely on the basis of low acute toxicity. As is illustrated by this compound, which is practically nontoxic acutely, rather profound functional changes can occur that directly or indirectly may lead to irreversible pathology, e.g., cancer.

Amide Herbicides

Several aniline derivatives esterified with organic acids are currently used as herbicides. These compounds also have relatively high oral LD50s for rats. A typical example is the herbicide propanil, which is used extensively to control noxious weeds in rice crops. The rice plant is selectively resistant to the herbicidal action of propanil because it contains an acylamidase that hydrolyzes propanil to 3,4-dichloroaniline and propionic acid. An interesting case of herbicide potentiation was observed in field studies in which propanil was applied to rice following the application of organophosphate insecticides. This procedure resulted in damage to rice plants and was subsequently explained on the basis that the organophosphates inhibited the hydrolysis of propanil, and thus the parent compound was preserved and exerted its herbicidal action in the rice. Williams and Jacobson (1966) demonstrated that mammalian livers also contained an amidase that hydrolyzed propanil, and they speculated that organophosphates and carbamates might potentiate the acute mammalian toxicity of this herbicide.

Studies of interactions did not reveal a significant potentiation, however. Further investigation demonstrated that inhibition of liver acylamidase by triorthocresyl phosphate (TOCP) prevented the cyanosis that was observed when mice were given toxic doses of propanil. The cyanosis was due to methemoglobin formation following hydrolysis to 3,4-dichloroaniline. Other signs of poisoning, i.e., CNS depression and death, were not prevented by inhibiting the hydrolysis of the herbicide. It appears, therefore, that aromatic amides that are hydrolyzed to aniline derivatives may produce methemoglobin, but that the acute lethal action is due to a different mechanism.

Much more extensive discussion of the toxicology of herbicides may be found in Dalgaard-Mikkelsen and Poulsen's review (1962) and comprehensive summaries of the toxicity and ecologic effects of herbicides are contained in the report by House and associates (1967).

FUNGICIDES

Fungicides like other classes of pesticides comprise a heterogenous group of chemical compounds. With a few exceptions, the fungicides have not attracted the detailed toxicologic research as have insecticides. A detailed review of their action on the target organisms (fungi-toxicity) has appeared. Although many of the compounds used to control fungus diseases on plants, seeds, and produce are rather nontoxic activity, there are some notable exceptions. The mercury-containing fungicides comprise the group that has been of greatest concern for hazard to health, and they have been responsible for many deaths or permanent neurologic disability resulting from the misdirection of mercury fungicide-treated seed grains into human and animal food.

Captan and *Folpet* because of some structural similarities to thalidomide were suspected as being possible teratogens, and this effect was confirmed in the developing chick embryo. Robens (1970) reported teratogenic effects in hamsters with doses of 500 mg/kg to pregnant females on days 7 and 8 of gestation. Other studies in rabbits, rats, and hamsters failed to reveal teratogenic effects from Folpet but in one study nine malformed offspring were observed out of 75 implantations in nine pregnant rabbits given, 75 mg/kg/day of captan orally on days 6 through 16 of gestation. Rats fed a low-protein diet were reported to be much sensitive to the acute oral toxicity (LD50, 480/mg/kg) of captan than rats receiving a normoprotein diet (LD50, 12,500 mg/kg).

Pentachlorophenol production and use are of the order of 50 million lb per year. It is used as an insecticide and herbicide as well as a fungicide, with major application as a wood preservative. Several cases of human poisonings have resulted in association with these uses. It acute toxic action in men and experimental animals resembles that produced by the nitrophenolic herbicides, i.e., marked increases in metabolic rate as the result of uncoupling of oxidative phosphorylation. It is readily absorbed through the skin. Two cases of fatal poisonings and several non-fatal cases occurred in a hospital nursery in which pentachlorophenol had been used as fungicide in the laundry room (against the labeled instructions) and ultimately contacted infants through their diapers. Several infants died before the cause and source of poisoning were identified. The fatal dose of pentachlorophenol for laboratory animals ranges from 30 to 100 mg/kg, and it is readily absorbed through the skin. In recent years it has become apparent that many commercial samples of pentachlorophenol with polychlorinated dibenzodioxins and dibenzofurans. These contaminants are generally hexachlorinated or octachlorinated dibenzodioxins or dibenzofurans, and they are less toxic than the tetrachlorodioxin contaminant in 2,4,5-T. Nevertheless, some isomers of hexachlorodibenzodioxin have LD50 values in guinea pigs of the order of 60 to 100 μg/kg, ranking them as extremely toxic chemicals. The octachlorodioxins are much less acutely toxic, in the order of 1 g/kg. Although pentachlorophenol is highly toxic in its own right, some studies suggest that contaminants may be responsible for some of the toxic effects of technical grade. A comparison of effects of technical versus purified pentachlorophenol indicated that only the technical produced grade produced chlorance, chick edema, hepatic porphyria, and increased relative liver weight. Technical grade was also much more active as a liver enzyme inducer.

Another fungicide, hezachlorobenezene (noted that this is distinct from hexachlorocyclohexane or lindane), produced more than 3,000 cases of acquired toxic porphyria autanea tarda, which was characterized by severe skin manifestation including photosensitivity, bulbae formation, deep scarring, permanent loss of hair and skin atrophy. The poisonings were traced to the consumption of wheat that had been prepared for planting by treating it with hexachlorobenzene for its fungicidal effects.

Dithiocarbamate fungicides have enjoyed rather widespread use in agriculture. They have a low order to acute toxicity, with oral LD50 values in rats ranging from several hundred milligrams to several grams per kilogram. There is little evidence of human injuries from exposure to the compounds; however, recently some of these compounds have been reported to have teratogenic and/or carcinogenic potential. Two groups of dithiocarbamates have been used, the dimethyldithiocarbamates and the ethylenebisdithiocarbamates. Their respective general structures are as follows:

Dimethyldithiocarbamates

Metal cation

Diethydithiocarbamates

The names of the fungicides are derived from the metallic cations. For example, when the cation is zinc or iron, the respective dimethyldithiocarbamates are ziram or ferbam. With manganese, zinc, or sodium as the cation in the diethyldithiocarbamates, the respective fungicide is maneb, zineb, or nabam. Some dimethyl-dithiocarbamates are reported to be teratogenic in animals, and they can be nitrosated to form nitrosamines *in vitro* and *in vivo*. The ethylenebisdithiocarbamates maneb, nabam, and zineb are also reported to be teratogenic. Furthermore, this group of compounds breaks down to form ethylene thiourea (ETU) *in vivo*, in the environment, and during cooking of food containing their residues ETU is carcinogenic, mutagenic, and teratogenic as well as antihyroid. A scheme for the degradation of maneb is as follows:

$\xrightarrow{H^+}$ $[CH_2NH_2]_2 + CS_2$

1 2

SO_4^{2-}

$C=S + CS_2$

3 4

Maneb is hydrolysed by acids to ethylenediamine and carbon disulfide. Carbon disulfide is also produced when ethylene bisthiuram monosulfide is transformed into ETU. Maneb produced an increased incidence of lung tumors in only one of four strains of mice that have been tested and studies in rats were equivocal. However, because of its conversion to the much more active ETU, it and other fungicides of this class require further study and evaluation of hazard.

Rodenticides

A wide variety of chemicals, which defy classification, have been used in the control of rats and mice. Although they are used to kill mammals, which resemble man in their physiology and biochemistry, there are wide differences in degree of hazard to man. In some case the rodenticidal selectivity of these compounds is based on the peculiar physiology of rodents, which differs from that of primates and other desirable species, and in some cases it is merely a question of taking advantage of the habits of rodents as opposed to species that are to be protected. In addition to potential widespread destruction of food and fiber by rodents, another primary reason for attempting their control is to eliminate intermediate hosts in the transmission of various vectroborne diseases, e.g., bubonic plague. Since rodenticides can be used in baits and placed in inaccessible places their likelihood of becoming widespread contaminants of the environment is much less than that associated with the use of insecticides and herbicides. The toxicologic problem posed by rodenticides, therefore, is primarily acute accidental or suicidal ingestion.

Warfarin

Warfarin, 3-(alpha-acetonylbenzyl)-4-hydroxycoumarin, is one of the most widely used rodenticides. Its safe usage is based on the fact that it requires repeated dosing for toxicity to develop. Thus, placed in baits accessible to rodents, repeated ingestion results in fatalities to rodents with little likelihood that pets or children would be repeatedly exposed.

The mechanism of action of warfarin is as an anticoagulant. It is an antimetabolite of vitamin K, and hence it inhibits the synthesis of prothrombin. Multiple doses are usually required to maintain inhibition of synthesis until prothrombin levels are sufficiently depleted to result in hemorrhage throughout the whole body, which is the cause of death. In addition to its anticoagulant action, direct capillary damage has also been attributed to warfarin. Single fatal doses in common laboratory animals range between 200 and 400 mg/kg. Basing estimates of toxicity to man on values for single lethal doses for animals, it has been suggested that an adult man would have to eat 1.5 lb of a warfrain concentrate or about 30 lb of a strong rat bait to result in fatality. On the other hand, daily ingestion for six days of as little as 1 to 2 mg/kg has produced severe illness in an attempted suicide. Two members of a Korean family of 14 persons lived for 15 days on a diet of cornmeal containing warfarin that was intended as a rat bait. All became severely ill with hemorrhage. The estimated dosage was 1 to 2 mg/kg/day. Symptoms of poisoning, which begin after a few days or weeks of repeated ingestion, include epistaxis and bleeding gums, pallor, and sometimes petechial rash leading to hematomas around the joints and on the buttocks, ultimately blood in the urine and feces, and occasionally paralysis due to cerebral hemorrhage, and finally to hemorrhagic shock and death. The principal diagnostic test for excessive repeated exposure to warfarin is a markedly reduced prothrombin activity, and therapy is directed to correcting this by the administration of vitamin K. Additional details concerning the toxicity and treatment are given by Hayes (1963).

Related anticoagulants used as rodenticides are coumafuryl (3-[1-furyl-3-acetyl-ethyl]4-hydroxycoumarin), diphacinone (2-diphenylactetyl-1,3-indandione), and pindone (2-pivalyl-1,3-indandione). These have the advantage over warfarin of being more readily soluble in water.

Red Squill

The bulbs of red squill (Urginen maritima) have been used for many years as a relatively safe rodenticide. The active principles are glycosides scillaren-A and scillaren-B. These glycosides have cardiotonic actions like the digitalis glycosides. Crude red squill also contains a central-acting emetic, which causes vomiting in animals other than rodents. This emetic action is the main factor that contributes to the safety of the rodenticide to humans. Symptoms that are associated with ingestion of large doses of red squill include vomiting and abdominal pain, blurred vision, cardiac irregularity, convulsions, and death from ventricular-irregularities. Quinine sulfate is used in treatment of reduce mild cardioirritability. The selective rodenticidal usefulness of squill, then takes advantage of the physiologic peculiarity of the rat's inability to vomit.

Norbormide

Norbormide is another rodenticide that takes advantage of a physiologic peculiarity of the rat for its selective toxicity. This compound acts directly on the smooth muscle of peripheral vessels causing them to constrict irreversibly resulting in widespread ischemia leading to death. The receptor sites for norbormide in the vascular smooth muscle apparently are different from the vasoconstrictive receptors for epinephrine. Since the compound is lethal to rats in dosages of 5 to 15 mg/kg and is essentially nontoxic for cats, dogs, chicken, ducks, primates, sheep, or swine, it must be assumed that the norbormide receptors in smooth muscle of peripheral vessels exist uniquely in the rat.

Sodium Fluoroacetate and Fluoro-acetamide

These rodenticides, whose use is largely restricted to licensed pest control operators, are among the most potent rodenticides known and are also highly toxic to other animals.

Fluoroacetate produces its toxic action by inhibiting the citric acid cycle. The fluorine substituted acetate becomes incorporated, as a normal acetate, into fluoroacetyl coenzyme A, which condenses with oxaloacetate to form fluorocitrate. Fluorocitrate inhibits the enzyme aconitase and thereby inhibits the conversion of citrate to isocitrate. As a result there is an accumulation of large quantities of citrate in the tissue, and the cycle is blocked. As might be excepted, the heart and central nervous system are the most critical tissues involved in poisoning by a general inhibition of oxidative energy metabolism. Thus, the symptoms following fluoroacetate poisoning, in addition to nonspecific signs of nausea and vomiting, include cardiac irregularities, cyanosis, generalized convulsions, and death from ventricular fibrillation or respiratory failure.

Estimates of the means lethal dose of fluoroacetate in man range from 2 to 10 mg/kg, and there have been a number of human fatalities. There are apparent species differences in the quality of symptoms that lead to death. Dogs die of convulsions or respiratory paralysis, but in man, monkeys, horses, and rabbits central nervous system actions are usually incidental, and the dangerous fatal complication is ventricular fibrillation. Provision of large quantities of acetate appears to antagonize fluoroacetate poisoning in a competitive manner in that monkey have been successfully protected from fluoroacetate poisoning by the administration of glycerol monoacetate.

Alpha Naphthyl Thiourea (ANTU)

ANTU was developed as a rodenticide following the observation that phenylthiourea kills rats but is not toxic to man. The thiourea derivative ANTU provide to be effective as a rodenticide because it lacked the bitter taste associated with phenylthiourea. However, some species of rats are not sensitive to it, and others develop resistance. There is a wide range of susceptibility to the acute toxicity of ANTU among mammals. The LD50 to rats is a few milligrams, approximately 3 mg/kg. Dogs appear to be next most sensitive with LD50s of 10 ml/ kg. Pigs, horses, and cows require 30 to 50 mg/kg for fatalities, and guinea pigs require 400 mg/kg. A mean lethal dose in monkeys was 4 g/kg, and it is assumed that man would be similarly resistant. ANTU produces its principal toxic action in susceptible species by causing massive pulmonary edema and pleural effusion, apparently due to action on pulmonary capillaries. Resistant animals do not show pulmonary edema. Biochemical changes occurred in poisoned rats that suggested effects of ANTU on carbohydrate metabolism may be secondary to adrenal stimulation since adrenal demedullation blocked these biochemical changes. Altered thyroid function also alters the toxicity of ANTU. Tolerance to the acute effects of ANTU in rats can be induced by administering progressively increasing doses, and pleural effusions are not present in tolerant animals that die from large doses. ANTU produces a cross-tolerance to several other edemagenic agents, including inhaled irritant gases such as ozone and NO_2. Reaction of ANTU with sulfhydryl groups may be a necessary part of the mechanism of toxic action, since it has been reported that sulfhydryl group blocking agents are effective in rats in some experimental conditions.

Strychnine Sulfate

This alkaloid of the nux vomica plant is a potent convulsant poison with a lethal dose of a few milligrams per kilogram of body weight for most animals. It lowers the threshold for stimulation of spinal reflexes by blocking inhibitory pathways exerted by Renshaw cells over the motor cells in the spinal cord. As a result, poisoned animals go into tetanic convulsions in response to rather minimal sensory stimuli. Nux vomica was introduced into Germany in the sixteenth century for use as a rodenticide. Although its use has declined, it is still used in poisoned baits in control of vermin, and accidental poisonings in humans continue to occur. Strychnine nitrate has been used as a "bearicide" in Hokkaido, Japan. The minimal fatal dose for bears appears to be about 0.5 mg/kg.

Inorganic Rodenticides

A number of inorganic compounds are used in rodent control. Most of these are nonselective in their toxicity and are generally hazardous to man and domestic animals so that their use has declined in favour of more selective or less hazardous organic compounds.

Zinc phosphide reacts with water and HCl in the gastrointestinal tract to produce the gas phosphine (PH_3), which causes severe gastrointestinal irritation. Apparent insensitivity of dogs and cats has been attributed to the emetic qualities of zinc phosphide, in the presence of moisture, may evolve phosphate, which inhaled in sufficient concentration can cause fatal pulmonary edema.

Thallium sulphate is lethal to most animals in doses of 10 to 20 mg/kg. It apparently acts by reacting with free sulfhydryl groups, but the precise mechanism of poisoning is uncertain. Acute poisoning is accompanied by gastrointestinal irritation, motor paralysis, and death from respiratory failure. Lower, sublethal doses taken over a period time result in reddening of the skin and loss of hair. Pathologic changes include perivascular cuffing around blood vessels and degenerative changes in brain, liver, and kidney. Neurologic symptoms are prominent in repeated subacute poisoning and include tremors, leg pains, paresthesias of the hands and feet, and polyneuritis especially in the legs. Psychoses, delirium, convulsions, and other kinds of encephalopathy may also be noted. Dimercaprol (BAL) is of litt'e benefit as a chelating agent in removal of absorbed thallium. Diethyldithiocarbamate has been demonstrated to accelerate the rate of excretion of thallium in experimental animals and to aid in the treatment of thallium-poisoned children. Use of 1 per cent thallium sulfate to control ground squirrels has resulted in outbreaks of thallotoxicosis in humans. In a 20-year period between 1935 to 1955, 778 persons were reported to have been poisoned by thallium-containing insecticides, rodenticides, and therapeutic chemicals, resulting in 46 fatalities. Because of its high, cumulative toxicity the use of thallium has been restricted to applications by qualified personnel, with a resultant marked decline in its use as a rodenticide.

White or yellow elemental phosphorus has caused poisoning because of the practice of spreading pastes containing this element on bread as a rodenticide bait. A dose of 15 mg of phosphorus can cause severe poisoning in humans and as little as 50 mg may be fatal. Shortly after ingestion phosphorus produces severe gastrointestinal irritation, and if a sufficient dose is ingested, hemorrhage and cardiovascular failure may prove fatal within 24 hours. The vomitus after phosphorus ingestion is luminescent and has a characteristic garlic odor. If the patient survives the initial gastrointestinal irritation phase, secondary systemic poisoning due to liver necrosis may ensure. Severe acute yellow atrophy of the liver is one delayed sequela that may ultimately prove fatal.

Barium carbonate and arsenic trioxide have also been used as rodenticides, but currently have little application for this purpose. Barium produces severe colic, diarrhea, and hemorrhage. It has a direct action on smooth muscles of the arterioles and cardiac muscle, which can result in increased blood pressure, cardiac irregularities, and death.

A variety of other compounds have some occasional application in rodent control. Carbon monoxide, methyl bromide, and hydrogen cyanide have been used as fumigants to kill rodents in enclosed spaces. These chemicals are generally toxic to all species. DDT, commonly thought of as an insecticide, is used as a poison for the house mouse and for bats. The principle of this treatment is to treat inaccessible areas where mice travel so that they will pick up a sufficient amount of DDT on their feet and fur, and ultimately, in preening, ingest the DDT and become poisoned. At best this seems an inefficient means of rodent control. Further discussion of action and therapy for poisoning by various rodenticides may be found in Hayes (1963).

Fumigants

Fumigants are used in the control of insects, rodents, and soil nematodes. They have in common the property of being in the gaseous form at the time they exert their pesticidal action and are used because they will penetrate to areas otherwise inaccessible for pesticide application (e.g., grain storage areas, rodent runways). Fumigants may be liquids that readily vaporize, solids that release a gas by chemical reaction (e.g., HCN from $Ca [CN]_2 + H_2O$), or gases contained in cylinders or ampules (e.g., methyl bromide). Thus they provide a potential hazard from the standpoint of inhalation exposure as well as in the case of solids and liquids, accidental ingestion or dermal exposure. Fumigants used in the protection of stored foodstuffs include acrylonitrile, carbon disulfide, carbon tetrachloride, chloropicrin, ethylene oxide, hydrogen cyanide, methyl bromide, and phosphine.

These chemicals have many other applications in industry and their toxicology has been discussed in other sections. In connection with pesticides it is worthy of comment that methyl bromide is said to have been responsible for more deaths in recent years among occupationally exposed persons in California than all of the more publicized organophosphate group of insecticides. During the period of 1957 to 1964, 62 systemic poisonings with five deaths were reported. In the usual case the early symptoms are malaise, headache, visual disturbances, and nausea and vomiting. Pulmonary effects included acute pulmonary edema, and neurologic effects in fatal poisonings included clonic and toxic convulsions. Several nonfatal cases resulted in persistent neurologic and psychiatric complaints ranging from muscular soreness and headache through decreased libido, mental depression, phobias, and paranoia. Although the neurologic and psychiatric symptoms resemble chronic poisoning by inorganic bromides, the serum bromide levels achieved in serious cases of methyl bromide poisoning are considerably lower than those required for poisoning by inorganic bromides. It has been suggested that this may be due to greater lipoid solubility of methyl bromide and hence greater penetration into the brain. However, since methyl chloride produces many of the same neurologic symptoms, it seems unlikely that the neurotoxicity of methyl bromide is due only to bromide ion. Methyl bromide methylates SH groups of cysteine, glutathione, and several SH-containing enzymes. Methylation of SH groups essential to cellular oxidation can be suggested as a possible mechanism for neurologic effects of methyl bromide and methyl chloride, and therefore BAL has been considered to possible usefulness in therapy. BAL given before exposure protected against lethal exposures in animals but had much less effect when given after exposure.

Phosphine, released from aluminum phosphate, although more acutely toxic than methyl bromide, is said to be safer for use as a grain fumigant under practical conditions. Use of acrylonitrile as a fumigant is limited by its flammability and high cost. Its toxicity has been attributed to release of CN ion *in vivo*, however, differences in symptoms and CN blood levels associated with poisoning by inorganic cyanides and acrylonitrile have led to some question about that mechanism. Chloropicrin (CCl_3NO_2) is a strong irritant, and sensory irritation gives early warning of its presence. It is, therefore, sometimes added in small amounts of other comparatively odorless fumigants to act as a warning agent. Ethylene oxide toxicity is also primarily due to its irritant actions in the lungs.

Ethylene dibromide in high concentrations (>200 ppm) produces primarily lung inflammation and edema is laboratory animals while repeated exposures to low concentrations resulted in histopathologic changes in their livers and kidneys as well. No abnormal signs were observed in rats and guinea pigs given 40 to 50 mg/kg/day for four months. A dose of 2 mg/kg/day given to bulls was reported to have resulted in impaired spermatogenesis within two weeks. Ethylene dibromide residues in fumigated cereal grains have been observed for up to two months after fumigation, and laying hens fed diets containing 10 ppm (daily dose of 1 to 2 mg/kg) had a decrease in egg weights. Investigation of the possible mechanism of this effect led to observation of impaired follicle growth apparently arising from impaired permeability of the follicular membrane to protein transfer. In a case of fatal human poisoning resulting from ingestion of 4.5 ml of ethylene dibromide, massive centrolobular necrosis of the liver and proximal tubular damage in the kidney were observed. Ethylene dibromide and 1,2-dibromo-3-chloropropane (DBCP), another nematocidal fumigant, were both found to rapidly produce highly malignant gastric squamous cell carcinoma in rats and mice.

DBCP also received considerable notoriety as a result of its being the probable cause of sterility and/or abnormally low sperm counts in workmen engaged in its manufacture. This resulted in a drastic reduction in its production and use. Studies in laboratory animals 16 years earlier had suggested the potential for this toxic effect when it was observed that repeated inhalation exposure to as little as 5 ppm of DBCP has an adverse effect on the testes and on reproductive function of male rats. Although the investigators, in that report, warned of the potential hazard, this warning was apparently not strong enough to prompt appropriate warning to workers and/or improve industrial hygiene practice sufficiently to protect workers. The future use of both ethylene dibromide and DBCP as fumigants will likely be served curtailed because of their strong carcinogenicity and their adverse action on reproductive function.

Special Problems

Interactions

Organophosphate potentiation

For several years following the observation by Frawley and coworkers (1957) of marked synergism of acute toxicity of EPN and malathion, the Food and Drug Administration Act required that all safety evaluations on anticholinesterase insecticides for which food residues were established should include tests of the toxicity of combinations. This led to routine tests for toxic interactions among this class of compounds. Most of these were acute toxicity tests using simultaneous administration. In 1961 DuBois reported studies in which the acute toxicity of various combinations of 13 different organophosphorus (OP) insecticides were tested in rats. Twenty-one pairs were additive in toxicity, 18 pairs less than additive, and four pairs synergistic. Since that time a few more pairs, involving new compounds, have been shown to be synergistic in acute toxicity tests. Combinations of several OP insecticides fed at recommended tolerance levels failed to produce significant synergistic toxicity in chronic feeding studies.

Malathion is one of the insecticides that has been observed most frequently as one constituent of a potentiating pairs of organophosphorus insecticides. This, normally, relatively safe insecticide is detoxified by carboxylesterases that are inhibited by other OP insecticides. The mechanisms of synergism among OP insecticides have been reviewed by DuBios (1969) and Murphy (1969). Two major mechanisms appear to be involved: (1) inhibition of detoxication by tissue carboxylesterase (aliesterases) and amidases, and (2) competition for nonvital binding sites that normally act as a buffer system to spare the vital acetylcholinesterase enzyme. Methods for screening for potentiating OP compounds by testing their potency as carboxylesterase inhibitors have been suggested as useful tests in acute studies and subacute feeding experiments. Compounds for potentiating OP compounds by testing their potency as carboxylesterase inhibitors have been suggested as useful tests in acute studies and subacute feeding experiments. Compounds that have a high potency as inhibitors of carboxylesterase relative to their anti-cholinesterase potency are likely to potentiate other OP insecticides or to alter the toxicity of other drugs and chemicals containing carboxylester or amide linkages. Pellegrini and Santi (1972) have demonstrated that impurities present in technical grade samples of malathion and phenthoate potentiate that toxicity of these compounds, thus accounting for the greater toxicity of technical samples as compared to highly purified samples. Synergism of malathion toxicity by impurities was offered as a possible explanation for the poisonings of malathion spraymen in Pakistan. This may account for the apparent "self-potentiation" of malathion reported by Murphy (1967). Noninsecticidal organophosphorus esters such as triorthotolyl phosphate are also potentiators.

These mechanism studies have demonstrated that simultaneous administration of compounds may not be the most suitable method for testing for interactions among OP insecticides, that carboxylesterases are much more sensitive than cholinesterases to inhibition by some compounds and that tissue carboxylesterase essays are suitable for detecting this subtle action in relatively short-duration feeding studies. The mechanism of competition of OP insecticides for nonvital binding sites has received less attention and should be subjected to further investigation. Measurements of relative carboxylesterase/cholinesterase inhibitory potencies may be a useful method of predicting potentiators, but they should also be corroborated with some *in vivo* toxicity tests.

Organochlorine insecticides

Tests of interaction among two or more pairs of organochlorine (OC) insecticides have usually involved measurements of the effects of one OC compound on the storage, excretion, and metabolism of another. Street's work on rats suggest that the storage of DDT and dieldrin in adipose tissue is reduced when they are fed in combination. This was attributed to accelerated rates of metabolism and excretion. Other indices of the toxicity of these compounds were not tested. A study of Diechmann and associates (1971) yielded the opposite effect with dogs; i.e. DDT fed with aldrin or dieldrin resulted in greater-than-expected residues of these compounds in fat and blood. Obviously additional work is required to determine if these represent true species differences, or if the discrepancies can be explained on the basis of differing experimental procedures.

Keplinger and Deichmann (1967) determined LD50s for over 100 mixtures containing two or three different insecticides. Most of the mixtures contained at least one OC insecticide. More than additive toxicities in mice were reported for endrin plus chlordane or aldrin, methoxychlor plus chlordane and dieldrin, and aldrin plus chlordane. Aldrin and chlordane were additive only in rats. Other potentiated mixtures included OC compounds with certain OP insecticides. The potentiations observed in this study were not striking (usually about twofold). It is possible that simultaneous administration of the compounds precluded the detection of some types of interactions.

Organochlorine insecticides protect against the acute toxicity of several OP insecticides. The mechanism of this protection appears to be due to the capacity of the OC insecticides to stimulate the enzymatic detoxification of OP compounds by liver microsomes or to increase noncatalytic binding sites for the OPs.

Other pesticides, drugs, and hydrocarbons that induce microsomal enzymes will, after an appropriate period of treatment, reduce the storage level of OC insecticides in rats and protect rats against acute poisoning by OP insecticides. Microsomal enzymes catalyze both the activation and detoxication of OP insecticides. In most cases it appears that the dynamics of the enzyme reactions and inductions favour detoxification. However, at least a few OP insecticides are potentiated by pretreatment with certain microsomal enzyme inducers. Caution should be exercised, therefore, in making broad generalizations concerning the effects of microsoma enzyme inducers on the toxicity of various classes of pesticides. Additional research is necessary to determine the specificities of various inducers (or inhibitors) on the several alternate pathways of metabolism of complex organic pesticides.

Although the above remarks have been primarily restricted to pesticide—pesticide interactions, they apply as well to other pollutant or drug effects on pesticide toxicities. In most cases where such interactions have been detected they appear to have been mediated through altered microsomal enzyme activities. Since at least 200 drugs and chemicals are known inducers of these enzymes, the number of possible interactions is tremendous. Relatively few have been subjected to toxicity tests in intact animals. Durham (1967) has reviewed many additional factors that may affect the toxicity of pesticides.

Pesticide-drug interaction

The capacity of organochlorine insecticides and certain herbicides to induce increased activity of liver microsomal enzymes that metabolize a variety of drugs is well established. However, attempts to correlate the increased capacity of tissues from pesticide-induced animals to metabolize drugs with effects of the pesticides on the intensity and duration of pharmacologic (or toxic) actions of the drugs are relatively few. Hexobarbital sleeping times or zoxazolamine paralysis times are often used as pharmacologic indices of altered drug metabolism *in vivo*, and in a few cases altered blood levels of drugs given to pesticide-treated animals have served as an *in vivo* index of pesticide-drug interactions. Conney and coworkers (1971) found that workers in a DDT factory had significantly higher excretion of 6-β-hydroxy-cortisol and a significantly reduced phenylbutazone half-life. This study suggests that at least occupational exposures can alter drug and steroid metabolism in man as well as experimental animals.

Unlike the organochlorine insecticides, OP insecticides have been shown to inhibit steroid metabolism by rat liver microsomes. Pesticide synergists of the methylenedioxyphenyl type such as piperonyl butoxide have been shown to inhibit or induce microsomal drug-metabolizing enzymes and to prolong or reduce hexobarbital sleep time and to potentiate or antagonize phosphorothioate insecticides depending on the dose and time of pretreatment with the synergist. When mice were pretreated with piperonyl butoxide, under conditions favourable to inhibition of microsomal oxidases, they were slightly more susceptible to the diethyl-substituted phosphorothionates, parathion and aziphosethyl, but were markedly resistant to the corresponding dimethyl-substituted compounds. The mechanism for this appeared to be, in part, due to the fact that glutathione alkyl transferase could serve as an alternate (to oxidation) pathway of detoxification of the dimethyl but not the diethyl-substituted compounds. Additionally, a rapid rate of reversal of dimethylphosphorylated cholinesterase (as compared to the diethyl compounds) allowed for reversal of injury to keep pace with the piperonyl butoxide-induced oxidative production of the active anticholinesterase metabolites.

The effect that microsomal enzyme induction or inhibition will have on the toxicity and action of a particular drug or chemical will depend not only upon the degree to which the enzyme activity is changed, but also upon the extent to which the enzymatic metabolism of the drug is the limiting factor in determining its intensity and duration of action and the relative influence on possible alternate pathways of metabolism.

Carcinogenic, Teratogenic, and Mutagenic Properties of Pesticides

Since other chapter have been specifically devoted to these pathologic processes, they have not, with a few exceptions, been considered in detail in this chapter. The report of the Secretary's Commission on Pesticides (1969) contains discussion and summaries of data on carcinogenicity, mutagenicity, and teratogenicity of pesticides.

Pesticides that the Panel on Carcinogenesis of the Secretary's Commission on Pesticides (1969) considered "positive" for tumor induction on the basis of tests conducted adequately in one or more species, the results being significant at the 0.01 level, included aldrin, aramite chlorbenzilate, p,p-DDT, dieldrin, mirex, strobane, and heptachlor (all registered for use on food crops), and amitrole, avadex, bis (2-chloroethyl) ether N-(2hydroxyethyl)-hydrazine, and PCNB. The recommendation of the panel was that human exposures to these compounds be minimized and that their use be restricted to purposes for which there was a clear health benefit. Many other pesticides were given priorities for further testing because the panel felt that they had not been adequately evaluated in experimental animals. Only three pesticides were considered to have been proven negative to tumor induction on the basis of "adequate" tests in experimental animals. Obviously this report has provoked much controversy, and the purpose of including these summary comments here is to make the reader aware of the problems. The situation for DDT is a case in point. The extensive use of this compound in industrial countries has not been associated with an increase in hepatic cancer in human populations, but many years ago Fitzhugh and Nelson (1947) reported that DDT fed in high doses to rats caused slight increase in hepatic cell tumors. Innes and associates (1969) reported a statistically significant increase in hepatomas in two strains of mice. Hepatic cell tumors in trout and tumors of several sites in F_2 and following generations of mice have followed DDT exposure. Additional studies sponsored by the International Agency of Research in Cancer confirmed the hepato-carcinogenicity of DDT in mice hepatomas were also increased in mice fed 250 ppm of DDE or DDD. While some oncologists feel that hepatoma induction is indicative of carcinogenesis, others feel that hepatomas are reversible lesions. The daily dosages ingested by animals in the experimental demonstrations of hepatomas are considerably greater than the dosage rate that man would receive, based on analyses of residues in typical meals. This, plus the failure of epidemiologic studies to demonstrate associations between DDT exposure and cancer in man, the controversy as to whether hepatoma production represents true carcinogenesis, and the fact that DDT has indeed been of great benefit in the control of malaria and other insect-borne diseases and in enhancing agricultural production, makes the administrative decision of whether or not to ban or greatly restrict its use especially difficult. It is not only a challenge to our scientific capabilities to adequately assess safety, but a challenge to social responsibility as well. Tomatis (1976) reviewed the program on the evaluation of the carcinogenic risk of chemicals to man of the International Agency for Research on Cancer. There were no pesticides among the 17 chemicals that he listed as having been found to have carcinogenicity in man or for which there was a strong suspicion of such action. Ten of the ninety-four chemicals, which the agency had determined to be carcinogenic in experimental animals only, were pesticides. These were amitrole, aramite, BHC, chlorobenzilate, DDD, DDE, DDT, dieldrin, lindane, and Mirex. The NCI bioassay program will not doubt continue to identify additional pesticides with carcinogenic potential and may exonerate some that IARC or others have branded as carcinogens. This is an area of great concern and one in which the compounds of greatest interest will likely continue to change.

Durham and Williams (1972) reviewed studies in experimental animals in which at least some mammalian species at some testable dosage of the following pesticides were reported to have produced teratogenic effects: carbaryl, captan, folpet, difolatan, organo-mercury compounds, 2,4,5-T, pentachloronitrobenzene (PCNB), and paraquat. Human consumption of organomercury compounds by pregnant women is known to have caused serious neurologic disorders in their offspring, which might be considered functional teratogenicity (or perhaps fetal toxicity). Other than this there is no confirmed relationship between exposure of pesticides and human terata. In the positive experimental studies the production of terata was usually demonstrated to be dose dependent, and the doses required were far in excess of what humans might be expected to receive under usual conditions. As with other toxic effects, pesticide teratogenicity and its relationship to human health must be considered from a dose-response standpoint and is subject to the same problems of interpretation and extrapolation as other dose-related effects, albeit a serious and tragic effect.

Recently proposed guidelines by the EPA for evaluating safety of pesticides include a battery of tests for mutagenicity. Durham and William (1972) reviewed the submammalian and mammalian tests available and commented on the problems of interpretation of these tests. Epstein and coworkers (1972) reported results of an extensive series of tests for mutagenic action of chemicals as determined by the dominant lethal assay in mice. Twenty-eight common pesticides were included in those tests. None of them was among the 16 chemical agents (out of a total of 174) that produced "unequivocal effects" on early fetal deaths and/or total implants, although TEPA (phosphine oxide, tris [1-aziridinyl]) and METEPA (phosphine oxide, tris [2-methyl-1-aziridyl]), which have been *proposed* as insect chemosterilants were positive. Durham and Williams (1972) reviewed reports of several pesticides that were mutagenic in nonmammalian systems (plants, bacteria, time culture, etc.), and they concluded that "from the present state of knowledge, it must be agreed that no firm conclusions can be drawn as to whether pesticides represent a mutagenic hazards."

Comparative Toxicity

A high degree of selective toxicity to target organism is a desirable goal in the development of useful pesticides. Metcalf (1972) has reviewed toxicity data for a large number of insecticides and calculated mammalian selectivity ratios, MSRs (mouse oral LD50/female housefly topical LD50). Considering only these two species and only acute toxicity it is apparent that there is an extremely wide range of relative toxicities. The situation becomes infinitely more complex when one considers a broader spectrum of non-target species.

Table 23.1. Relative toxicity of various insecticides to rats and houseflies.

Class	*Compound*	*MRS*
Organochlorines	DDT	59
	DDT	174
	Methoxychlor	668
	Chlordane	72
	Aldrin	27
	Dieldrin	24
	Endrin	2.4
	Heptachlor	72
	Lindane	107
Organophosphates	Parathion	4
	Methyl parathion	20
	Malathion	37.7
	Azinphosmethyl	4.1
	Chlorothion	85
	Dimethoate	390
	Ronnel	1,315
Carbamates	Aldicarb	0.175
	Carbaryl	0.60
	Zectran	0.60
	Propoxur	4.5
	Mobam	10.0

There are indeed occasional marked differences in susceptibilities of common laboratory test animals, but even more striking are species differences noted among wild animals of the same vertebrate class. For example, Hayes (1967a) compared reported single-dose LD50 values for 20 pesticides in five mammalian species commonly used in safety evaluation studies. The range of susceptibilities generally varied within a factor of less tenfold. All species were not compared for all 20 compounds, but in the majority of cases rats were more susceptible than mice, guinea pigs, rabbits, or dogs. Comparing the smallest single doses required to produce a serious effect in rats and man, man was more sensitive than rats (usually by factors of tenfold or less). In a similar comparison or reported acute insecticide toxicity values for five species of fish, Murphy (1972), calculated LD50 ratios of least to most sensitive of 2.7 for DDT, 4.7 for dieldrin, 246 for Guthion (azinphosmethyl), 49 for parathion, and 430 for malathion. A similar calculation for ten avian species gave least to most sensitive species ratios of 45 for dieldrin and 192 for parathion. The mechanisms of these species differences have received relatively little research, but there is evidence that they include both differences in sensitivity of target enzymes as well as differences in rats of biotransformation to either more or less toxic metabolites. Certainly, for a class of toxic chemicals that become as widespread in the environment as pesticides, for effects on a broad spectrum of nontarget species is reasonable. Since it is clearly unrealistic to except all pesticides to be tested for safety to all nontarget species that might be exposed, the only reasonable approach appear to be to attempt to understand basic mechanisms of species differences in susceptibility and, with this information base, to select or design compounds that will not only be safe for man but also be least likely to affect other nontarget organisms present in the specific areas in which they are applied. An impossible task? Perhaps. A worthwhile objective? Certainly.

INDEX

A

A. eriocarpa, 4
A. labriformis, 4
A. subverticillata, 4
Abrus precatorius, 12, 13
Acacia beriandieri, 20
Aconitum napellus, 20
Adagam, 225
Adaptogen, 178
Adaptogenic, 181
Adverse event reporters, 64
Aged garlic extract, 98
Agnus, 213
Agnus-castus, 213, 218, 221
Allii sativi bulbus, 98
Allium cepa, 17
Allium sativum, 98
Ambrosia psilostachya, 249
Apis mellifica, 196
Apium graveolens, 240
Aplopappus heterophyllus, 4
Ardisia, 237
Ardisia teysmanniana, 238
Ardisia villosa, 236
Argemone mexicana, 19
Aristolochia, 225
Aristolochia chrysops, 225
Aristolochia dabieshanensis, 225
Aristolochia debilis, 226, 227
Aristolochia heterophylla, 225
Aristolochia indica, 225
Aristolochia kaempferi, 225
Aristolochia longa, 226
Aristolochia mollis, 225
Aristolochia neolongifolia, 225
Aristolochia recurvilabra, 225
Aristolochia shimadae, 225
Aristolochia sinarum, 226
Arnica montana, 232
Artemisia judaica, 235
Artemisia loureiro, 235
Artemisia monosperma, 240
Asclepias, 4
Aspergillus, 22, 108
Atropa belladonna, 10, 257
Attention-deficit hyperactivity disorder, 183
Atypical, 185
Aurantii pericarpium, 33

B

Baccharis trimera, 233
Bacillus, 108

Baptisiae tinctoriae, 47
Beats per minute, 161
Benign prostatic hypertrophy, 191
Berloque dermatitis, 36
Blighia sapida, 16
Blood pressure, 161
Brassica napus, 17, 19
Brauneria angustifolia, 45
Brauneria pallida, 45
Bupleurum chinense, 242
Bupleurum falcatum, 241, 242
Bupleurum fruticescens, 242
Bupleurum octoradiatum, 241
Bupleurum togasii, 242
Bupleurum vanheurckii, 242

C

C. albicans, 48
C. aura ntium, 34, 37
C. aurantium, 32, 33, 34, 35, 36, 37, 38
Calendula officinalis, 232
Candida, 108, 118
Candida albicans, 47, 154
Candida kefyr, 47
Candida shehata, 47
Candida steatulytica, 48
Candida tropicalis, 48
Carum carvi, 240
Castitas, 213
Cathine, 55
Centaurea solstitialis, 20
Centella asiatica, 240
Central nervous system, 55, 122, 169, 182, 203
Centranthus ruber, 201
Chronic cystitis, 191
Chronic fatigue syndrome, 83
Chronic fatigue syndrome, 24
Chronic myeloid leukemia, 164
Chrysanthemum parthenium, 88
Cicuta maculata, 20
Cimicifuga racemosa, 222
Cirsium japonicum, 233
Citrus, 32
Citrus amara, 33
Citrus aurantium, 32
Citrus bigarradia, 33
Citrus vulgaris, 33
Class effect, 59
Claviceps paspali, 20
Claviceps purpurea, 20
Clostridium, 108
Clostridium botulinum, 114
Cnicus japonicum, 233
Cnicus spicatus, 233
Compositae, 96
Conium maculatum, 20, 240
Coriandrum sativum, 240
Crataegus, 142
Crataegus curvisepala, 142
Crataegus laevigata, 141
Crataegus monogyna Jacquin, 141
Crataegus oxyacantha, 141
Crithidia fasciculate, 109
Crossostephium artemisoides, 235
Crossotephium chinense, 233
Cryptococcus neoformans, 108
Cycas, 11
Cyclic adenosine monophosphate, 105

D

Daphne mezereum, 12
Daphnidium cubeba, 254
Datura stramonium, 19, 20, 257
De novo, 144
Delphinium, 15
Derris elliptica, 294
Descurainia pinnata, 19
Diastolic blood pressure, 107
Diastolic runoff, 59
Dieffenbachia, 13

Diervilla, 232
Digitalis purpurea, 13, 18
Doctrine of Signatures, 178
Dopaminergic effect, 222
Drosera, 248
Drosera burmannii, 247
Drosera indica, 247
Drosera madagascariensis, 248
Drosera peltata, 247
Drosera rotundifolia, 247
Dulcamara, 10

E

E. angustifolia, 44, 45, 47, 48, 49, 52, 53
E. coli, 41, 42
E. distachya, 56
E. equisentina, 56
E. geriardiana, 56
E. intermedia, 56
E. major, 56
E. pallida, 45, 47, 48, 49, 53
E. purpurea, 44, 45, 46, 47, 48, 49, 50, 52, 53
E. senticosus, 179, 186
E. vulgaris, 56
Echinacea, 52
Echinacea angustifolia, 44
Echinacea pallida, 44
Echinacea purpurea, 44
Electroencephalogram, 201
Eleutherococcus senticosus, 179
Endocomia macrocoma, 229
Entamoeba histolytica, 109
Enterococcus, 108
Ephedra sinica, 56
Ephedrine, 57
Ephedrine alkaloids, 59
Epidermophyton, 108
Epidermophyton fluccosum, 173
Equisetum arvense, 15
Escherichia, 107
Escherichia coli, 41, 108, 128
Essential fatty acid, 72
Eupatoirum volubile, 246
Eupatorium, 4
Eupatorium caudatum, 246
Eupatorium rugosum, 4, 21
Euphorbia esula, 12
Euphorbia pulcherrima, 5
Evening primrose, 71

F

Febrifugia, 88
Feverfew responders, 92
Fluorescence polarization immunoassay, 189
Foeniculum vulgare, 240
Food supplements, 56
French pharmacopoeia, 248
Fructus Agni Casti, 214
Fructus aurantii, 33

G

G. biloba, 154, 182, 183
Garlic burns, 117
General population, 258
Giardia lamblia, 109
Gibberella, 13
Ginkgo biloba, 131, 154, 182
Ginseng abuse syndrome, 184
Gossypium, 11
Gutierrezia microcephala, 22

H

H. perforatum, 148, 150
H. pylori, 107, 108
Halogeton glomeratus, 3, 12, 15, 18
Hangover, 170
Hangover effect, 201
Helicobacter pylori, 107
Herbal ecstasy, 56, 64
Herbicides, 259
Herpes simplex, 108, 154

Herpes simplex virus, 47
Herpes zoster, 118
Horsfieldia, 228
Horsfieldia amygdalinia, 228, 229
Horsfieldia glabra, 228
Horsfieldia merrillii, 229
Horsfieldia oblongata, 229
Horsfieldia prainii, 229
Horsfieldia prunoides, 228
Horsfieldia thorelii, 228
Horsfieldia tonkinensis, 228
Hospital Anxiety and Depression, 157
Humulus lupulus, 210
Hydrocotyle asiatica, 240
Hyoscyamus niger, 257
Hypericum, 147, 151, 152, 153, 157, 160, 166, 238
Hypericum erectum, 238, 239
Hypericum perforatum, 17, 147, 238

I

I. opaca, 10
Ilex, 10
In vitro, 17, 271, 272, 273
In vivo, 17, 268, 271, 273
Index of ulceration, 25
Insecticides, 259
International normalized ratio, 164, 187
Inula britannica, 250, 251
Inula chinensis, 233
Inula japonica, 250
Inula viscosa, 251
Ishvara, 225
Isotrema chrysops, 225
Isotrema heterophyllum, 225
Isotrema iasiops, 225

K

Kava, 167
Kava dermopathy, 172
Kava lactones, 169
Kawaism, 172
Klebsiella, 108

L

L. cubeba, 255
Lathyrus odoratus, 17, 18
Laurus cubeba, 254
Laurus nobilis, 252
Leishmania enrietti, 48
Leishmania major, 109
Leptomonas colsoma, 109
Leucaena glauca, 22
Leucanthemum parthenium, 88
Lipocortine, 224
Listeria monocytogenes, 48
Litsea citrata, 254
Litsea cubeba, 255
Litsea zeylanica, 253
Lonicera affinis, 230
Lonicera brachypoda, 230
Lonicera chinensis, 230
Lonicera confusa, 230
Lonicera japonica, 230, 231
Low-density lipoprotein, 144
Lupinus sericeus, 11, 19
Luteinizing hormone, 217
Lycopersicon esculentum, 10
Lycopodium, 4

M

Macbeth, 7
Magnoliopsida, 71
Matricaria, 88
Matricaria chamomilla, 88
Melampodiinae, 243
Melilotus, 11, 17
Methyl allyl trisulfide, 105
Mickania scandens, 246
Microparticle enzyme immunoassay, 189
Microsporum, 108

Mikania chenopodifolia, 247
Mikania cordata, 244, 247
Mikania volubilis, 246
Mucor pusillus, 108
Mycobacterium tuberculosis, 108
Mycobacterium tuberculosis bacilli, 127
Myocardial infarction, 36
Myristica amygdalina, 228
Myristica glabra, 228
Myristica prainii, 229
Myristica valida, 229
Myrtales, 71

N

Natural flavoring, 38
Negundo, 214
Neolitsea zeylanica, 252
Nicotiana tabacum, 4

O

O. biennis, 72
Oenothera, 71, 72
Oenothera biennis, 71
Onagraceae, 71
Onoclea sensibilis, 20

P

P. ginseng, 178, 179, 180, 181, 182, 184, 185, 186, 188, 190
P. methysticin, 173
P. methysticum, 168, 173
P. sepium, 187
Panax, 179, 180, 186
Panax ginseng, 178, 179, 196
Panax pseudoginseng, 179
Panax quinquefolium, 179
Panax quinquefolius, 178
Paraquat, 298
Paspalum dilatatum, 20
Passiflora, 210
Periploca sepium, 187
Pesticides, 259
Philopon, 55
Philosphy of opposites, 178
Physalis, 257
Physalis alkekengi, 257
Physalis angulata, 257
Phytolacca americana, 9, 11, 16, 18
Pimpinella anisum, 240
Piper methysticum, 167
Plantae, 71
Platelet-activating factor, 135
Postfeverfew syndrome, 96
Premenstrual dysphoric disorder, 221
Premenstrual syndrome, 72, 157, 214
Prosopis juliflora, 14
prostate-specific antigen, 192
Proteus, 108
Prothrombin time, 137
Prunella vulgaris, 250
Prunus, 21
Pteridium aquilinum, 11, 18
Pygeum africanum, 196
Pyracantha, 11
Pyrethum parthenium, 88

Q

Quercus, 16, 18

R

Radioallegosorbent test, 117
Radix valerianae, 201
Randomized controlled trials, 83
Rapid eye movement, 203
Rheumatoid arthritis, 95
Rhizoma valeriana officinalis, 201
Ricinus communis, 11
Rudbeckia purpurea, 45

S

S. aureus, 156
S. intrusum, 5
Sabal serrulata, 191

Saccharomyces cerevisiae, 47
Salmonella, 107
Sambucus hookeri, 231
Sambucus javanica, 230
Sambucus sieboldiana, 230
Sambucus thunbergiana, 231
Samonella typhimurium, 128
San guinea, 47
Santolina chamaecyparissus, 233
Saponaria, 16
Sarcoplasmic reticulum, 127
Seasonal affective disorders, 147
Secale cereale, 20
Second component, 197, 198
Selective serotonin reuptake inhibitor, 162
Senecio, 11, 16
Serenoa repens, 191
Serenoa serrulatum, 191
Serotonin syndrome, 70
Shabu, 55
Shigella, 108
Siberian ginseng, 179
Sigesbeckia glabrescens, 246
Sigesbeckia orientalis, 233, 244, 245
Skin prick tests, 116
Slow-wave sleep, 201
Solanum, 10
Solanum intrusum, 5
Solanum nigrum, 5
Solanum pseudocapsicum, 10
Solanum tuberosum, 10
Species plantarum, 7
Staphylococcus, 107
Staphylococcus aureus, 108, 154
Stellaria media, 122
Stipa robusta, 20
Streptococcus, 108
Streptococcus mutans, 108
Suckleyea suckleyana, 14
Supplements, 109
Symplocarpus foetidus, 9
Systolic blood pressure, 107

T

T. canadensis, 9
T. parthenium, 93
Tanacetum parthenium, 88
Taxus, 9
Taxus cuspidata, 18
Tetradenia zeylanica, 253
Tetradymia, 17
Thrusting, 185
Thujae occidentalis, 47
Thyroid-stimulating hormone, 162
Thyrotropin-releasing hormone, 217
Tracheobionta, 71
Transtorines, 54
Trichophyton, 108
Trifoliata, 214
Trifolium repens, 20
Trifolium subterraneum, 16
Triterpenoids, 224

U

Uncariarhyncophylla, 210
Upper respiratory infections, 45

V

V. agnus castus fructus, 215
V. agnus-castus, 213, 214, 215, 216, 217, 218, 219, 220, 221, 222, 223
V. agnus-castus group, 218
V. fauriei, 205
V. mexicana, 209
V. myrtillus, 24, 26
V. officinalis, 202, 203, 204, 208, 212
V. wallichii, 209
Vaccinium, 42
Vaccinium macrocarpon, 39
Vaccinium myrtillus, 24

Valeriana alliariifolia Vahl, 201
Valeriana officinalis, 201
Valeriana sambucifolia, 201
Valeriana wallichii, 201
Valerianae radix, 201
Veratrum californicum, 11, 21
Veratrum viride, 9, 18
Verbenisa, 240
Verbenisa turbacensis, 240
Viscum album, 210
Visual analogue scale, 220
Vitex, 213, 214, 216
Vitex agnus-castus, 213

W

Weigela floribunda, 230

Z

Z. officinale, 128
Zea mays, 14, 21
Zingerberis rhizoma, 121
Zingiber capitatum, 121
Zingiber officinale, 121
Zingiber zerumbet, 121